THE SEVEN AGES

OF WOMAN

by ELIZABETH PARKER, M.D.

Edited by Evelyn Breck

THE JOHNS HOPKINS PRESS
Baltimore and London

The Johns Hopkins Press, Baltimore, Maryland 21218
The Johns Hopkins Press Ltd., London

ISBN-0-8018-0521-x

Originally published, 1960
Second printing, 1967
Third printing, 1971

AUTHOR'S PREFACE

ANY ATTEMPT to "explain" femininity with its countless shades of meaning and its multitudinous facets of reflection requires some justification from the person who has the temerity to assume so formidable an undertaking. Two questions need to be answered at the outset: What are the foundations in fact on which such an exposition is to be made? What purpose is to be served?

The source material for *The Seven Ages of Woman* is derived from the search for an understanding of female physiology and function, which stretches back through the centuries. The first glimmerings came long before the Christian Era when the Chinese used seaweed to treat goiter, the Egyptians tested for pregnancy by germination of seed, and the Romans guarded their maidens' virginity with a necklace. The factual material has been provided by medical research, which has so brilliantly revealed some of the mysteries of female endocrinology. Any author on the subject of female function or femininity owes a tremendous debt to the investigators who have contributed to our great wealth of knowledge. I wish here to acknowledge my debt and for a particular and important reason.

The Seven Ages of Woman has been written for women. The scientific technicalities and language have been eliminated as far as possible. The names of those who have provided the scientifically established facts have been omitted to facilitate the narrative form. Full acknowledgment would mean the history of endocrinology—an exciting and fabulous story that has yet to be written and deserves its own telling. In such history would be related the work of the great scientists whose vision, dedication, ability, ingenuity, and unrelenting toil have opened new pathways and set milestones. It would also include the recognition of the thousands who have done the spade work and provided the bricks by which the roadway was built, but whose names have slipped into oblivion even in scientific writings.

There is a second and personal obligation which I would like to acknowledge here. This is the debt I owe to the many women who through a quarter of a century have honored me with their confidence as their physician, friend, and sometimes mother-confessor. They have provided me with the means of understanding the scientific facts of female endocrinology and, perhaps even more important, the human aspects of femininity—woman's ideals, her hopes, her fears, her sorrows, and her triumphs.

Furthermore, it has been women's eagerness to know, as exemplified by their searching questions, their appreciative attention to explanation, and their omnivorous reading that convinced me of the need for a book to which they could turn not only for fuller answers but for the whole wonderful story of feminine function. This also convinced me that they are far more capable than they are often given credit for not only of understanding scientific information if properly presented (shorn of the language that makes specialized scientific writing an unknown tongue except for its own initiates), but also of making good use of it.

As we look back through all history, it is obvious that woman has never been the dominant sex in government or commerce, war or exploration, science, or even the arts. Rather she has been cast in a role, which some choose to call inferior, over which man has exercised a dominance to which she was forced to submit. In the light of present-day knowledge, we might well ask why this is so. She has intelligence, imagination, and determination. While physically she does not have equal strength, she possesses a greater durability. The one quality for success in these areas of human endeavor that she seems to have lacked is interest. Perhaps, therefore, she occupies her position from choice. To her, fulfillment was not to be measured in terms of success and the furtherance of what we are pleased to call progress and civilization but in the intangibles of human relationships, and she found it good to be a woman. Her eagerness, her interest has always been directed toward this—the perfection of her femininity.

When it comes to citing the assistance that others have rendered in bringing *The Seven Ages of Woman* into book form, it would be impossible to list them all. One does not just sit down and write a book (at least I did not). It is the outgrowth of life experience. Thus during the years this book was in the making, there have been many who have helped, some by their interest and enthusiasm for such a book, some by suggestions and criticisms, and some by words of encouragement. Even the doubting Thomases have served by making it a challenge. To all I express my thanks. And there are those who have contributed greatly in specific ways.

Dr. Barton Richwine has always been generous with his time and knowledge in the discussion of problem cases. He was equally generous in the care with which he read the manuscript. His corrections and comments were very helpful.

Miss Evelyn Breck, Editor at The Brookings Institution, occupies a very special place in my list of thank-you's. It was her unwavering enthusiasm and confidence matched with her professional editorial skill that have contributed so greatly to the finished product.

And last there is P. B., whose forbearance with the "mood for authorship" and gentle but insistent prodding when other pleasures threatened to divert, provided the continuing impetus that has made *The Seven Ages of Woman* a reality, not something that I would do tomorrow.

Elizabeth Parker Bartsch

"LEBANON," Lorton Va.
December 1959

CONTENTS

THE SEVEN AGES OF WOMAN

CREATION OF WOMAN

Then one day, as they rested at noon beneath the thick shade of a Kadamba tree, the King gazed for a long time at the portrait of his mistress. And suddenly he broke silence, and said, Rasakosha, this is a woman. Now, a woman is the one thing about which I know nothing. Tell me, what is the nature of woman? Then Rasakosha smiled and said: King, you should certainly keep this question to ask the Princess; for it is a hard question. A very terrible creature indeed is a woman, and one formed of strange elements. I will tell you a story: listen.

In the beginning, when Twashtri came to the creation of woman, he found that he had exhausted his materials in the making of man, and that he had no solid elements left. In this dilemma, after profound meditation, he did as follows: He took the rotundity of the moon, the curves of the creepers, and the clinging of tendrils, and the trembling of grass, and the slenderness of the reed, and the bloom of the flowers, and the lightness of leaves, and the tapering of the elephant's trunk, and the glances of deer, and the clustering of rows of bees, and joyous gaiety of sunbeams, and the weeping of clouds, and the fickleness of the winds, and the timidity of the hare, and the vanity of the peacock, and the softness of the parrot's bosom, and the hardness of adamant, and the sweetness of honey, and the cruelty of the tiger, and the warm glow of fire, and the coldness of snow, and the chattering of jays, and the cooing of the kokila (Cuckoo), and the hypocrisy of the crane, and the fidelity of the chakrawaka; and compounding all these together, he made woman, and gave her to man. But one week, man came to him, and said; Lord, this creature that you have given me makes my life miserable. She chatters incessantly, and teases me beyond endurance, never leaving me alone: and she requires incessant attention, and takes all my time up, and cries about nothing, and is always idle; and so I have come to give her back again, as I cannot live with her. So Twashtri said: Very well; and he took her back. Then after another week, man came again to him, and said: Lord, I find that my life is very lonely since I gave you back that creature. I remember how she used to dance and sing to me, and look at me out of the corner of her eye, and play with me, and cling to me; and her laughter was music, and she was beautiful to look at, and soft to touch: so give her back to me again. So Twashtri said: Very well; and gave her back again. Then after only three days, man came back to him again, and said: Lord, I know not how it is; but after all, I have come to the conclusion that she is more of a trouble than a pleasure to me: so please take her back again. But Twashtri said; Out on you! Be off! I will have no more of this. You must manage how you can. Then man said: But I cannot live with her. And Twashtri replied: Neither could you live without her. And he turned his back on man, and went on with his work. Then man said: What is to be done? for I cannot live either with or without her.

A Digit of the Moon, translated from Sanskrit by F. W. Bain (published by G. P. Putnam & Sons, New York, London, 1907)

THE MEANING OF THE SEVEN AGES

WOMAN—THE ETERNAL MYSTERY!

What constitutes femaleness? What is the essential nature of woman?

This has been the mystery that has challenged the minds of mankind throughout the centuries. All manner of men—poets, novelists, philosophers, teachers of religion, and scientists—have been intrigued by it. And they have given to the world, at least to that part which cared to listen, their theories about women—in song and verse, in novels good and bad, and in learned treatises. How right each or any one of them may have been is still a matter of opinion, for their answers are as diverse as the men who proposed them. There has been among them hardly a meeting of the minds, much less a single body of thought.

The controversy remains, as it always will, a lively one. Woman is interpreted as the lost sex, the second sex, the inferior sex, the superior sex, the mystical sex, and sometimes only sex! But whatever the adjective used to qualify her, the important thing is that she is never denied her sex. Perhaps it is here that the answer will be found.

Woman today is just what she has always been—a feminine personality, a feminine mind in a feminine body. The feminine mind, her psyche, is mysterious because the minds of all humans, male or female, are mysterious. How is it that we learn, store knowledge, remember, and forget; that we "think" of ourselves, of others, and of the world about us as we do? That we are far from having the final answers is apparent in the fact that there are different schools of psychology, which give us widely different answers for "why we behave like human beings." Even more revealing of this diversity or lack of unanimity are the different schools of thought in psychiatry, which tell us "why we misbehave like human beings."

There will never be one answer, for woman has behaved and mis-behaved, thought and acted, believed and disbelieved, hoped and feared, according to the culture in which she lived. She has acted as she was taught to act, believed what she was taught to believe, feared what she was taught to fear, according to the knowledge, customs, and ethics of the times. Mostly she has done what was expected of her; occasionally, what she thought she could "get away" with; and rarely, she has revolted. This is important to remember when reading of "sexual behavior" whether it be of "modern woman" or the "savages of another land."

Feminine behavior has meaning only when it is viewed in relation to both the time and the place in which the woman lived. It would seem unlikely that Scheherazade had any feeling of "inferiority" after one thousand and one nights of successfully protecting both her virginity and her life. Anne Boleyn, who was not so successful, probably regretted the "guilt" of poor judgment and the misfortunes of her life rather than felt "shame" for the expression of her sexuality.

Patterns of feminine behavior are never static. For example, if you were asked who are the modern American women, you would answer—they are the women living in America today. That is true, but they include three generations—the teen-agers, the mothers, and the grandmothers. And no one has to be told the difference between what a grandmother and her granddaughter think about such matters as "woman's place," "dating," "going steady," "sex," and "marriage." Multiply this difference by the variations that result among families from differences in education, in religious and racial backgrounds, and in the life of a rural community and of a big city, and it is evident that there is no such thing as "the modern woman" who thinks and behaves in one particular way.

The second part of woman's personality, her soma (or body)—its struc-ture and function—is no longer a mystery. It is now known that the physical basis of femaleness is the same without regard for race or color, whether she be primitive or modern. Furthermore, the mechanisms that produce the physical characteristics of womanhood—her feminine curves, the sweetness and softness of her voice, the fine texture of her skin, and the feminine functions of menstruation and pregnancy are well understood. This knowledge is the result of the unraveling by scientists of the mystery of her endocrine glands. They are the forces responsible for the changes in her body that characterize each of the ages of her life.

The story of *The Seven Ages of Woman* tells of the structure and functions of her mind and body and how these change to meet the needs of life at each age. At first thought, life divided into ages might appear artificial or even false. Life is a continuing process, each day leading to and preparing for the next, and each day what it is partly because of what has gone before. But from day to day there is change, and when the life cycle is viewed in its entirety, there are "ages" that have characteristics of mind and body that set them apart.

The fact that these changes occur is obvious and age old, but the knowledge of the mechanisms that bring about these changes is recent. We now know something of the how and why of a woman's structure and function because we know something of the functions of her endocrine glands. These tiny structures scattered through the body influence, and in many instances completely control, her life processes. Indeed, a woman's life consists of seven ages because of the action of her endocrine glands. The division of woman's life into seven ages is valid and meaningful from one other standpoint—each age marks a change in her view of the world and in her relationship to her fellow travelers.

The first, the Age of the Unborn, is the most clearly defined as to time. It begins with the union of the two parent cells in the mother's body to make one single cell. In just nine months this single tiny cell, by the processes of growth and differentiation, becomes a little armful of humanity. It is the protective and directive action of the mother's endocrine glands that makes this possible.

The second, the Age of Infancy and Childhood, is primarily one of growth and development. It is concerned with increase in body stature, in development of skills in physical control of the body, and in growth of knowledge and understanding.

The third, the Age of Youth, is a continuation of the growth period but is modified by the development of sex function. The little girl changes to a woman.

In the fourth, the Age of Maturity, the body has attained its growth and sex function and is developed for the fulfillment of the fifth age, Marriage and Motherhood.

The Age of Marriage and Motherhood is the active reproductive period with its problems of marital adjustment, child spacing, fertility, and sterility. It is a time when a woman is called upon to hold a successful balance between the development of her own talents and the fulfillment of the needs of her husband and children. Woman of today has more on her shoulders than at any other time in history. She has far greater freedom to express herself, and with this comes a greater responsibility because she must also meet her inherent duties of childbearing and child-care.

The sixth, the Age of the Menopause, is a period in which the reproductive (not necessarily sex) function is waning. It is not a fearsome period but merely the beginning of release from childbearing and child-care.

The seventh age has never been accurately named. What shall this age be called—the life remaining after fifty? It is almost a new age because the American woman of today can expect hers to be longer and healthier than ever before in the history of womankind. It can be rich and full in human experience. The old medical terminology, the Age of Senility, is no longer acceptable because it is untrue, unfair, and misleading. A better term is the Age of Serenity. These years, which constitute about one third of life, can be the happiest of a woman's life if she has built properly for them and has stored up within herself resources for activity. The burden and responsibility of child-training and child-care are past, and she is free to devote her time and energy to further develop her talents and pursue her interests.

The development or unfolding of the seven ages is a slow, gradual, and orderly process not marked by cataclysmic or climactic changes. It is brought about by varying levels of function of the endocrine glands. In the Age of Infancy and Childhood the dominant glands are those concerned with growth and development of the body. To these are added in the Age of Youth the function of the sex glands. By maturity the sex glands have achieved dominance with activity to ensure a succeeding generation, the prime motif. Sex glandular function recedes through the menopause, leaving in the final age only those glands concerned with maintaining normal, nonreproductive body functions.

Interesting though this story may be, what is to be gained by the recounting of it? Is the knowledge worthwhile from the standpoint of the woman's health and happiness? The answer is definitely "Yes."

This glandular mechanism of body control is intricate and delicate. It is not surprising that there are many mishaps along the way; but usually they are not too serious. A woman should be able to recognize significant symptoms of abnormality and separate them from those that are not significant. She should be able to do this not for self-diagnosis and self-treatment; that is the most dangerous error into which she could possibly fall. But a basic knowledge of structure and function will enable her to know when something is wrong, to discuss her symptoms intelligently and without embarrassment with her physician, and finally to follow medical advice most intelligently. After all, understanding what is wrong and how to help nature correct the fault constitutes a large percentage of medical practice. Nowhere in medicine is this more true than in the field of female endocrinology.

Women are being deluged today with "medical information" by newspapers, magazines, and radio. So much is being written about the abnormal with especial emphasis on neuroses, sex, and cancer, that in the minds of many women, confusion has been created and fear instilled. A basic knowledge of the normal will enable woman to evaluate what she reads and to separate facts from fancies and half-truths. She will not be so easily convinced that she is a neurotic, that she is frigid, or that every blemish is a cancer.

Modern woman has assumed equal status with man in all phases of modern life. If she is capable of understanding and contributing to world politics, atomic research, medical science, and all the other elements that make up our world of today, surely she can and should be able to understand her individual world—herself. Understanding herself, she will come to the realization that being a woman and fulfilling efficiently a woman's mission, that of wife and mother, will not only need the exercise of all her talents but also will bring her the greatest reward—true happiness and peace within herself.

The story of *The Seven Ages of Woman* opens with the Age of Maturity because maturity is the vantage point for a survey of all the ages. Here woman is at the peak of her physical development and function. When she knows how her body functions at its greatest efficiency and fullest capacity, she will have more interest in knowing, and will better understand, the purpose and significance of the changes in the ages leading to maturity. Perhaps more important, she will have a basis for anticipating what the future has in store for her in those years which, in fact, can be the most meaningful period of her life.

THE AGE OF MATURITY

I

SIGNPOSTS TO MATURITY

THE PATHWAY OF life's journey has often been likened to a trail across a single mountain. The traveler emerges from the nebulous unknown of the Age of the Unborn and begins the climb, which continues through infancy, childhood, and youth to reach the peak of maturity. Here, the traveler may pause only a moment and then must start the downward trail—the sunset road.

This picture is false, because this concept of maturity is false. Life's journey is better characterized as an upward climb along a trail that is a little different for every traveler. The trail may have sharp rises and falls, sometimes meaningless meanderings, sometimes long stretches through pleasant mountain meadows. Occasionally, it passes through dark forests or ascends to dizzy heights. For some, it opens out on breath-taking vistas. But always the trail is upward and onward. When the traveler ceases to climb because no higher goal is perceived to lie ahead, the end of the trail is near.

This is the true picture because maturity is not a single fixed goal that is achieved at a specific time. Rather, it is a quality of the traveler herself, involving her total personality, and it has a different meaning for each of the attributes of her personality—for each characteristic function of her mind and body. Some attributes of maturity she achieves quite early in the journey, some quite late, and still others she strives to perfect all her life.

How then can it be said that woman's life is marked by stages—that there is an Age of Maturity? While it is true that this journey is progressive and that the qualities of maturity are ever changing, there is one definitive aspect of her personality the changes in which mark quite clearly the ages of her life. That is the quality of her relationship to others as expressed in the degree of her dependence or independence and of her particular kind of responsibility. The Age of Maturity stands out as the age wherein she achieves independence and assumes the responsibilities of being not only an adult but also a woman. How she may choose to assert her independence as an adult, or whether she chooses to assert it at all, will be contingent on the fact that physically she is now a woman with woman's particular obligations. The ages before are marked by the transition from complete dependence to independence with foreshadows of her feminine responsibilities. After maturity and its fruition in motherhood, another transition brings a different phase of maturity in which she is relieved of most of the physical responsibilities of being a woman, and she may then devote her efforts to exploiting her potentialities as a person.

The Age of Maturity for woman in our modern world is vastly different from that of previous generations and other cultures. In the early days of America, the responsibilities of maturity were mainly marriage and motherhood, and they were placed on woman's shoulders very early. She married at sixteen, even fourteen, proceeded immediately to produce a family, sometimes at the rate of a child a year, and she was old before she was forty. Today, she is usually older when she assumes the full responsibilities of maturity, and the age holds for her the promises of longer duration, better health, and richer experiences. As it passes, she still has many years of active life ahead, which were denied the majority of women of preceding generations. With these changes in her life expectancy, her economic and social emancipation, and the complexities of everyday living, the nature of modern woman's responsibilities of maturity has changed.

Woman in becoming "modern" has a particularly difficult job in also becoming "mature" because she has assumed a dual role in society, new in the history of womanhood, which she has not yet learned to integrate. She has achieved the rights to help run the world's business, to pursue a career, to earn a living, to make her own decisions. In many instances, the necessity for her to do these things is thrust on her whether she wants it or not. At the same time, she must continue to fulfill the age-old duties peculiar to her sex—childbearing and homemaking. It is no wonder that at times she appears a little bewildered about how best to fulfill these major roles successfully or that her actions sometimes appear contradictory. It is not an easy task to achieve maturity both as a female and as a person.

What then is a "mature woman"? There is, of course, no single definition, for woman is a very complex creature indeed. The meaning of maturity in woman is to be found in the blending of the physical and psychological elements of her personality. The main concern of this book is with the physical aspects, but what she is physically can never be divorced from what she thinks about herself. In order to arrive at a meaning of maturity in modern woman, some standards must be set up by which to measure it. For this purpose, maturity may be examined as to three qualities—the psychological, the physical, and the sexual.

The process of maturing has a different time of starting, a different rate of developing, and specific goals for attainment for each of these phases. But each phase is dependent on the other two if a fully matured personality is to be achieved. Maturity in one phase promotes maturity in the others.

The interrelationship among the three phases of maturity is evident in menstruation. As a physical phenomenon, it means only periodic bleeding; but, to a woman, it is never without emotional significance. Its first appearance signals the dawn of womanhood. If this occurs at too early an age, her childhood is cut short, and she may be confronted with physical drives with which she is unable to cope. If it fails to occur at the expected age, she feels that she is "different." During the Age of Maturity the regular occurrence of menstruation signifies to a woman that she is normal, but her plans of activity frequently must be adjusted to it. If she observes herself, she will note that her moods and emotions vary with her cycle. Sudden cessation of her cycle, announcing the start of a new life, may be the fulfillment of a great longing, or an added burden, or, if she is unmarried, will bring shame and sorrow. Such is the impact that the physical has on the psychological. The reverse may also be true. Emotional disturbances can result in either failure to menstruate or abnormal types of menstruation.

PSYCHOLOGICAL MATURITY

There is here no intention of explaining the psyche of woman, but some recognition of the psychological attributes of maturity must be established. There are two components of psychological maturity—emotional and mental. Woman's emotional maturity is not mysterious, devious, or uncontrollable. Nor is it something that she is destined to have or not to have. Rather, it is an achievement toward which she must continuously strive. Some may arrive at a degree of emotional maturity at an early age, some later, and some never. For some, the road to achievement is smooth, and progress is steady. For others, many obstacles are thrown in the way, and the going is rough and slow.

How mature a woman is emotionally is shown by her attitude toward herself and the world about her. A mature woman accepts her place in life, and life has a meaning and a purpose. She has respect for herself but is not self-centered. She gets along well with others and respects their rights. She has work to do, exerts herself to do it well, and derives satisfaction from it. She accepts responsibility and is dependable. She makes mistakes, but acknowledges her errors and seeks to correct them. She has problems, disappointments, grief, and sorrow, but she does not give way to self-pity. She can forgive and forget. She can look back, without living in the past, and she looks forward with confidence and optimism, but her main energies are devoted to her world of today. The crowning attribute of her maturity, which gives meaning to all the others, is love. This she can freely give and graciously receive. To be such a woman at all times would be perfection and not of this earth, but she is an ideal toward which all may strive.

This concept of maturity and the means by which it may be attained, even the fact that training and guidance are necessary to attain it, has been obscured in recent years. We seem to have lost our perspective. By emphasizing the negative aspects, those that contribute to failure of maturity, and dwelling on "immaturity," "insecurity," "inferiority," "frustration," "complexes," "neuroses," "ego-protection," "shame," and "guilt," we lose sight of the true goal. Emotional maturity then comes to mean the ability to get what one wants for one's self in a hostile world.

Emotional maturity should mean the ability to be a contributing member of the world of people, an outgoing, outgiving personality concerned with the welfare of others. To be such a member of our modern culture requires also the ability to live within the rules and standards of the everyday world. Such positive aspects of personality as honor, courage, modesty, decency, compassion, loyalty, diligence, thoughtfulness, unselfishness, integrity, responsibility, tolerance, and humility should be emphasized. They should be taken out of the category of old-fashioned virtues and made a living part of our striving for maturity. These are the qualities a woman needs to meet the problems of her adult years, whether they be of a profession, work, or those of her sex—marriage, home, and children. Everyone has some of these attributes some of the time. But as we are confronted with new problems that require new solutions, we are not always able to meet them in a "mature" way.

Maturity is not based on self-deprecation, but on a healthy respect and high regard for one's own self. Its goal is not conformity, but growth of one's personality through the recognition of individual potentialities and determination to make the most of them. Nor is maturity expressed only as a member of society. It requires a degree of self-sufficiency and inner resourcefulness whereby one may retreat into privacy and not be bored by one's own company and emerge from the aloneness refreshed.

Mental maturity, the other component of psychological maturity refers to the development and use to its greatest capacity of the brain power with which a woman is endowed. It means the acquisition and use of knowledge, and it is a process that should be continuous throughout life. American woman today has greater opportunity to achieve higher goals than ever before in history. No field of learning is denied her, and better and higher degrees of education are open to her. Travel, books, radio, and television have opened vistas once accessible to only a favored few. In turn greater mental maturity is demanded of her. It is no longer sufficient to have only a beautiful face and figure; she must have "personality," which implies intelligence, training, and knowledge. The merits of such training and knowledge should not be measured in terms of dollars and cents— that is, earning a living—or in the ability to acquire a husband; but rather in the degree of maturity she achieves in whatever career she may choose, and how much she contributes to and enjoys the complex world in which

she lives. One important part of this knowledge is an understanding of
and confidence in herself.

PHYSICAL MATURITY

Psychological maturity deals with the intangibles. It is, and probably
will continue to be, a subject of discussion and controversy. But physical
maturity can be seen and measured, and we have scientific facts to explain
the biological mechanisms that underlie it.

A physically mature woman has attained her full body growth. Her
height falls within the range of normal for her sex and race, her weight
is proportionate to her height, and her body has the typical feminine
contour. But women are not satisfied with just being normal. They want
to be attractive and would like to be beautiful. Here again standards
change. In the gay nineties the small-waisted, full-bosomed, broad-beamed
lady was the height of fashion. In the wild twenties, she was flat-chested
and had no waist at all! But the abiding standard of beauty is found in
the harmony and perfection of the normal features of the body—rounded
breasts, adequate waist, slender hips, dignity and grace of carriage, and
freedom of motion. Women of today accept these standards with a few
exceptions. There is, however, overemphasis on breast development, a
glorification of slenderness, and an extravagant evaluation of cosmetics.

SEXUAL MATURITY

Sexual maturity is not merely a phase of physical maturity. It is rather
the result of blending the psychological and physical phases as they
relate to sex. Physical sexual maturity is attained by woman when her
sex organs have reached their full growth and are capable of fulfilling
their definitive function—reproduction. This, nature accomplishes for her
at an early age, fourteen to sixteen years, and sometimes much earlier.
Psychological sexual maturity is attained when a woman has not only
knowledge of the physical aspects of sex, but also a healthy emotional attitude toward being a woman. This she must achieve for herself.

How sexual maturity is attained is an important part of each of the ages as we shall see. Through these ages she learns to accept sex as a normal, natural part of her life. She recognizes in it a force for her to use with joy and confidence in making her life richer and fuller; not a force to be dreaded or feared. She recognizes sex as one of the compelling forces that give direction and meaning to her life, but not the only one.

A healthy, happy, emotional attitude toward sex is predicated on sound factual knowledge of the physical basis of sex. Some of this knowledge she will get by observation in her daily personal relationships through the years when she is growing up. Some will come from actual experiences as her body changes from that of a child to that of a woman. These alone are not enough; she must know the basic facts of the structure and functions of her reproductive organs. These facts she must be taught—and the unfortunate truth is that, even in this generation, she rarely is taught.

Most women arrive at the age of sexual maturity with only vague ideas concerning their sex anatomy and physiology, and many women are completely innocent (or, to put it more bluntly, ignorant), of the simplest facts on this exceedingly important phase of her personality. To make matters worse, they have been given an overdose of misinformation. In place of truth, she has fears, superstitions, and taboos.

That she suffers from this lack of sex education—ignorance, misinformation, and lack of understanding of the attendant responsibilities—is apparent on every hand. The high frequency of illegitimate pregnancies and births is one example. In 1956, one of our major but not largest cities reported that at least one hundred junior high school girls were excused from attendance because of pregnancy. There are no accurate statistics for other groups of girls and women, but there are many such cases. The incidence of criminal abortion, with its attendant heartache, physical suffering, and occasional death, is appallingly high, and the most frequent victims are young married women.

Divorce affords another example of this lack of knowledge—on the part of the husband or the wife, or both. Failure in marriage is too frequently the result of their immaturity in the concept of what marriage means and lack of knowledge of how to meet and overcome its problems and determination to do so. A large and important part of this failure is lack of sexual maturity. These examples could be multiplied if we considered the unhappiness and mental and physical suffering that are the lot of so many women because of their ignorance and fear related to problems of woman's sexuality.

Another stumbling block in woman's pathway to sexual maturity is the false standards provided for her. What chance has she to attain the ideals of maturity when attention is directed only to perfection of face and figure and the one basis for marriage is physical attraction? It is tragic that the physical attributes of beauty, youth, and sexuality are the ideals set for womanhood in all the media of communication and entertainment. Even many books, offering guidance in the problems of daily living (such as marriage manuals) and purporting to be scientific analyses of woman, overemphasize the physical. These, of course, have a rightful place in woman's life and thoughts, but only a fraction of her energies should be directed toward them. If she accepts these standards and directs her life accordingly, she is destined to unhappiness and to failure as a mature woman.

Our main concern in *The Seven Ages of Woman* will be with the physical aspects of her personality. But it is hoped that with the knowledge of the wonderful mechanism that is her body, woman can make it the instrument for a full and happy life and will never allow it to become her mistress.

II

THE WONDERFUL MECHANISM OF THE BODY

THE HUMAN BODY is the most wonderful mechanism in existence. Nothing that man has ever invented, even radar, the outerspace missile, or the mechanical brain, can compare with it. Its component parts are not only designed for definite purposes, but they are exquisitely adjusted to work in perfect harmony to maintain the welfare of the whole body under all kinds of conditions. We can see this every day in ourselves and in others if we pause to observe and analyze this marvel of creation. A single incident, which might happen to anyone, will demonstrate the working of this mechanism.

It is dusk in springtime at the seashore. A young woman is walking along the beach with an easy graceful swing; not hurried, but every movement expressing the very joy of being alive. The wind, causing her light garment to cling to her, reveals the graceful feminine lines of her body. Her face, fresh and lovely, is lifted to catch the soft breeze blowing from the ocean. She pauses a moment to gaze out over the peaceful waters. Perhaps she is remembering the boisterous pleasures of the seashore as a child; or she may be dreaming of the future. Whatever her thoughts, she releases them and resumes her contented, unhurried pace.

Suddenly she stops as an unseen hand is placed on her shoulder. Her whole body tenses. Her face loses its rosy hue and becomes deathly white. She gasps for breath. Her heart pounds. The sudden pressure on her shoulders, because it was unexpected and of unknown identity, is instantly interpreted as danger. Her body automatically readies itself for action— either to flee or to turn and fight. A voice known to her and trusted speaks, and her fright vanishes as quickly as it came. She trembles with relief, or perhaps with resentment at being startled. It will take her body a little time to recover from the quick mobilization of its forces, which so changed the pattern of her body function. This whole incident, simple and common-place, lasted only a few minutes, yet it epitomizes the mechanism of body function.

SYSTEMS OF CONTROL

Women's body may be analyzed in terms of a machine for a better understanding of the meaning of both its structure and its function. Whether it be the electric stove in the kitchen, an automobile, or Univac, a machine has three components: first, there are a certain number of parts, each of which has a definite purpose, and these parts must be put together properly so the machine can work; second there must be a system of controls that direct and co-ordinate the work of each part so the machine will work efficiently as a whole; finally there must be a source of power to make it work.

The human machine consists of parts put together in systems, each specialized to meet one or more of the body's needs. Examples include: the digestive system, which takes food in and changes it to simple chemical substances that the body cells can use; the respiratory system, which extracts the oxygen from the air; and the circulatory system, which carries this food and oxygen to every cell of the body. We have glimpses of these in the incident mentioned above in the woman's apparent good health, in the texture and color of her skin. The muscular system is the one we see working, and it does so, smoothly and efficiently, because it is adequately supplied with food and oxygen. These systems and all others that make up her body are working harmoniously, each making its contribution to the welfare of the whole, and in turn receiving the benefits of the work accomplished by the other systems.

Like other machines, the body must have a means of communication and control that will direct and integrate the activities of all the parts under varying conditions. The body's control mechanism consists of three systems each of which is highly specialized but all efficiently integrated—the central nervous system, the autonomic nervous system, and the endocrine system.

The central nervous system is exceedingly complex and beyond our purpose to discuss further than a simple sketch to round out the picture of total body regulation. It consists of the brain, the spinal cord, and the nerves to all parts of the body by which the conscious control of the body in relation to the external environment is effected. Sensory nerves such as those of the eyes, the ears, and the hands send messages to the brain of what is going on in the world outside the body. The brain receives, interprets, and records this information and sends out messages of appropriate action along the motor nerves to the muscles. This handling by the brain of information, we recognize as reason, judgment, memory, emotions—all the facets of the mental activity of the individual.

The action of the central nervous system was represented in the instance above in the woman's contemplation of the world about her—its present beauty bringing memories of the past and hopes for the future; and by her enjoyment and sense of well-being as she walked along, derived from the fact that her body was working harmoniously both within itself and within its environment. When danger threatened, it was the central nervous system that detected it and sent out the "alarm." It was the central nervous system that recognized the voice of a friend and sounded the "all clear" signal.

The autonomic nervous system is less complex than the central nervous system. It consists of groups of nerve cells, or ganglia, and nerves distributed throughout the body. Its function is to regulate the activities of the body that are vital and must be continued at all times—the heart beat, blood pressure, breathing, rhythmic contraction of the intestines, and so on. These activities continue without our thinking about them. We cannot directly change them by any conscious or deliberate act, and they continue when consciousness is lost as in sleep, fainting, or anesthesia.

The action of the autonomic nervous system in our demonstration became apparent with the tensing of the woman's muscles, the blanching of her skin, the increased heart beat, and faster breathing. Her body automatically adjusted itself for increased physical activity.

The third system of control is the endocrine system, which does its work not through such physical structures as nerves, but by chemical changes within the body. To analyze the part it played in our example, we must direct attention not to the activities of the woman's body but to the structure of the body itself. She is of adult size, feminine proportions, straight and sturdy because the endocrines of growth and sex maturation have functioned normally. Her skin is soft and of fine texture, her body is well nourished and full of energy because the chemical processes within her body have been efficiently handled by her endocrine glands.

A machine, besides being of a definite structure with a system of controls, must also have power. In the body this, of course, is the mysterious force we call life, which resides in every cell, and the summation in all cells of this force makes us thinking, feeling, and acting human beings.

The nature of the control mechanism of the body has always been an intriguing question. The ancient scientists described it in terms of magic, spirits, humors, and vapors. Knowledge of the nervous system as a directing force had its birth many centuries ago when anatomical dissection was first practiced. The endocrine glands were discovered then also, but no useful purpose other than filling space was attributed to them. Their secrets were not revealed until modern chemical analysis and animal experimentation, joined in the science of biochemistry, furnished the effective method of study—an accomplishment of the present century and largely of the past thirty years.

This knowledge of endocrine mechanism has solved many mysteries of certain phases of body function. It has revolutionized our whole concept of the meaning of health—and in turn of disease. It has brought insight, understanding, and appreciation of two important characteristics of body function, which no man-made machine could ever possess—the "wisdom of the body" and "adaptation to stress."

THE WISDOM OF THE BODY

The term "wisdom of the body" means the ability of the body to maintain stability while it is performing many diverse functions, and in the presence of an ever-changing environment. It was coined more than a quarter of a century ago to express what has become the basic philosophy of modern medicine—the concept that the body possesses the power of exquisite adjustment, and the way to health and mastery of disease is through understanding this wisdom of the body. "Nature" (or natural forces) and "normal," terms we frequently use as applied to our well-being, are in reality expressions of this basic physiologic concept. An understanding and appreciation of the details as applied to our special field of interest—female function—is the purpose of this book. At present, let us see what is meant by "stability."

The body is composed of many millions of living cells, and a large proportion of each is fluid. Each cell is constantly undergoing chemical change, yet the stability that is normal is maintained. There are many familiar examples of this. We weep salty tears because all body fluids maintain in health a constant salinity. All the chemical tests of body fluids for such substances as sugar, cholesterol, and sex hormones are useful because in health they are maintained at a stable level (within a small range of variation). The cells have a limited life span, some no more than a few weeks, but the over-all or total number is kept stable or constant. A blood count is normal when it has the usual number of red blood cells and of the different types of white blood cells. When these tests vary from the range of "normal," they indicate that something has happened to disturb the internal stability. For each internal function of the body, stability is maintained by a specific regulatory mechanism. We shall meet these later as "endocrine mechanism of the menstrual cycle," "weight-regulatory mechanism," and the "forces of labor." For the body as a whole, internal stability is maintained by drives such as hunger, thirst, and sleep.

Stability, however, does not mean rigidity. It means balance, at varying levels, which is optimum for body needs in varying circumstances. The speed of each system is so timed that it will perform most efficiently for a particular activity. All are synchronized for smooth, efficient functioning of the body as a whole. The individual speed of each system will be changed for different activities. In sleep all would be slowed down (heart beat is slower, blood pressure is lower, digestion slows down, muscles are relaxed). In strenuous activity some would be greatly accelerated and others would be slowed (pulse is faster, blood pressure raised, breathing more rapid—but digestion stops). In our demonstration the mechanism of the body was at first functioning at a speed best suited for the particular activity at the moment—a quiet stroll. But the speed was also adjusted to the environment—the cool of the evening at the seashore.

The body must function in an ever-changing physical environment and be able to make adjustments so that the body itself is not changed and stability is maintained. It must adapt to various degrees of heat and cold, moisture, and amounts of oxygen in the air. It must maintain the same normal temperature in the heat of the tropics or the icy blasts of the arctic. It must maintain its fluid balance in the drying winds of the Sahara, the fog of London, or in the high humidity of a rain forest. It must supply the same amount of oxygen to each cell whether the supply is abundant as at the seashore or scarce as at the mountain top. This is accomplished by "adaptation," that is, change in speed of certain systems of the body.

The maintenance of stability and adaptation of function to body needs is dependent on not one or the other systems of control, but on the co-ordinated action of all three—the central and autonomic nervous systems and the endocrine glands. But the body can change its pattern of activity suddenly and efficiently when danger threatens; it can adapt to stress.

ADAPTATION TO STRESS

So far we have been speaking of adaptation within a favorable environment. But the body rarely finds itself within such a happy situation. There are always dangers lurking—pressures within the mind and body of the individual and threats and assaults from the world without. The body possesses a built-in mechanism of defense, which it uses against these various types of assault.

Stress is a word heard frequently today with many different shades of meaning. Usually reference is to everyday events that threaten a person's peace of mind, self-respect, or well-being, such as worry, fear, or overwork. But we also speak of stress as applied to surgical operations, which may include the person's emotional reaction to her situation or the body's response to the physical and chemical trauma incident to surgery. In all such situations, the common denominator is the state within the body induced by something that threatens its integrity of structure, its stability, its health. Stress thus comes to mean any condition—any assault on the body on either the physiologic or psychologic level or both—which calls into play (and may throw out of balance, damage, or exhaust) the body's defense mechanism. The body's defense reaction is always the same, but the causes that produce stress are such diverse things as extreme heat or cold, nervous tension, emotional strain, infection, excessive physical activity, traumatic injury, or irradiation.

The body's defense mechanism that sounds the alarm and mobilizes its forces for resistance involves all the systems of control, but the endocrine system is responsible for the physiological changes that make resistance possible. If the defense mechanism is effective, the danger is met, injuries are repaired, and health is restored. If it fails, illness, disease, or death may ensue. In our demonstration we saw only the superficial evidence of the initial stage of stress—the alarm reaction, when the woman was frightened. Had she been injured, her body would have been able to make the necessary repairs to maintain her life and restore her to health.

The ability of the body to meet these ever-changing needs and to respond and adapt itself to an ever-changing environment, to defend itself against assault, to make repairs after injury are the attributes that make it more wonderful than any invention of man's mind.

The wisdom of the body is an attribute that everyone possesses but not according to one rigid pattern. Each woman has her own individual differences—in the quality of her structure, intensity of her needs, character of stability, and the meaning of stress—derived from her heritage and shaped by her experience, which makes her a woman different from all other women.

MUTUAL DEPENDENCE OF THE
NERVOUS AND ENDOCRINE SYSTEMS

The three systems of communication share in the control of body function, but each is dependent to a certain extent on the others for its efficient and normal function. When something happens to disturb the function of one, it has repercussions in the others and alters their function also. That is to say, the endocrine system can be rendered inefficient by a disturbance or stress that primarily affects the function of the nervous system. The reverse is also true. This is an important fact, which will be apparent as we learn more of female endocrine function. Two examples will serve to clarify what is meant by this mutual dependency and emphasize its importance.

Jean had been unable to conceive during the ten years of her marriage, and her desire for a child had become an obsession. One month she failed to menstruate and was convinced that she was pregnant. In the following months she experienced all the signs and symptoms of pregnancy—absence of menstruation, morning sickness, gain in weight. She even thought she "felt life." It was a severe blow when, after several months, her obstetrician told her she was not pregnant. Her disappointment was intense, but in a few weeks all the symptoms of pregnancy had vanished. Jean is an example of the effect emotional stress may have on glandular function. Her intense desire for pregnancy resulted in suppression of ovarian function. This is not a unique case but is of fairly frequent occurrence. History tells us that Mary, Queen of England, kept all England and her Consort, Prince Phillip of Spain, in suspense while she awaited the heir who never arrived. She too was a victim of false pregnancy.

Isabel, age 46, had noted a peculiar and frightening change in herself. She had always been placid, cheerful, and energetic, but she had recently become depressed for no apparent reason and would burst into tears on the slightest provocation. Her teen-age children irritated her almost beyond endurance, and her body was acting queerly also. Her hands would get numb and tingle, her heart would suddenly start beating rapidly. At times sudden waves of heat swept over her body and were followed by drenching perspiration. A careful medical survey showed that there was nothing wrong with her heart nor was she losing her mind as she feared. The primary fault was in her endocrine system. She was experiencing the menopause, which occurs when the ovaries go to sleep and lose their ability to function as endocrine glands. The hot flushes, sweats, numbness, and tingling were due to disturbances of the autonomic nervous system. The mental depression and irritability were due to disturbances in the central nervous system, as a result of the glandular deficiency. Relief of the stress on the glandular level by the administration of ovarian hormone restored the normal balance within the other two systems of control.

The endocrine system thus plays a role, directly or indirectly, in every phase of body function, contributing greatly to our health and happiness.

This is particularly exemplified in female physiology where it plays a dominant and dramatic part. Woman's mind and body and sex function are expressions of her normal endocrine function. So, if we are to know her, we must know her glands. So far, we have met the endocrine system only as a chemical means of control. Every woman should be introduced to each of these glands and understand the part each plays in the great endocrine symphony. This introduction must wait until we become acquainted with the instruments on which they play—particularly woman's reproductive organs.

WOMAN'S REPRODUCTIVE ORGANS

To understand female sex physiology, we must first know what organs make up the reproductive system, where they are located, and what part each one plays in reproduction. Scientific names must of necessity be used because in most instances there are no others. This should not be too difficult, for the names are euphonious, and every woman should know this much of scientific anatomy.

The reproductive organs of the female consist of two groups of structures. The external genitalia are those visible from the outside of the body, and the internal are those concealed within the pelvic cavity. The external organs are the mons veneris, the labia majora and labia minora, clitoris, vestibule, vaginal opening, and hymen. The internal organs are the vagina, Bartholin glands, cervix, uterus, tubes, and ovaries.

The mons veneris (Mount of Venus) is a pad of fat covered with skin and hair situated over the pubic bone. Extending downward from either side are two other thick soft pads of fat covered with skin and hair called the labia majora (large lips). Between the two major lips and partly concealed by them are two long thin folds of soft moist tissue with no hair, called the labia minora (small lips). These are frequently dark brown in color. These inner lips are rarely of uniform size. They may be quite small in some individuals and almost completely concealed by the major lips. In others, one or both of the lips may extend an inch beyond the major lips. Such variation is not abnormal and has no significance, although women are sometimes frightened by it.

Where the labia minora come together in front just below the mons veneris and completely concealed by these structures is the clitoris. This is a small rounded structure of soft tissue and is very sensitive. It corresponds to the penis in the male. The valley between the two pairs of lips is called the vestibule. There are two openings in the vestibule, a small one about a quarter inch in diameter behind or below the clitoris which is the opening of the urethra—the canal that extends to the urinary bladder. Below this is the larger opening of the vagina. Just within the opening of the vagina is a thin soft membrane or fold of tissue, the hymen.

The hymen varies considerably in size, shape, and consistency in different individuals and in the same individual in different ages. In the virgin it usually consists of a half-moon, or crescent-shaped fold puckered across the lower part of the vagina. It is soft and easily stretched. Its opening allows the admission of one finger. After marriage only a little ridge, or a few little tags of tissue, are all that remains of the hymen. Occasionally, the hymen is thick and tough and must be cut before marriage relationships can be consummated. Very rarely, the hymen completely closes the vaginal opening and must be removed or punctured to allow the escape of the menstrual flow.

The vagina is a canal about six inches in length. It extends upward and backwards with a slight curve into the pelvic cavity. Its walls are soft, moist and elastic, and are usually thrown into folds. The vagina is the organ of sexual intercourse. It is the canal through which the menstrual flow passes from the uterus to the exterior, and it is also the birth canal. On either side of the opening of the vagina where the lips fade out is a small gland, the Bartholin gland, which secretes a lubricating fluid at times of sexual excitement. Ordinarily it cannot be felt, but when it becomes infected or filled with fluid, a woman may be quite conscious of it.

The uterus (womb) is the organ that houses the baby during pregnancy and is the source of monthly periods. It is a pear-shaped organ with the narrow part, cervix or neck, extending downward into the vagina and the large part, corpus or body, extending upward into the pelvic cavity. The membrane lining the cervix contains glands that secrete a heavy mucus, the purpose of which is to moisten the vaginal canal, which has no glands of its own.

The walls of the uterus are composed of layers of muscle, the contractions of which cause labor pains and delivery of the child. The lining of the uterus is a soft velvety membrane called the endometrium the function of which is to form a nest and furnish nourishment for the embryo during pregnancy. It is the source of menstrual bleeding.

The Fallopian tubes, two in number, extend outward from either side of the upper portion of the uterus, and their cavities are continuous with that of the uterus. The function of the tubes is to transport the ovum from the ovary to the uterus. This is accomplished by the rhythmic contraction of the muscle in the walls of the tube, aided by the waving of small hair-like structures (cilia) on cells in the lining membrane, which set up a current to carry the ovum along. It is in this tube that the ovum and sperm meet and unite and then move downward into the uterus. The tubes are not directly attached to the ovaries, but the outer end of each tube has many finger like projections (fimbriae) directed toward the ovary, which effect the movement of the ovum from the ovary to the tube. The cavity of the tube varies in diameter. At its largest part, it may be the size of the lead of a pencil, but in the smallest part, it is no larger than the shaft of a pin. Closure of the tubes by disease is one of the most common causes of sterility.

The ovaries have a double function. They produce the germ cells or ova, and they elaborate the all-important sex hormones. They are two almond shaped bodies on either side of the pelvis. If the ovary is cut across, it is seen to be studded with little rounded structures called follicles situated mostly near the surface. These are in all stages of development—immature follicles, mature Graafian follicles, and corpora lutea (yellow bodies).

All the internal reproductive organs of the female are safely housed in the pelvic cavity. The walls of the pelvis are made up of a complete circle of bones, the pelvic girdle, cushioned on the inside with soft tissue and muscle. Also in the pelvic cavity are the urinary bladder, which is in front of the uterus, and the rectum, which is in back of it. The upper opening of the pelvic cavity is continuous with the abdominal cavity. The lower opening is closed in with layers of strong muscle, soft tissue, and skin, which support all these structures.

These then are woman's particular organs—well developed and ready to function as a part of the wonderful mechanism that is her body. The spark needed to bring it to life is furnished by her endocrine glands.

III

THE ENDOCRINE GLANDS

THE ENDOCRINE GLANDS are chemical laboratories, ever busy each minute delivering to the body their products, which not only keep the flame of life burning with a steady and purposeful glow but also give it warmth and brilliance. They are tiny organs, as compared with others, but they have a mammoth function. In size, they vary from a small cluster of cells scarcely visible without the aid of a microscope to the largest, which is no more than half the size of a fist. Yet from these small structures come secretions of chemical substances that play a vital part in every function of a woman's body and in every age. Her body cannot do its work without them—it cannot live without them.

The secretions of the endocrine glands, because they are so important for the welfare of the whole body, not to one particular part, are poured directly into the blood stream, which carries them to all parts of the body. That is why they are called endocrine (or ductless) glands—meaning secreting internally. This distinguishes them from all other glands of the body, which are called exocrine or glands of external secretion.

The exocrine glands deliver their secretions by means of ducts (little tubes) into one particular place in the body—mostly the surface and hollow organs, as the stomach and intestines, where they serve a particular function. The sweat glands of the skin keep the surface of the body moist, and the salivary glands of the mouth secrete saliva to provide moisture and prepare food for further digestion.

The endocrine glands, pouring their secretions into the blood stream, thus constitute a system of communication and control that extends to every cell in the body. It is a chemical system that is concerned with maintaining the chemical balance of the body. This over-all balance consists of many chemical processes carried on by many kinds of cells to serve specific functions. By this communication system every cell is directed to function, according to its abilities, at the time and speed that will maintain an internal state that is optimum for the health and welfare of the body as a whole.

The secretion of each endocrine gland contains at least one specific substance of definite chemical structure called a hormone. Some endocrine glands produce several hormones. The word "hormone" means "to arouse" or "to set in motion," which is exactly what a hormone does. Each hormone is a chemical messenger, which is sent to some particular organ with specific instructions. The hormone does not tell the cells of the organ how to do their work, but just how much and how fast the work must be done. Neither does the hormone take any part in the performance or the process. Sometimes the message carried is a positive one—it says "get busy" or "speed up." Scientists speak of this as the "stimulating action" of hormones. In other instances, the hormones may carry the message "slow down" or "stop," which is called "depressing action." Each hormone has its "target" organ whose activity it directs, but as it circulates through the body, it also affects other organs. Thus hormones may have both "specific" and "generalized" actions within the body.

The term "hormone" is a generic term applying to all the chemical messengers sent out by all the endocrine glands. To have meaning, it must be made specific. Usually this is done by preceding it with the name of the endocrine gland from which it comes, as ovarian hormones and thyroid hormone. Scientists have determined the exact chemical structure of some hormones and have given them specific names. Thus certain ovarian hormones are known as "estrone" and "progesterone." Other hormones are known only by their physiological properties and are identified in that manner, such as the "thyroid stimulating hormone."

We know what hormones do—that they are regulators of cell activity—but we do not know very much about how they accomplish this. Nor do we know the complete story of how endocrine glands manufacture their hormones, what they use as basic substances, how they are synthesized to the active product, or what happens to many of the hormones after they have served their purpose.

When the endocrine glands are producing their hormones in normal amounts, they constitute a system of checks and balances, which keep all the body functions at the optimum level of activity—that of good health. Sometimes a gland does not produce its hormone as it should, and the particular function it fosters becomes disturbed. This condition doctors recognize as a "functional disease." If the gland for some reason produces too much hormone, scientists call it "hyperfunction"; if it produces less than it should, it is called "hypofunction." These abnormal states of excessive and deficient function of the endocrine glands were recognized by doctors long before they understood how such conditions were produced; but this first suggested to doctors what the normal function of the endocrine glands might be.

Woman's endocrine glands are: the pituitary, the thyroid, and the two adrenals, which are vital to her general health. They also contribute to her sexuality, and we shall consider them in some detail for that reason. The two ovaries are, of course, her own specific sex endocrine glands. The pancreas and several pairs of parathyroid glands are important to specific metabolic function, which need not concern us. There are other structures such as the thymus and the pineal body, which some think are endocrine glands, but we still do not know very much about their purpose.

THE PITUITARY GLAND

The pituitary gland occupies an exalted position in the body anatomically (it is the only endocrine gland situated in that most important part of our anatomy, the head), from which it exerts dynamic authority on physiology. The facts that the pituitary lies just below the brain and is connected to the base of the brain by a small stalk or stem and that it is protected by its own little bony case (the sella turcica or turkish saddle), which conforms to its own size and shape, are suggestive of the important role that it plays in the control and welfare of the body.

Ancient scientists, who first discovered this little structure hanging like a cherry by its stem, were more impressed by the fact that it was placed just above the throat. They considered it an important gland, which secreted phlegm (pituita) to moisten the throat, and so they named it the pituitary gland. Others called it the hypophysis cerebri (undergrowth of the brain). Neither name gives any hint of the true function of this gland. It would be exceedingly difficult to devise a word to describe the multiplicity, intricacy, and importance of the activity of this tiny organ.

The pituitary might be likened to the control tower of a vast communications center. Here, messages originate and are sent out that direct the activities of various substations, and here also are received messages of the activities and needs of the various outposts. These messages, out-going and in-coming, must be co-ordinated to the end that the whole endocrine system will function efficiently, harmoniously, and effectively. The pituitary is the control tower of the system of the body that is concerned with maintaining the chemical balance of the body. In this manner, the pituitary exerts a regulatory action on most of the chemical processes of the body. This is one general function, but it is far from the whole story.

The chemical system, made up as it is of many diverse processes, is never set at a fixed state of equilibrium, because the internal needs of the body are constantly varying. They vary with the change in body activity and with changes in the external environment. Therefore, adjustments to maintain the optimum are constantly necessary. There are the usual adjustments that take place in the everyday activities of waking and sleeping, of being hungry and eating, of rest and exercise. But frequently the body is subjected to greater stress, such as exposure to excessive heat or cold, to infection or injury, and adjustments must be quickly made to maintain the integrity of body function. So we may say further that the pituitary controls the adjustment of body function to the changing needs of both the internal and external environment.

This adjustment to change and stress is an exceedingly complex function, but it is no more than is accomplished in certain man-made mechanisms. The human body is more than a mere machine—it is a living organism, which means that it grows and is constantly making repairs and replacements of worn out parts. Furthermore, a living organism has the unique characteristic of reproducing itself. The pituitary plays a regulatory role in both growth and reproduction.

In the light of these general facts concerning pituitary function, it is easy to see why the pituitary gland is often referred to as the master gland, the "conductor of the endocrine symphony," and sometimes as the "brain of the endocrine system." The means by which these functions are accomplished are not simple. With one exception, the pituitary does not perform the functions directly or independently. Rather, its hormones stimulate other endocrine glands to produce their galaxy of hormones. In turn, the pituitary function is affected by the other hormones and by the nervous system.

The hormones concerned with these functions are secreted by one portion of the pituitary—the anterior lobe or adenohypophysis (glandular). There is a second portion, the posterior lobe or neurohypophysis, which is more closely related to the nervous system and need not concern us.

The exact number of hormones produced by the anterior pituitary has not been definitely established. This arises from the fact that the pituitary hormones are complex protein substances, which are difficult to obtain in pure form and to identify positively by chemical means. However, enough is known about the activity and chemistry of some (about six) substances derived from the gland to give each of these a name that describes its function.

The pituitary hormones are called "tropins," which means that they are stimulating to their target organs, which are (with one or two exceptions) other endocrine glands. What is equally important to note is that these glands are dependent on pituitary stimulation to enable them to adequately produce their own specific hormones. The interactions of the pituitary and its target endocrine glands are exceedingly complex mechanisms, which we shall consider in more detail later.

One of these tropins is the thyreotropic hormone or thyreotropin that stimulates the thyroid to normal function. Without it, thyroid hormone production is not completely lost, but it is inadequate for body needs.

The tropins that stimulate the ovaries are called gonadotropins, meaning sex-gland stimulators. There are two or three (authorities differ on this) gonadotropins produced in the human female. The rhythmic function of the ovaries, which is responsible, among other things, for the rhythmic function of the uterus (menstrual cycle), is the result of the rhythmic production of these several gonadotropins.

And there is ACTH. This has become almost a household word since the substance has been used so extensively in the treatment of many human illnesses, such as arthritis, severe burns, and nephrosis in children. It is a pituitary tropic hormone. Its target is the outer part (the cortex) of the adrenal gland and is therefore called *adreno-cortico-tropic-hormone* or by the initials ACTH. It is primarily by ACTH, and the thyreotropic hormone, that the pituitary controls body function in relation to environment and stress.

The pituitary produces one hormone that acts directly on a single organ—the breast. The mammotropic hormone initiates the secretion of milk by the breast after the delivery of a child or the termination of a pregnancy. This hormone is more often called prolactin or the lactogenic hormone. Some authorities consider it a gonadotropin and call it luteotropin.

Finally, the pituitary produces a hormone that acts directly on the body as a whole—the growth hormone. This hormone, somatotropin, is concerned with the growth process in the young. It cannot be said that somatotropin completely controls growth because there are other factors necessary for normal growth, including the action of other endocrine glands, nutrition, and freedom from disease. But in general it is true that the growth hormone must be present at the right time and in the right amount for the achievement of normal growth of the body.

Woman's pituitary gland thus controls by its many hormones her growth to adult proportions, the development of her feminine characteristics of body structure and function, her fertility, and her ability to meet the stresses and strains encountered in each age of her life. As a rule it performs its role quite well. But occasionally it does not, and hypofunction or hyperfunction results. It would be difficult at this point to portray what a woman's symptoms might be in either of these conditions—for two reasons. In the first place, the abnormality may involve one, any combination of two or more, or even all of the tropic hormones, which makes possible an almost limitless variety of symptoms. Second, these symptoms are expressions of other endocrine gland disturbances. We need to know more about the normal function of these glands before undertaking the description of their abnormalities.

There are, however a, few situations that may be briefly described, such as marked deficiency of all the hormones (pan-hypopituitarism) and either hypofunction or hyperfunction in just one panel, for example, the growth factor.

Pan-hypopituitarism occurs when something drastic happens that destroys normal anterior pituitary structure making any function impossible. The destructive agent may be thrombosis of the main artery, which produces necrosis of the gland, pressure of a tumor against the gland or irradiation (administered to control tumor growth). But destruction of the gland must be almost 100 per cent. Nature has provided a wide margin of safety here (as she has in most other vital organs). One-half of the gland can be destroyed and cause no symptoms; destruction of three fourths produces only mild symptoms.

Pan-hypopituitarism is rare, but it occurs four times as frequently in women as in men. It usually has its onset after a rapid succession of pregnancies (five or more), and in most instances the immediately preceding pregnancy was complicated by severe post-partum hemorrhage and collapse. The symptoms are rapid loss of weight to extreme emaciation with a comparable loss of strength. The general appearance deteriorates similar to that of rapid aging to the point of senility. The skin is wrinkled, dry, loses its pigment, and takes on a peculiar waxy palor. The hair of the head and the body fall out, the nails become brittle and dry. All body functions fail. There is a loss of appetite and inability to retain food; the menstrual function is lost; mental processes are slowed down, with apathy and depression. Available tests show marked deficiency in function of all the endocrine glands, particularly the adrenals, the thyroid, and the ovaries. The usual outcome without treatment is death.

The results of abnormal production of only one pituitary hormone is most easily demonstrated by the growth hormone. When there is an excessive production of this hormone in a young person (before maturity), the result is an individual of excessive height, a victim of giantism. This is almost exclusively confined to males. The excessive production after maturity, which occurs more frequently in females, produces distortions of appearance, a condition called acromegaly. The features become large and coarse due to increase in size of the bones of the face, and the hands and feet are grossly enlarged.

Deficiency of the growth hormone in childhood results in stunted growth or dwarfism. This is rare, for deficiency is usually accompanied by deficiency in other hormones as in the gonadotropic and thyreotropic. These are extreme conditions and are very rare. They are described not to suggest that they might happen to you or your children but merely to point up the general function of the pituitary. This will also be true of the other grotesque humans that will be described for other endocrine gland abnormalities.

THE THYROID GLAND

If the pituitary is the "master gland of the endocrine system," the thyroid is the pacemaker. If the pituitary is the "conductor of the endocrine symphony," the thyroid is its "metronome"—it sets the tempo at which the symphony is rendered. In the intricacy and delicacy of the feminine endocrine symphony, the thyroid is especially significant, determining whether the rendition of each of its movements or ages shall be confused and apathetic or purposeful and vigorous, for it is the pacemaker or metronome not only for the endocrine glands but also for every other cell in the body.

The thyroid, because of its position in the neck, was known to early, even ancient, scientists. To them this soft mass of tissue, shaped like a butterfly hovering around the larynx or voice box, seemed to serve no useful purpose unless it might be a packing to fill out space or to keep the neck warm. The protective function attributed to it is implied in its name "thyreos," meaning "shield."

The early physicians recognized that the thyroid was always larger in women than in men and that in women it swelled to even larger size at puberty, menopause, menstruation, and pregnancy. Some thought that it must in some way be related to her sex function, but the best explanation they could give was that the gland shunted the blood from the brain—and women had greater need for this protective device, or so they thought, because she had more "irritation and numerous causes of vexation of mind than the male!" Or a larger gland was assigned to the female to make "her neck more even and beautiful." Many of the paintings by the old masters are of women with goiterous (enlarged thyroid) necks.

The association of the thyroid with beauty is not as farfetched as it might seem. The most grotesque and misshapened of human creatures is the "cretin"—a human born without a functional thyroid gland. They are dwarfs whose every feature is distorted, whose minds are dull and stupid. In adults, more frequently in women than men, whose thyroids for some unknown reason cease to function, the appearance becomes that of an "old hag." The face is bloated, the skin thick, wrinkled, and dry; the hair sparse, coarse, stringy, and brittle; the muscles flabby and weak, capable only of slow and clumsy movements. The mind is dull and apathetic or gives way to madness.

Why does thyroid failure result in these caricatures of a human? The answer lies in the vitalizing ability of the one hormone the thyroid produces, and in the fact that this hormone acts on not just one organ, not just another endocrine gland, but on every cell, of every tissue and organ of the body. Modern scientists who have ferreted out the secrets of the thyroid hormone, summarize its function by saying that it "controls metabolism." This is what they mean:

The routine work of living, as carried on within the body, is accomplished by chemical processes. By these chemical processes, food and oxygen are transformed into living matter, heat and energy are released, waste products are cast off, and the wear and tear of constant activity is repaired. Thus, there are different chemical processes for breathing, digestion, muscular activity, glandular secretion, and so on for every body function. The sum total of all these chemical processes going on within the living body is called "metabolism."

The body can live, which means it can do all these things, without the thyroid hormone. It does them well only when the thyroid hormone tells each chemical system how fast to work under different conditions of body need for the maximum efficiency and health of the body as a whole. Thus the thyroid controls the tempo of life. By what mechanism is the thyroid able to vary the tempo as occasions demand? The answer lies in a delicately balanced interaction between the thyroid and the pituitary gland.

The thyroid gland is able to speed up metabolism by increasing the amount of hormone it pours into the blood stream. Metabolism slows down when the amount is decreased. If the thyroid were uncontrolled and undirected and could pour out as much hormone as it could make, an excess would accumulate in the blood stream and the body would be speeded up to a state that would be dangerous. This does not happen because the thyroid is controlled and directed.

The thyroid is not independent—a master mind. It is in fact very dependent. It cannot work at all unless it is stimulated by the thyreotropic hormone from the pituitary gland. But that does not answer the question how the amount of thyroid hormone is kept within healthy limits. It merely removes the point of origin of the driving force from the thyroid to the pituitary. Something must be acting to tell the pituitary when there is enough thyroid hormone in circulation and therefore to slow down. That something is the thyroid hormone itself.

The thyroid hormone has a particular kind of action on the pituitary, different from its stimulating action on the rest of the body. It inhibits the ability of the pituitary to produce the thyreotropic hormone. Thus between the pituitary and thyroid, there is a self-regulatory mechanism of check and balance that works in a cyclic manner. It starts by the thyreotropic hormone stimulating production of the thyroid hormone. The amount of thyroid hormone increases, and as it increases, it inhibits the further production of the thyreotropic hormone. With a leveling off and drop in thyreotropic hormone, the thyroid is unable to maintain its high level of production. With the resulting drop in the thyroid hormone, the pituitary is released from its inhibiting action and starts again to produce thyreotropin, and the cycle starts all over again.

This same self-regulatory mechanism exists in the relation of all the pituitary tropic hormones and those of their target glands. We shall meet with it again in the regulatory mechanism of the gonadotropic-ovarian hormones in the menstrual cycle.

This then is the function of the thyroid gland—to control metabolism—and the mechanism by which it is kept within the bounds necessary for normal body function. When the thyroid is functioning normally, in the environment of a healthy body, the result is efficiency, vitality, spark. Just what this means is better appreciated if we see what happens when the thyroid produces too little hormone (hypothyroidism) or too much (hyperthyroidism).

The symptoms of hypothyroidism are diverse and variable. They are diverse because the thyroid hormone affects every tissue of the body, and deficiency may show itself by disturbance in function of any part of the body. They are variable depending on the degree of deficiency. The picture presented earlier is that of profound failure in adults called myxedema, which is not common. But mild to moderate degrees of hypothyroidism are exceedingly common, especially among women.

Moderate hypothyroidism in woman may show itself in many symptoms.

Her mental activity is lower, she finds it hard to concentrate, she is forgetful. She is less interested in her work, her home, her friends, and her husband. She is irritable and subject to headaches. Although she requires and usually gets more than the usual amount of sleep, she is tired all the time. She gets up in the morning exhausted, but her energy may speed up somewhat later in the day. Simple exercise exhausts her. She has poor tolerance for cold, she shivers all winter and is comfortable when others find the summer heat excessive. Her skin is dry and thickened. Her hair is coarse and dry and may come out excessively. Constipation is a source of much worry and discomfort. One of the most characteristic symptoms of hypothyroidism is disturbance of ovarian function. She may stop menstruating or her periods become too profuse and prolonged. Sterility and abortions are frequently the result.

The symptoms of hyperthyroidism are just the opposite. The woman is overstimulated. As a result she is nervous, irritable, and on the move all the time. She cannot be still. She cannot stand heat and perspires profusely. Her hands shake. Diarrhea is troublesome and contributes to loss of weight. Her heart is very rapid—and she is conscious of it. In one type of hyperthyroidism (exopthalmic goiter) the eyeballs bulge, giving her the appearance of being startled or frightened. Here too the sex function is disturbed, the usual result being loss of menstruation and sterility.

Normal thyroid function is important in all ages. It contributes to growth and sex maturation, fertility, mental development, emotional stability, the enthusiasm for living. Failure of the thyroid to function may produce an idiot. A properly functioning thyroid may not make a genius, but there could be no genius without a normal thyroid. While it is not essential to life, that is, mere existence, as is the case with the adrenals and pituitary—life would hardly be worth living if denied the vitalizing influence of the thyroid.

We come now to the third of woman's endocrine glands that contribute to the female sex function, the adrenals. Their role, however, is not as clear cut as that of the pituitary, thyroid, or the ovaries. We really know very little of their part in the sex cycle.

THE ADRENAL GLANDS

The adrenals derive their name from the fact that they are perched on the kidneys, each like a "cocked hat," where they are cushioned in a mass of fat and protected by the lower ribs. They were also called suprarenals (above the kidneys) as more appropriate for humans with their upright position. Either name is misleading, because proximity is their only direct relationship to the kidneys.

These two little structures have a unique place in the history of endocrinology. They seemed to have had a peculiar fascination to early physicians, whose only tools, before the day of scientific investigation and laboratory experimentation, were observation of structure and speculation. They ascribed to the adrenals such functions as the production of "black bile," a ferment that made the heart beat stronger, or as padding to support a more important structure—the stomach. Even in those days, the many theories were not taken too seriously but were put aside with the hopeful comment that perhaps some day the truth would be revealed. Such revelation was a long time in the making.

The results of the first scientific investigation of the adrenals, which consisted of observing the effects of removal of the gland and the administration of crude extracts, were more confusing than revealing, until it was realized that each adrenal was not a single gland but two glands with completely independent functions.

Each adrenal is like a bonbon (of a peculiar shape to be sure!), the thickened outer coating representing the cortex and the soft filling the medulla. The cortex is a true glandular structure, while the medulla is more closely related in structure and function to the autonomic nervous system. The realization that these were two glands led to the early discovery of the function of the medulla. Its hormone, adrenalin or epinephrine, was the first of all the hormones of the body to be identified chemically and synthesized.

The first scientific information on cortical function came from biological experimentation that nature herself performed in the destruction of the gland by disease and the astute observations of an English physician, Dr. Thomas Addison, of the resultant changes in body structure and function.

He recognized the cause-and-effect relationship of this form of human adrenalectomy. His description, in 1855, of the symptoms that occurred when the adrenal was destroyed by a then prevalent disease—tuberculosis—is a medical classic not only because of its lucidity but also because it is remarkably complete and valid in the light of present-day endocrinological knowledge.

"The leading and characteristic features of the morbid state," he wrote, "are anaemia, general languor and debility, remarkable feebleness of the heart action, irritability of the stomach and a peculiar change in color of the skin occurring in connection with a diseased condition of the supra-renal capsules. This singular dingy or dark coloration usually increases with the advancing disease; the anaemia, langour, failure of appetite and feebleness of the heart become aggravated;—the pulse becomes smaller and weaker, and without any special complaint of pain or uneasiness the patient at length gradually sinks and expires."

In Addison's Disease the victim thus suffers a steady deterioration of the total body vitality, which ended inevitably in death before the present-day available help of the adrenal hormones.

The adrenal cortex has been the most difficult of all endocrine glands for scientists to solve the secrets of its functions and relationships—to ascertain the identity of its hormones and what they do. This accomplishment is one of the most brilliant in the history of endocrinology and was achieved by ingenuity, imagination, and perseverance—not by just one person, but by many investigators using varied chemical and biological methods of experimentation. And they are still searching for further understanding. From the days of Dr. Addison it was known that the adrenals were absolutely essential to life, but it has been only in the past twenty years that the hormonal mechanism has been explained.

The first successful step was the production of a cortical extract, called "cortin," which could maintain life in an animal deprived of its adrenals. Since then a large number (thirty or more) of chemical substances of the "steroid" family (which also includes the sex hormones, cholesterol, vitamin D, bile salts, etc.) have been isolated from the adrenal cortex. Only a few of these, about six, are capable of replacing one or more functions of the adrenal cortex. But no single known hormone can perform all the functions. These biologically active cortical steroids fall into three groups according to the type of function they serve. The first are the glucosteroids, which play an important part in the metabolism of organic substances such as carbohydrates, fats, and proteins, and include cortisone, corticosterone and hydrocortisone. The second are involved in the metabolism of inorganic materials, as minerals, sodium, potassium, and chloride, and in water balance. They are called mineralocorticoids. Aldosterone is an example. The two groups are antagonistic to each other in some ways, an important one being in relation to inflammation. The glucosteroids inhibit inflammation, while the mineralocorticoids enhance the process. The third group includes both male and female steroids whose function in health is still an enigma, but they are known to play an important role in certain adrenal abnormalities.

The specific functions performed by these adrenal hormones are exceedingly complex, involving many metabolic processes. It would lead us too far astray to pursue them in any detail, so we shall confine ourselves to generalities.

Life, Work, Stress: these are the key words of adrenal cortical function. They sum up the ability of the body to live and perform effectively and safely in the changing environment for which the cortical hormones are essential.

The adrenal cortex is essential to life. In the function of maintaining life, it enters into many of the vital metabolic processes, including carbohydrate, protein, and fat metabolism, fluid and salts balance, and immunilogical reactions. An animal or human deprived of its adrenals will surely die unless the vital hormones are administered. This can now be done.

The adrenal cortex is essential to the ability to work. Deficiency of secretion leads to such weakness of the neuromuscular basis of physical exercise that the organism can perform only a short period and even then ineffectually.

The adrenal cortex is essential to meet stress. We speak of the stress of living today, recognizing that it plays an important role in our health—both physical and mental—but perhaps without recognition of its full significance. "Stress," as used in physiology, is a condition that threatens the health of some function or group of functions or even the whole body. It may come from changes within the body or from external agents. Single stressors (conditions that produce stress) are such things as excessive heat or cold, injury, toxic agents, infections, or emotional tensions such as fear and anxiety. A surgical operation is a condition of stress. The body must be able to adapt—to mobilize its defenses to meet the stress, promptly and effectively. It does so—it adapts—in a stereotype fashion, whatever the threatening agent may be. Adaptation is effected through the pituitary-adrenal axis, and the nervous system, and the corticoids play an indispensable role. If the body is able to adapt to stress, health is maintained or restored. If it fails, disease and sometimes death is the result.

Stress has acquired a new and revolutionary meaning in medicine in the past decade. The general symptoms of any illness—malaise, elevation of temperature, rapid pulse—are part of the body's way of meeting stress, whatever the cause may be. There is considerable evidence that illness and diseases the causes of which are unknown, and therefore incurable, represent the breakdown in the ability of the body to meet stress. In acute situations when stress is overwhelming and adaptation is absent or inadequate, death occurs promptly. In chronic conditions that represent a lesser degree of stress over a longer period of time, the process of adaptation is distorted due to hormone imbalance. Some hormones overdo their job causing changes in function and structure that are harmful. Essential hypertension and arthritis may be examples.

This concept of stress—the part it plays in disease and the role the adrenals play in meeting stress—is the basis on which cortisone and ACTH have come to be used in so many different conditions. They are used to block, prevent, or relieve the harmful reactions within the body, regardless of what the cause of stress may be. They do not remove the cause nor do they effect a cure. This should in no way detract from the marvel of their performance. Cortisone and its kindred steroids and ACTH (which makes the adrenal of the patient produce its own cortisone in increased amounts) have performed miracles. They have saved the lives of thousands in critical emergencies and others doomed by a previously hopeless disease. They have restored arthritic cripples to normal activity. And they have made life more comfortable for millions by the relief of minor irritations such as the discomforts of allergic reactions and the pain of bursitis.

The adrenal is not an autonomous organ performing these vital actions alone and unaided. It must fit into the endocrine symphony with other glands and is aided by these in many of the complex metabolic processes.

But most important, it is also dependent on the anterior pituitary stimulation by corticotropin to perform adequately and effectively. The balance is maintained in much the same manner as the thyro-pituitary relationship.

The functions of the cortex, which have just been briefly and oversimply described, are performed for the most part by the first two types of corticoids. There remains the third group, whose known action pertains to sexual characteristics of body structure and function.

Woman's adrenal cortex plays the role of accessory to her ovaries in that it produces sex hormones, but it differs from the ovaries in two important ways. In the first place, the adrenal produces not only her own female sex hormones, estrogen and progesterone, but also the male hormone androgen. And second, it starts this function early, before birth, and continues throughout her life. What purpose these hormones serve is not entirely known. Undoubtedly they play an important part during the Age of the Unborn in the differentiation of her primary sex characters—her reproductive organs. Later in the Age of Youth they play a minor role in the development of the secondary sex characters. When the ovaries go to sleep at menopause, the adrenals take over as a steady source of the sex steroids, which woman still needs as a source of strength and stability.

The relation of the adrenals to the sexuality of an individual was recognized long before anything was known about hormones. Early scientists noted that an individual's masculinity or femininity was changed in the presence of overgrowth or tumor of the adrenals. "Infant Hercules" was the name given to a male child with such a tumor because his body rather suddenly acquired adult male characteristics—hair on the face and body, deep voice and particularly muscular development like an athlete's. "Virilism" was the name applied when a tumor of the adrenal developed in an adult woman and was accompanied by the appearance of male characteristics and the loss of her female ones. This condition caused hair to grow on her body as in a male, complete with beard and mustache, her voice became deep and masculine, and she lost the typical feminine contour of her body—the breasts became small, the fatty pads on hips and shoulders disappeared and her muscles became enlarged. Menstruation ceased and she became sterile.

These conditions we now know are due to the excessive androgen produced by the tumor. If the tumor is successfully removed, the male traits recede.

Hyperfunction of the adrenal in the sex sphere of function may involve the overproduction of either male or female sex steroids, and such excess may occur at any time in life. The hypersecretion may be the result of a tumor or hyperplasia (overgrowth) of the adrenal or of overstimulation in this panel by the pituitary. We may cite a few examples.

There are occasionally infants whose sex cannot be determined at birth by observation. Such bizarre conditions are frequently associated with adrenals of abnormal structure. In childhood, sex is marred depending on which sex steroid is produced in excess. For some reason, it is usually androgen, which results in masculinization of the young girls. Rarely, the female hormone is produced excessively, and the little girl undergoes a form of precocious puberty.

A more common situation is virilism in the adolescent or young woman. This is due to adrenal hyperplasia (overgrowth without tumor formation) with increased production of the male sex steroid.

In looking back on the enodcrine symphony with the pituitary as the conductor and the thyroid the metronome, the question arises: What role shall we ascribe to the adrenals? From their versatility and indispensability, they would seem to constitute the orchestral instruments of many of the sections. And what is the music they play? It is the harmony of life and good health. But something is lacking to make the performance exciting, momentous, and complete. That something is supplied by the ovaries.

THE OVARIES

What part does the ovary play in the life symphony of the endocrines? It would seem that the major roles are very well performed by the pituitary, the thyroid, and the adrenals. There is only one role unaccounted for— that of the prima donna, for which the ovary is a natural. She is late in taking her part, but the overture is building up for it. She begins perhaps by a subtle introduction of new harmony or sometimes on a stridulent note, but her entrance is always dramatic. Thereafter, she holds the spotlight, dominating and dramatizing each theme and passage with richness, variety, and delight. When her role is finished, she leaves the stage, and the symphony goes serenely on—but the impact of her performance lingers and is re-echoed by less dramatic performers. The symphony could have been rendered without her, but it would have been a dull, monotonous performance indeed.

To translate this flight of fancy to the reality of physiology, let us note only some of the highlights of ovarian performance in the life cycle of a woman and leave the details for each of the ages. This may best be done by recounting what happens when ovarian function does not conform to the normal.

The ovaries may be completely unable to produce hormones at the appointed time in the young girl. Life goes on, the body continues to grow, she may achieve adult height or even be quite tall—but she can never be a normal woman. She will lack the feminine contour of well-developed breasts, curvaceous hips, and rounded shoulders. She will fail to achieve the feminine functions of menstruation and fertility. With this failure in achieving her physical basis of womanhood and maturity, she will have difficulty, although not insurmountable, in attaining a mature personality.

At the opposite extreme, the ovaries may start to function some years before the normal time. Her body then takes on the adult female characteristics including menstruation and fertility, but growth in height ceases early, and she is confronted with physical sexuality long before she is able to cope with it.

The ovaries may be removed surgically early in the Age of Maturity. She will retain her feminine contour, but menstruation ceases and her fertility is lost even though the uterus is left in place. She will experience the symptoms of menopause usually of more violent nature than when they appear at the appropriate time.

The ovaries perform these—and many other functions—by the two hormones that they produce, estrogen and progesterone.

Progesterone plays little part in woman's own body economy. She can be quite healthy without it, but it is profoundly important as a factor in her fertility. Estrogen and femininity are almost synonymous, for estrogen is the guardian angel of all the attributes of her sex throughout her whole life.

If we recount the characteristics of the seven ages of woman, we may substitute "estrogen" for "endocrine glands" as the causative agent for the changes she experiences and still be correct. In infancy and childhood, she develops along the same lines as boys because her ovaries have not yet started to produce estrogen. Her femininity unfolds in youth to attain maturity because of estrogen. The hallmarks of physical maturity, menstruation and pregnancy, are dependent on estrogen. In menopause, the cyclic rise and fall of estrogen is lost, but estrogen is still adequate to maintain her "serenity."

Estrogen is important to woman in ways other than those directly concerned with reproduction. Her outward appearance—the texture of her skin, the distribution of fat, and the distribution of hair are distinctly feminine because of estrogen. Even her size is dependent on estrogen, for estrogen is a controlling factor in the growth and sturdiness of her bones.

Estrogen is important in over-all control of her body because it affects both the way her other endocrine glands function and the way her nervous systems function. Emotional stability of maturity is dependent on the stability of estrogen production. The waxing and waning of estrogen in her life cycle is the cause of the emotional instability of youth and menopause.

"Estrogen" is a familiar term. Most women have heard of it in the treatment of many female problems, especially menopause, and have seen it advertised as a magic ingredient in creams to restore a "youthful complexion"—or to increase the size of the breasts. Some articles praise it to the skies, a boon to womankind; and others damn it as dangerous, to be left strictly alone because it may cause cancer. Wherein does the truth lie?

What is this magical substance—estrogen? First let us see what the name itself means. Estrogen is a general term under which are grouped many substances. All of these have the same physiological action, that is they produce the same response when they are administered to a woman's body or to laboratory animals. Chemically, they may be similar, but they can be quite different. It is the biologic activity, not the chemical structure, that makes them estrogens. The name estrogen came to be applied to these substances in this way: When scientists were trying to identify the hormones of the ovary, they studied reproduction in laboratory animals, particularly female rats and mice. They found that the female periodically went into heat or "estrus"—that is, she became receptive to the male. This reaction of estrus or heat (which holds for many other animals) was accompanied by a definite series of changes in the animal's body. Finally, scientists were able to demonstrate that these changes were the result of an ovarian hormone. They called it estrogen, meaning estrus-producing. With this "estrus-producing" action as a means for testing the ovarian hormone, scientists were then able to search out its occurrence and to determine its chemistry. They found that there was not just one estrogenic hormone, but several. These estrogenic hormones were found in fairly large quantities not in the ovaries but in the blood and urine of female animals and in much greater quantity during pregnancy. Woman does not have an estrus cycle, but her hormones are still called estrogen. They are three in number: estrone, estriol, estradiol.

The estrogens have been available for many years for doctors to use in treating many of woman's problems. Most of them are derivatives of one kind or another of the three basic structures and are marketed under such proprietary names as premarin, amnestrogen, estinyl, or just estrogenic hormone. Stilbesterol is an inexpensive synthetic product, which is quite different chemically from the natural estrogens but has similar biological action and the added advantage of being very potent when taken by mouth.

The role that the ovaries play is a distinct part of each of the ages of woman. It can best be understood by turning first to how the ovaries function in maturity when they are responsible for the typical feminine function—menstruation.

IV

FEMININE FUNCTIONS

THE EPITOME of feminine functions is expressed in menstruation—the normal, precise, and unique physical evidence that a woman has achieved maturity in this phase of her being. In modern times, this significance is recognized and appreciated, and the woman does not allow it to interfere with the even tenor of her life. But this has not always been so.

There is probably no occurrence in nature or the physical aspect of human life that has been so surrounded with myths, superstitions, and taboos as the process of menstruation. This periodic flow of blood from the woman's body has been interpreted by every group of people, primitive and civilized, as something that makes the woman "different" at the time of its occurrence. Many of these superstitions are still implied, when menstruation is designated as "sickness," "sick time," being "unwell," and the "curse."

Among most primitive people, in many parts of the world, who in this century are still living according to the customs of their ancestors, woman is even now considered unclean, sometimes even dangerous during the period of menstruation. Therefore, she is isolated in one way or another for its duration. In some tribes, "houses of blood" are set apart in their villages, and to these women must go and stay during the time of menstruation. In others, she is barred from community activities such as religious ceremonies, cooking, and bathing. Certain tribes require her to wear special apparel to mark her as unclean and therefore not to be approached. She is not allowed even to cross the path of cattle because, some believe, she would cause the milk cows to go dry and the pregnant ones to abort. She cannot tend the fields, or the plants will wither.

Even in the traditions of civilized, more cultured peoples, the concept of menstruation rendering the woman unclean still is accepted. Perhaps it stems back to the Mosaic Law, which stated that when a woman was menstruating "she shall be put apart seven days; and whosoever toucheth her shall be unclean until the even." In the early Christian Church, communion was forbidden to menstruating women. More recently, in farming communities, woman could not go into the dairy during this period, because it was believed that she would cause milk to curdle. Nor could she work in the winery because her presence would change wine to vinegar. Even today, it is a common belief that the touch of a woman menstruating will cause flowers to wither.

The true significance of menstruation remained an unfathomable mystery until quite recently, but not because physicians and scientists were not interested. From ancient times, they believed that the purpose of menstruation was twofold: that it was a form of purification or cleansing process; and that it was in some way essential to conception and pregnancy. They were intrigued by the question of its mechanism, and many theories were advanced to explain it. Perhaps the oldest and the one most obvious is the "Lunar Theory." In this the similarity in the time cycle of the waxing and waning of the moon and the monthly occurrence of the bloody discharge led to the belief that this womanly function was due to some influence exerted on her by the moon. The "Theory of Plethora" originated with Galen (about 160 A.D.) and held sway for many centuries. He thought that women were more full-blooded than men, and that a periodic relief by bleeding was necessary for a healthy life.

The present-day concept, which we may call the "Endocrine Theory," had its beginning in the middle of the nineteenth century, when it was first stated that the menstrual flow was a secretion of the uterus under control of the ovaries. This was based on the case history of a young girl from whom the ovaries had been removed by mistake. Previously, she had been a normal-appearing young woman who had regular menstrual periods. But after the operation she never menstruated again. Prior to this case, scientists knew that menstrual bleeding came from the endometrium, which showed differences in structure at different times of the month, but they had no idea what caused it. When this case demonstrated that these changes in the endometrium did not occur when the ovaries were removed, scientists began to study the ovary and found to their surprise that it too had a different structure at different times in the month.

Here was something entirely new—cyclic changes in two related organs. No organs in other systems of the body behaved in such manner. The heart, the kidneys, the liver looked the same and functioned the same day after day throughout the months and years. What was the mysterious force behind the cyclic changes in woman's reproductive system?

The first glimmer of truth came in the 1870's in the suggestion that the whole cyclic process was under some form of "central control," the nature of which was unknown, and that this cycle was not confined to the reproductive organs. According to this theory, for no proof could be offered, the menstrual cycle was depicted as a wave in which the metabolic processes in woman followed a distinct rhythm. The wave, it was postulated, started at a low intensity just at the end of the bleeding period, gradually increased through the month to reach a peak at the onset of menstruation, when it suddenly broke and the level of activity dropped to another low level. It was not until fifty years later that the identity of this "central control" was established.

This was the stage of our knowledge during my first year in medical school in 1926. I recall that one textbook, in discussing the menstrual cycle, stated in a footnote that Ascheimm and Zondek (who later devised the pregnancy test that bears their name) had recently presented data which indicated that the pituitary gland was probably the "motor"— the driving force—of these rhythmic changes. Thus, practically all of our knowledge of the mechanism of the menstrual cycle has evolved in the last thirty years. It has been a story much more thrilling than any novel, to follow this fitting together of facts as they have been discovered, to reach the solution of the age-old question, why do women menstruate?

Woman has always had an answer that was meaningful and satisfactory to her (even if not to the scientists). Menstruation signifies that she is a normal woman, and, if and when the right time comes, she will be able to conceive and have a child. When menstruation is normal, she accepts her potential fertility as a matter of fact. It is only when she does not have normal periods that she has misgivings and is apt to feel that she is less a woman because she will not be able to conceive.

In a way she is right, for there is a direct correlation between normal menstruation and fertility. But the actual flow of blood each month is not important because it is only a lamentation for a pregnancy that did not occur. Rather, significant events occur unseen and unnoticed (to a certain extent) in weeks preceding the flow when nature goes through an elaborate process of getting the body ready for pregnancy and preparing a nesting place for the baby-to-be. When conception fails to occur, nature must tear down and throw away her handiwork. This discarding of the nesting place is menstruation. Nature, not easily discouraged, starts all over again, even before she is quite through clearing away, to rebuild for another anticipated pregnancy the next month. This recurring cycle of building and tearing down is the menstrual cycle.

THE MENSTRUAL CYCLE

The menstrual cycle, in point of time, extends from the first day of menstruation to the beginning of the next period of flow. From the standpoint of physiologic change, it involves not just the uterus—the source of the flow—but the woman's whole body, her whole personality. It is a delicately balanced endocrine mechanism that changes from day to day. No two days are alike. No wonder women are changeable and unpredictable! The endocrine glands (the ovaries directed by the pituitary) have as their primary target the reproductive organs. All parts of the reproductive tract—ovaries, tubes, uterus, vagina, and breasts—have cyclic changes, because each has a vital part to play in the event of pregnancy. But these glands also have an effect, more subtle perhaps, on other parts of the body, such as skin, hair, blood, basal metabolism, blood pressure, nervous system, mind, and emotions. This ebb and flow, this changing level of endocrine function, with its resultant changes in body structure and function, is the basis of all the significant aspects of health and well-being that characterize the Age of Maturity.

Since we are now concerned only with menstruation—how and why it occurs—let us concentrate our attention on just those parts of the body that play a direct part in it. They are the uterus, the ovaries, and the pituitary gland.

The mechanism of the menstrual cycle is exceedingly complex. If you find it hard to follow, do not be discouraged. Just remember that it took medical scientists all the ages down to the present to grasp it. It will be more easily understood if we follow first the changes that occur in the endometrium (the lining of the uterus) during the month, then go back to those occurring in the ovaries, and finally retrace the cycle to see what the pituitary has been doing. When we understand what each has done separately, then we can put it all together to get the rhythm.

CYCLIC CHANGES IN THE ENDOMETRIUM

The endometrium at the end of the period of bleeding is very thin, not much more than the thickness of a heavy piece of paper. It is then a raw oozing surface, which looks very much like a brush burn on the arm when the skin has been scraped off. The blood becomes congealed in order to close the oozing surface, and bleeding stops. The lining begins to grow and continues to do so throughout the cycle. The surface acquires a soft velvety appearance. Just before bleeding starts again, the lining has grown to a thickness of about one quarter of an inch.

What happens to the structure of the lining of the uterus during this process of growth? It is well to keep in mind what the purpose of the whole process is. The lining is undergoing changes to make it a suitable place for the fertilized ovum to find lodging and to grow. Therefore, it must be thick and soft so that the ovum can burrow in, and it must have an abundant supply of food to nourish the ovum. If we look at a piece of the endometrium for each week of the cycle through a microscope, we can follow the changes in structure.

In the first week, it contains glands that are like little tubes extending from the base to the surface. They are straight and have a smooth lining. Between them are many small, coiled blood vessels, all held together by a loose connective tissue. Growth during the first two weeks consists only in an increase in the size of these structures resulting in increased thickness of the endometrium. At the beginning of the third week (in a twenty-eight day cycle), there is an abrupt change. The glands become coiled and their lining is thrown into the folds. The cells of the glands begin to manufacture a secretion, which will serve as food for the ovum.

The blood vessels also change. This phase is called "progestational," meaning preparation for pregnancy. The endometrium has now become a soft bed for the ovum to rest in and is full of secretion to nourish it. If at the end of these two weeks a fertilized ovum has not become embedded, the endometrium begins to crumble and bleeding starts.

The third stage, that of menstruation, is more than just bleeding, because it involves the whole endometrium. Bleeding starts as small hemorrhages from little blood vessels. This is followed by crumbling of the glands and connecting tissues, which opens up larger blood vessels and results in heavier bleeding. There is great variability in the time required for bleeding to be established. There may be only slight bleeding in the beginning so that in the first day the woman notices only a light flow. There may be only oozing for twenty-four to forty-eight hours so that she notices only a brownish discharge. It is brown because the amount of blood is only a trickle, moving slowly toward the outside, thus exposing it for a longer time to destructive influences which change its color. (A brown or black discharge always indicates old blood.) On the other hand, at the very beginning, the breakdown or crumbling may involve wide areas of the endometrium and extend deep into this lining so that larger blood vessels are involved. In this case the bleeding from the very start is heavy and bright red. Bleeding continues until almost all the lining has crumbled away.

There is one interesting characteristic of menstrual blood. It is the only instance in normal individuals that blood does not clot immediately after leaving the body. This is because the blood, while in the endometrium, has been subjected to a change that prevents clotting. When clots, especially abundant and large ones, occur in menstruation, it means that the endometrium has been remiss or unable to perform this duty.

An understanding of this monthly change in the lining of the uterus will dispel many old wives' tales. Menstruation is quite obviously the destruction of a tissue for which there is no use. It is not a cleansing process. It is not a way to get rid of poisonous substances. So, if for some reason the menstrual cycle and bleeding has not occurred, there is no retention in the body of poisonous substances. The question is frequently asked: If menstruation does not occur, where does that blood go? There is no excess of blood built up in the woman's body each month.

Rather she suffers a small loss at menstruation which must be replaced, and this is usually accomplished very quickly.

CYCLIC CHANGES IN THE OVARY

The cyclic changes in the ovary accomplish two objectives as a part of the preparation for pregnancy—the production of a mature ovum (fertile egg cell) and the manufacture of the hormones that bring about the changes in the endometrium.

If we took an ovary and cut it across, we would see many little areas varying in size from a pin point to a pea. These are little sacs or cavities containing fluid called the Graafian follicles. They are the most important functional element of the ovary, for it is here that the ovum grows. It is also the tiny chemical factory that manufactures the ovarian hormones. There are thousands of these follicles. Some authorities believe that all a woman will ever have are present in the ovary at birth. Recent work indicates that ova and follicles are being developed all through the life of the individual and that the life span of a single ovum is limited to about the same duration as that of the blood cell—a matter of weeks. Whichever may be the case, we do know that usually only one follicle goes through the process of full development each month with extrusion of an egg cell to be fertilized and the production of hormones to ensure a successful pregnancy. Let us follow the development of one follicle during a cycle.

At the end of menstruation, a follicle that is to develop is a little sac filled with fluid, lined with a single layer of cells. At one point, the lining cells are piled up, and in the middle of this little hill of cells is a single cell much larger than the others—the ovum. A follicle now looks like a signet ring. During the first two weeks of the cycle, the follicle grows by increasing the number of cells lining the sac and by increasing the amount of fluid, so that the structure bulges out on the surface of the ovary like a blister. During this period, important changes are taking place in the ovum. It is undergoing changes in structure by the process called "maturation" so that it will be able to unite with a sperm cell. We shall see the significance of this process in the Age of the Unborn.

The process of maturation is finished at the end of the second week, and the ovum is ready to start on its journey in quest of a sperm. The follicle breaks, and the ovum is floated out from the ovary in the fluid of the follicle. This launching of the ovum on its hopeful quest is called "ovulation." The sac now collapses because a good part of its wall and all of its fluid are gone.

What was previously a sac or follicle is now only a solid mass of cells. These cells increase in number and become filled with a yellow pigment. This characteristic color gives the structure its new name—corpus luteum, meaning "yellow body." The corpus luteum continues to grow until the end of the cycle is approached. If the ovum has found its mate and pregnancy is established, the corpus luteum continues to grow and to exert a protective influence on the pregnancy. But if pregnancy does not occur, the corpus luteum begins to shrink and finally disappears. Thus the changes in the ovary each month produce the female sex cell, which is ready to unite with the male cell, should one be available. Usually only one follicle goes through the full cycle each month. But many are called into readiness, increase in size and function, thus contributing their hormones to the over-all mechanism of the menstrual cycle. Let us go through the cycle again and see how the hormones are secreted and what purpose they serve.

HORMONE CONTROL OF THE MENSTRUAL CYCLE

Remember that we said the wall of the follicle consists of several layers of cells. These are the secretory cells. They manufacture the hormone "estrogen." They start making this hormone at the very beginning of the cycle and continue to do so in increasing amounts. After ovulation, when the follicle is transformed into the corpus luteum, it continues to make estrogen but also adds another hormone, progesterone. These hormones are not stored in the ovary but are discharged immediately into the blood stream and carried to all parts of the body. They have their specific action on the uterus. Estrogen stimulates the endometrial growth during both the first and the second halves of the cycle. Progesterone, which comes in the second half of the cycle, transforms the endometrium into a nourishing bed for the ovum.

Estrogen and progesterone, therefore, are the chemical messengers sent out by the ovaries, which cause the lining of the uterus to go through the changes necessary in preparation for pregnancy. What is the force that stimulates the ovaries to go through their cycle?

The ovaries go through their cycle of hormone production because they are directed to do so by the pituitary gonadotropic hormones. We do not know the exact chemical identity of these hormones, but most scientists agree that there are three: follicle stimulating hormone (FSH); luteinizing hormone (LH); the luteotropin. These are produced, not all at the same time or in a constant amount. They are sent out in swelling waves, one after the other. Each wave of gonadotropin occupies a certain number of days. It starts as a small amount of hormone, increases some each day to reach a peak, and then decreases and disappears. Just before it disappears, the wave of the second hormone starts. After the second hormone has reached its peak and is decreasing, the third wave starts. The first wave causes the follicle to grow. The combination and overlapping of the first and second wave causes ovulation, and the third wave transforms the collapsed follicle into the corpus luteum. The succession of pituitary gonadotropic hormones therefore accounts for the changes in the follicle, ovulation, and the secretion of the ovarian hormones.

There are still two questions to be answered: What causes the rhythm of the cycle? What causes menstruation (i. e., bleeding)?

The rhythm of the waves is a result of interplay between the ovarian hormones and the pituitary hormones. It is a see-saw action. The pituitary hormones stimulate the production of ovarian hormones, but the ovarian hormones depress the production of specific pituitary hormones. The first wave of gonadotropin causes the follicle to produce estrogen. As estrogen increases, it depresses the first pituitary hormone and allows the second to appear. The third wave of pituitary hormone stimulates the production of progesterone, and it, in turn, depresses the third pituitary hormone.

What then causes menstruation? To explain this, we must see what the situation is in the third week of the cycle in the three parts of the mechanism—the endometrium, the ovary, and the pituitary. The endometrium is at the height of the secretory phase because the ovary is supplying it with an abundance of estrogen and progesterone. The corpus luteum is at its height because the wave of the third pituitary hormone is also at its height. This is the crucial moment. As long as the corpus luteum is functional, the endometrium will maintain its secretory function and will not break down and bleed. And the life of the corpus luteum can be prolonged only by the beginning of a pregnancy. If conception has occurred, this is the time the ovum becomes embedded in the endometrium and starts the production of another pituitary-like hormone, which maintains the corpus luteum. When no pregnancy is present, the corpus luteum shrinks and ceases the production of estrogen and progesterone. It is the loss of adequate estrogen and progesterone that causes the endometrium to break down and bleed. This is an oversimplification of a complex mechanism, but it should be adequate for a general understanding of how the endocrine mechanism of the menstrual cycle works.

OVULATION

Ovulation is really the highlight, the most significant event in the menstrual cycle, for it starts the mature ovum on its way. What triggers the release of the ovum? How is it timed? Ovulation is thought to occur as the result of the combined action of the follicle-stimulating hormone and the luteinizing hormone, in a very delicately balanced amount, on the follicle. Its actual time of occurrence is as variable and unpredictable as the length of the cycle itself, because ovulation is more closely correlated with the period to follow than with the one that precedes it.

Ovulation usually occurs without symptoms so that a woman has no idea when she ovulates, but, occasionally, the rupture of the follicle and the accompanying discharge of some fluid and blood into the pelvic cavity may cause some pain. When ovulation involves the right ovary, such pain may be suggestive of a mild appendicitis. It is probable that ovulation occurs from one ovary one month and the opposite ovary the next, which would account for the differences in duration of the cycle and amount of flow from month to month. When one ovary has been removed, the remaining ovary takes on the full-time job and functions each month.

Ovulation however, does not have to occur in every menstrual cycle.

As a matter of fact, "anovulatory menstruation" is a common occurrence in adolescence for as long as the first two years. Anovulatory cycles may also occur later in life and may be an important factor in the problem of sterility since they may be clinically indistinguishable from ovulatory cycles.

OTHER FACTORS

Although the menstrual cycle seems to be self-regulatory, it is by no means an independent mechanism. It must harmonize with the body function as a whole. When it fails to do so, there are repercussions in other systems of the body. But more important to us at present is the fact that the menstrual cycle is affected by other phases of body function.

The thyroid gland is of tremendous importance in the mechanism of the menstrual cycle. This is not because the thyroid plays a specific part as the pituitary gland does, but rather because it has an over-all regulatory function. When the thyroid is underactive, the whole body slows down. The delicate mechanism that is the menstrual cycle is especially susceptible to this deficiency. One of the most frequent causes of menstrual irregularities is an underactive thyroid.

The menstrual cycle is also subject to disturbances emanating from the central nervous system. We have seen in the case of false pregnancy, how emotional stress can interfere with the normal sequence of the cycle. This is effected through the connection between the pituitary gland and the brain. You will recall that the pituitary was described as being "like a cherry" with its stem attaching it to the base of the brain. This stem is not just tissue that holds the gland in place; it contains structures vital to normal pituitary function—nerves and blood vessels. Furthermore, the stem connects the pituitary in a functional way to the hypothalamus (base of the brain) whereby the hypothalamus exerts a regulatory action on the pituitary gland. Some scientists believe there is a "sex center" in this region of the base of the brain that regulates the sex cycle, just as there are centers that control respiration, heart action, etc. Equally important, this hypothalamus-pituitary connection provides a means of direct communication from the higher centers of the brain to the pituitary, which accounts for the fact that emotional stress (and other kinds of stress as well), can profoundly change the pattern of pituitary function including that of ovarian stimulation. There can be no doubt that mental health and emotional health play an important part in the normal mechanism of the menstrual cycle.

Finally, in considering the elements of the normal menstrual cycle, there is one very important consideration that is often overlooked. This delicate glandular mechanism, to function normally, must exist in a normal environment—a healthy body. And a healthy body does not mean just freedom from disease. It means a body that is well nourished, treated to a well-balanced routine of adequate physical exercise and adequate rest, and not subjected to repeated or prolonged overstimulation, tension, or stress. These are the simple and basic facts of everyday living for which the woman is responsible. She cannot abuse her body and expect it to function normally. And there is a corollary to this: a doctor cannot adequately treat functional abnormalities without consideration of the elements of total body health.

WHAT IS "NORMAL MENSTRUATION"?

If one word could be used to describe the outstanding characteristic of menstruation, it would be "variability." Menstruation varies in the length of the cycle, in the duration and amount of flow, and even in the kind and amount of discomfort associated with it. It also varies not only from one woman to another but also in the different cycles of the same woman.

The myth of the twenty-eight-day cycle has been accepted for centuries, probably dating back to the Lunar Theory. Even today many women think that a twenty-eight-day cycle is the normal one. This is not true, and the fact has been demonstrated by many studies of carefully recorded calendar dates of the flow of many women. These studies have proved that there is no one specific length of cycle that is usual for all women. The twenty-eight-day cycle merely represents an average and is of no more frequent occurrence than the twenty-seven-day cycle or the twenty-nine-day cycle. Furthermore, the length of the cycle may vary from month to month in the same individual, even though she may consider herself to be regular and consistent. This variability is more marked in young girls and in women approaching menopause. A woman whose cycle falls within twenty-five to thirty-five days is normal and does not require treatment to make the periods more regular.

The duration of the flow is also variable to a certain extent. For any one woman, the duration and amount of bleeding she experiences each month is more constant than the length of her cycle. Each woman has her own pattern of flow, which is normal for her although it may be long or short, scanty or profuse as compared with other women. The average duration of flow for most women is about four and a half days, but it may range from three to seven days. There is no correlation between the length of the cycle and the amount and duration of the flow. Thus, one woman may have a heavy flow that lasts three to four days, another a scanty flow for six to seven days, and another a heavy flow for six to seven days. All of these are normal for each particular woman. The important point is that while the time of onset of menstruation may vary from month to month by several days, once the flow starts, for any woman, it will usually be like her other menstrual periods.

Menstruation, as already noted, is not a hemorrhage—that is, a flow of pure blood. It is rather, a bloody discharge, which means that it consists of blood mixed with other elements. Actually, blood constitutes only one half to three quarters of the total discharge. Since menstruation has its origin in the crumbling of the endometrium, this tissue in the form of small bits adds considerably to the flow. As the flow passes from the body of the uterus, it is mixed with mucus from the cervix and the fluids and desquamated cells of the vagina.

The menstrual flow is preceded by a flow of mucus, which is colorless, cream colored, or slightly yellow, and which may gradually become tinged with blood. Then follows the period of bloody discharge, which usually is at its maximum on the second day and thereafter tapers off, ending with a mucus discharge tinged with old blood that gives it a brownish color. Thus an increased white discharge, bloody flow, brownish discharge, and finally white discharge is the sequence of events in the normal menstrual period. But the continuity of flow can be affected by such things as chilling, emotional upsets, or exercise, which may either stop the flow or increase it.

While menstruation is a normal physiological process, a large percentage of women experience some discomfort at that time. The kind and degree of discomfort, just as in any other aspect of the cycle, are variable. Some experience no discomfort at all and may even have an increased feeling of well-being, while to others menstruation is a limited period of acute illness, which may last a few hours to a few days. Pain is the usual symptom in relation to menstruation. This may be a dull heaviness in the abdomen, or sharp cramping pains, or backache. The feeling of lassitude or fatigue or its opposite—nervousness, irritability, and insomnia, depression or despondency—when present, usually precede but may accompany the flow. Digestive disturbances, constipation, diarrhea, or nausea may also be present. The breasts often become swollen and tender before the period. These symptoms disappear as soon as the flow is established. A mild acne of the face, dark circles under the eyes are frequent tell-tale signs of menstruation. These symptoms are all real and occasionally may be incapacitating. They are not the product of a woman's imagination. The multiplicity of the symptoms emphasizes the fact that menstruation is only a part of a series of changes that involve the whole body.

HYGIENE

Woman herself can, and indeed must, do her share in maintaining a normal menstrual function. The menstrual cycle is a part of her daily life; day in and day out she is in some phase of it. Therefore she should take proper care of her body as to diet, rest, exercise, and all the aspects of sane and healthy living every day and not confine her solicitousness to the days of actual flow. As a matter of fact, there is no reason physiologically why there should be any great change in her activities at this time. She is not "ill" or "unwell" but is merely experiencing the terminal events of a cycle that has been building up all month to this climax.

The old taboos surrounding the hygiene of menstruation have no foundation in fact. There is no reason why she should not bathe during her period—and every reason why she should. A short warm shower will not only make her feel better but will also give her confidence and assurance of her personal daintiness. There is also no reason why she should not indulge in all the physical exercises and sports to which she is accustomed. Swimming is possibly an exception, in pools for obvious aesthetic reasons, and in cold water because it may stop the flow.

The use of internal tampons instead of external pads during menstruation has recently come into vogue, and many women, especially the younger generation, have adopted them wholeheartedly. They have some obvious advantages. But the disadvantages or dangers from their use are more important. Whether they could actually impede the flow by back pressure is questionable, but certainly they are not adequate to control the flow when it is very heavy. It is, however, by the introduction of a foreign object into the vagina that harm can be done by irritation and the carrying in of infection.

Nature protects the internal pelvic organs from infection. The vagina is a collapsed tube guarded at the outside by the lips (labia minora), which are usually folded together in close contact. Moreover, there is a certain amount of fluid provided by the cervix, the flow of which is always outward, which thus keeps the tract clean. Within a few hours after the uterus has stopped bleeding, the vagina is clear of any evidence of blood. The introduction of a tampon breaks down this natural defense mechanism. This is made all the more serious because of the proximity to the vaginal orifice of the anus, which teems with all sorts of bacteria. The two openings are scarcely one inch apart, and few women are able to insert the tampon without first contaminating it.

Finally there is the problem of the "lost tampon." Many times a woman forgets whether or not she has removed the tampon; and because she cannot feel it or find it, she is both anxious and embarrassed and goes to her doctor to have it removed. Occasionally, she forgets that she has not removed it, and she goes to the doctor because of the resultant unpleasant discharge.

The question of douching—the when, the how, and the why—is one that woman frequently is puzzled about. She reads advertisements of products for "feminine hygiene" and wonders whether she is being remiss in not subscribing to their use. Most of their claims are quite misleading. In some instances, in a veiled reference to contraception (for which they are actually quite inadequate), these advertisements recommend such solutions, which may be fine to sanitize the bathroom plumbing but certainly have no place in feminine hygiene. They are too strong and harsh even for her hands to touch. They are injurious to the far more delicate and sensitive tissues of the reproductive tract. The milder douche powders are as a rule harmless and quite pleasant to use, but they are no more beneficial than just plain water. As a matter of fact, for a normal woman douching is unnecessary. A certain amount of moisture at all times is normal, and this increases at mid-period as well as before and after the period. When excessive discharge—leukorrhea— is present, douching is not the answer. The woman should see her doctor.

Leukorrhea (white flow) does not refer to a specific pelvic problem but is a symptom of several distinct conditions. Whatever its cause, it is a very disturbing symptom to women. They are annoyed and made uncomfortable physically by it, but just as important is their emotional reaction to it. Some are frightened by its sudden appearance and immediately jump to the conclusion that they have a venereal disease or cancer, which is rarely the case. Some are ashamed that such a thing should happen to them, that it belies their fastidiousness, and they are reluctant to seek medical advice. Most women feel uncomfortable, ill at ease, and unsure of themselves because they are constantly reminded of its presence and its implied insult to their daintiness.

The most important thing that women should know about leukorrhea is that it is just a symptom, which has many causes; and that it is a medical problem that she should feel no reluctance to report to her doctor.

So much for the hygiene of menstruation. What is proper hygiene for the remaining part of the cycle?

We have reviewed the mechanism of the menstrual cycle—the hidden changes that are occurring throughout the month. Every phase of this cycle has some outward manifestation the woman can and does observe— and there are things she can do to contribute to its normality. We shall examine the repercussion of endocrine gland function during the whole cycle on her general well-being in later chapters on health and beauty and on equanimity. But before we do, let us first examine conditions that affect the menstrual cycle itself and disturb the feminine functions.

V

DISTURBANCES OF FEMININE FUNCTIONS

WHEN WE CONSIDER the intricacy and delicacy of the mechanism of the menstrual cycle, it is not surprising that it gets upset at times. Really, it is a wonder that it ever works at all!

Menstrual abnormality is one of the most common complaints a woman takes to her doctor. She may be having periods at intervals of six weeks to two or three months or every two or three weeks. She may think the flow is too scanty or too profuse. She may be made ill each period with the symptoms of pain, headache, or nervousness. Or she may have stopped having any periods at all. All these complaints indicate that something has disturbed the normal mechanism of the menstrual cycle.

There are many different conditions that can disturb this intricate mechanism. Disease of one of the organs concerned—such as infection or tumor growth—may render that organ incapable of performing its function normally. This applies to the endocrine glands as well as to the reproductive organs themselves. Ill health that accompanies disease in another part of the body, such as tuberculosis, may depress the function of the endocrine glands. Mental and emotional illnesses may also have such a depressing effect. But by far the most common cause is a "functional glandular disturbance," which means that one or more of the endocrine glands is not working properly. The misbehaving gland may just be lazy and not producing enough hormone, or overactive and producing too much hormone. Such misbehavior, whether it be "hypofunction" or "hyperfunction," will throw the whole mechanism out of balance and result in abnormalities of menstruation.

Irregularity itself is usually not harmful to the woman, but it is important to find out why the irregularity occurs. The cause may be a condition that is or could be harmful or even dangerous to her health. So the doctor's first job is to find the cause. Sometimes that is easy; more often it requires a very careful study of the case.

The study starts with a medical history by which the doctor learns all that the patient can tell about herself and her health, past and present. Next is a physical examination, which includes not only an examination of the pelvic organs but of the whole body as well. Finally, the doctor will have laboratory tests for whatever further information is needed—blood count, tests for thyroid function, sex hormone assays, X-rays, etc.

Menstrual irregularities or abnormalities may be considered in three main groups—amenorrhea ("a"-without, "meno"-menstrual, "rrhea"-flow), hypomenorrhea (deficient menstruation), and menorrhagia (menstrual hemorrhage), usually called functional bleeding.

AMENORRHEA

Amenorrhea is the term doctors use when a woman has failed to menstruate for at least three months. It may be only a passing incident, or it may be a turning point in her life when it indicates pregnancy. Emotional stress such as arises in adjusting to a new way of life, to the physical factors in a new environment, or from fear of or desire for a pregnancy can cause amenorrhea. It is also common in chronic illnesses such as infections, hyperthyroidism, and in prolonged periods of malnutrition. Girls in concentration camps during the war frequently stopped menstruating but became regular when they returned to normal living conditions. It can also be due to some abnormality in the intrinsic glandular mechanism.

How the doctor finds the cause of amenorrhea in a particular case will be most easily understood by going to case histories and following them through. Let us consider the records of four young women, all unmarried, who sought medical care because of amenorrhea. Jane, Amy, and Sara had at one time experienced quite regular and normal periods. Claire had never menstruated.

Jane, age twenty-two, came for medical help because she had not menstruated for six months and because she was distressingly overweight.

This was her story: At the age of fourteen, when she had her first menstruation, she was a normal girl in all respects. She continued to be well, to have regular periods, and to maintain her normal weight until two years previously. She had an appendectomy at that time, which seemed to mark the onset of her difficulties. Thinking that she must make some effort to regain her strength after the operation, she ate more and was less active physically. The result was she started to gain weight. By the end of one year, she had gained forty pounds and her periods were becoming a little irregular—usually a few days and occasionally a week or so late.

Jane's solution of her problem at that time was radical but not wise. She practically stopped eating. For breakfast she had only black coffee; for lunch more black coffee and a clear soup; and for dinner she had only a hard boiled egg and a plain vegetable salad. She stayed hungry all the time, and when she felt that she must have something more to eat she indulged in what she craved most—sweets. She lost some weight at first, but as her sprees of eating became more frequent she began to gain. With this erratic dieting, her periods became more and more irregular and finally failed to occur. Six months later Jane was truly an obese, miserable girl and a case of amenorrhea to be solved.

A physical examination was done with several objectives in mind; (1) to see if the signs of physical maturity were present, which would indicate that her endocrine glands had been functioning normally before she started to gain weight; (2) to see if she had any bodily illness that might account for loss of menstruation; (3) to detect any signs of endocrine deficiency. She proved to have the normal signs of maturity. There were no evidences of physical disease. The only abnormalities noted were obesity (she weighed 180 pounds and was only 5 feet-3 inches tall); her skin and hair were coarse and dry; her blood pressure was low, and her pulse was slow. Examination of the pelvic organs revealed that the uterus and ovaries were well developed and normal in size. There was no evidence of cysts, tumors, or inflammatory masses.

So far no physical cause for amenorrhea was found. There remained the endocrine glands to be investigated. It will be recalled that when we sought to understand the mechanism of the menstrual cycle, we considered first the uterus, then the ovaries, and then the pituitary gland,

and their interrelated functions as the basic mechanism of menstruation. But we also found that this balance was affected by the efficiency of the thyroid function and a woman's general health, including physical and emotional factors. If these factors necessary for normal menstruation were examined, the reason Jane failed to menstruate should be revealed.

The uterus obviously was not at fault. It was normally developed, and as she had menstruated in the past, it had been, of course, responsive to ovarian hormones. It was safe to assume, therefore that Jane's ovaries were no longer secreting the necessary hormones to make the endometrium go through the cyclic changes. Why were the ovaries not producing the necessary hormones? Ovarian failure may be the result of two things: (1) either the ovaries have become incapable of doing their normal work; or (2) they are not being properly stimulated by the pituitary. The question was whether the glandular deficiency was primarily in the ovaries or in the pituitary or whether both were at fault. The ovaries were probably not the cause of the deficiency, because they had functioned normally in the past and there were no cysts, tumors, or infections that might interfere with their normal function. This left the pituitary as the starting point of the deficiency, but could pituitary deficiency be proved?

To establish the fact of pituitary deficiency, our story of glandular physiology will have to be anticipated, and one clue, which will be established later, will be stated: Primary ovarian failure, when the fault is in the ovary, leads to pituitary over-activity. An example of primary ovarian failure is the menopause. But as Jane had none of the symptoms of menopause, it may safely be assumed that the pituitary was not functioning properly. This could be confirmed by special laboratory tests for the pituitary hormones, but such tests are difficult and time consuming and were not necessary to solve this case.

A few simple laboratory tests were done, and the findings rounded out the picture. A blood count showed that Jane was moderately anemic and a low basal metabolism rate (BMR) pointed to thyroid deficiency. When these facts were fitted in with Jane's history, the solution was apparent.

First, Jane put on weight after her appendectomy. It is a common occurrence for a person to gain weight after a surgical operation. It has been suggested that the anesthetic produces some imbalance in the endocrine system, which leads to obesity. The more likely explanation is that the inactivity of convalescence accompanied by an increased appetite results in a person's eating more food than the body can use, so it is stored as fat. As fat accumulates, it becomes a burden to the body—to the heart, the kidneys, the skeletal system, and especially the delicate endocrine gland system. This burden of obesity eventually decreases the ability of these systems to maintain normal function. Even more important in Jane's case was malnutrition, resulting from a diet which was deficient in all the protective foods—proteins, minerals, and vitamins. Add to this the emotional factor of her unhappiness because of her size, and we have sufficient evidence to account for the failure of her delicate glandular mechanism.

What could be done to restore the endocrine balance and help Jane become a normal girl again?

Just as Jane's dilemma was of her own making, the correction of it depended on her own efforts. She had to correct her faulty habits of eating and go on a strict diet, which was high in proteins, minerals, and vitamins and low in calories, both to reduce her weight and to correct her state of malnutrition.

What could be done to make her pituitary and ovaries function normally again? The answer is, nothing directly. There is no specific hormone or any other means to stimulate pituitary function directly, nor are there any effective pituitary gonadotropic hormones available for clinical use to stimulate the ovaries. But indirectly her general health could be improved to the point where these glands might again resume normal function. She could be further helped by taking iron, vitamins, and the thyroid hormone, which would improve the efficiency of all her body functions, including her endocrine glands.

The ovarian hormones, estrogen and progesterone, are available in pure form and very potent and when used properly may prove very helpful. The symptoms of amenorrhea can be very quickly relieved by the administration of either large doses of estrogen alone given over a period of a few weeks; or by one or two large doses of progesterone. Either will induce the uterus to bleed once, but will do nothing to correct the cause or have a permanent effect.

If, however, these hormones are given in smaller doses, and in a cyclic manner, trying to imitate the way the ovaries produce them, then cyclic uterine bleeding can be established. This may be helpful in several ways. First, it will restore the uterus to its normal degree of activity whereby it will again be sensitive and responsive to the ovarian hormones. It has been inactive and therefore out of practice for its function of response to hormone stimulation. Second, as previously noted, the rhythm of pituitary function is due to the action of the ovarian hormones on it. Therefore, the use of the ovarian hormones in a cyclic manner may stimulate the pituitary to secret the gonadotropic hormones. The whole effect is a sort of pump-priming procedure, getting the system going by the addition of hormones and hoping that it can then carry on by its own power. Usually, it does. Even if the ovarian hormones are not used, with the reduction of weight, establishment of normal living habits, and the administration of thyroid extract, the menstrual function would probably return. But if these general measures were ignored and hormones alone were given, there would probably never be any improvement. The endocrine glands need a healthy body environment to function at their best.

Jane's case has been given in detail because it illustrates several important things, which will be true of all the endocrine problems in all the ages: Functional problems involve the whole person and not just the pelvic organs. The total personality must be considered in solving these problems. One of the most important means a doctor has of diagnosing any problem is a careful and thorough history. He must know his patient. On the other hand, the doctor should not be considered negligent because he does not order a lot of laboratory tests and X-rays. If he is skilled in female endocrinology, he will find most of the information he needs in the history and physical examination and will be selective in the tests that he orders. The solution of Jane's case was reached (with the exception of the BMR) in much less time than it has taken to tell it.

Functional problems are in part and sometimes wholly the result of violation of the basic laws of hygienic living and good health. If a woman has a functional problem, she is probably responsible in some way for its existence. She has violated some of the basic rules of health. Therefore, she must be prepared to do her part in finding the cause and effecting the cure when she seeks medical help. She must be frank with her doctor.

His questions are not aimless prying into her private affairs, but his way of finding facts which, the woman may not realize, are contributing to her problem. Furthermore, she must accept the fact that stressful living, emotional tensions, faulty eating habits, inadequate amounts of rest are all contributory factors to her problem, which she alone can correct.

Amy's story is short and is told because it represents the most common cause of amenorrhea within the Age of Maturity, and is therefore the first possibility that a doctor must consider regardless of the woman's age, the facts she relates—or does not relate.

Amy had started menstruating at twelve and had been regular until three months previous to her visit to the doctor's office when her periods suddenly stopped. Although only sixteen, Amy was very mature for her age. She was of medium height and had a feminine body with well-rounded, turgid breasts and graceful curves. Her skin was clear and fresh. She appeared alert, but a little nervous and on the defensive.

Her history and general physical examination gave no indication of illness. She was apparently a normal, healthy girl. Pelvic examination revealed an enlarged, soft uterus. Sufficient facts were now apparent to make a tentative diagnosis—she was probably pregnant. The facts were: cessation of menstruation in an otherwise normal girl, full turgid breasts, marital vagina, enlarged soft uterus. But these are only probable signs of pregnancy. They are also signs of other conditions, and a doctor must be sure of his diagnosis. A large ovarian cyst, for example, might be identified as the uterus and could also cause amenorrhea. Therefore, in Amy's case a pregnancy test was done and was positive for pregnancy. There was no question of medical treatment for Amy, but rather she presented a problem that she and her family had to work out.

Sara is a third case of amenorrhea in a girl who had previously had normal periods. Her problem proved to be the most serious and was due to a rare condition. She was twenty-six years old when she sought medical advice, partly because she had not menstruated for five months, but primarily because she did not feel well. She complained of headaches, dizziness, inability to concentrate, and disturbance of her vision.

No startling abnormalities were found on physical examination. She was of average build and normal maturity, and her pelvic organs were apparently normal. There was only one suggestive finding. Her facial features were coarse and her lower jaw appeared to be quite heavy for a woman. She also had large hands and feet. On questioning, she said that recently her gloves and shoes had become uncomfortable, necessitating the purchase of larger sizes. Her reactions were slow, and she appeared troubled and ill.

The significant clues in this case were: the regression of sex function (loss of menstruation); the symptoms of headache, dizziness, and change in vision due to increased pressure in the head, and the enlargement of her jaw, hands, and feet. The occurrence of growth after the body had attained its mature size suggested that the pituitary was producing too much growth hormone. The loss of ovarian function suggested that it was not producing enough gonadotropic hormones. Why should the pituitary be secreting too much of one kind of hormone and too little of another? There is only one condition capable of bringing about that state of affairs—a tumor. An X-ray showed that Sara's pituitary gland was greatly enlarged by a tumor. Further X-ray of the bones of the hands and feet confirmed the suspicion of their overgrowth. Sara was a case of acromegaly due to a pituitary tumor. She was referred to a neurosurgeon, who recommended that the tumor be removed. (Some other types of pituitary tumors are better treated by X-ray.) She was successfully operated on, recovered her general health rapidly, and many years later was still in comparatively good health. Her feet and hands were still large. She remained amenorrheic, however, and consequently infertile because there was not sufficient pituitary function remaining to stimulate her ovaries and maintain fertility.

Claire, the last girl, is of interest primarily from the point of view of what therapy did for her. She was twenty-four years old and had never menstruated. Physically, she was a girl who had grown tall but failed to mature. Her breasts were those of a child and her uterus was not much larger than it had been at birth. It was not possible to bring her to full maturity and fertility, but what was accomplished completely changed the course of her life.

When Claire first asked for help, she was a quiet, shy girl. She had finished high school and held a small government job. Because she felt that she was different, not a normal woman, she did not make friends with other girls and was shy with men, repulsing any who approached her. She was an unattractive, mousey young woman—destined for a life of loneliness.

Examination and tests showed no disease of her reproductive organs. The glands responsible for sexual maturation had not functioned, and her organs were no larger than those of a child. It was explained to her that while nothing could be done to make her ovaries work, it might be possible by prolonged therapy with ovarian hormones, to correct some of the results of this deficiency. She was unenthusiastic and quite skeptical, but agreed to start treatment.

After a few months, she began to blossom out. She gained a little weight and her body developed the feminine curves it had never had before. The breasts began to grow. Her skin and hair acquired new life. After six months of treatment, she had her first menstrual period. She was elated that at last she was truly a woman and as time went by, she came to enjoy normal social activities.

These cases demonstrate that amenorrhea is just one symptom in a chain of events. It may occur either as a result of normal change in glandular function or as a result of abnormal endocrine balance, which may be due to various types of physical abnormalities in the Age of Maturity.

It is important to find the cause and to treat the amenorrhea, not because amenorrhea in itself is harmful to the woman, but because it is a symptom of a serious glandular deficiency. It is important to restore menstruation whenever possible to help maintain a woman's general good health and her fertility. Just as important, it reassures her that she is a normal woman.

HYPOMENORRHEA

There are various types of menstrual abnormalities in which the deficiency is less severe than in amenorrhea. This gives rise to a multitude of menstrual patterns due to the fact that there are three variables: length of the cycle; duration of the flow; and amount of the flow. Thus the interval may be abnormal—too short (less than twenty-one days), or too long (more than thirty-five days), the duration may be more than seven days or less than three, and the flow can be scanty sometimes amounting to little more than spotting or be so profuse as to be hemorrhagic. These may occur in any combination. All indicate some deficiency in the mechanism of the menstrual cycle.

For the sake of simplicity, we shall include under hypomenorrhea all the patterns in which one or more element is deficient: the frequency of the flow; the amount of flow; the duration of the flow; and the loss of a regular cycle. Most of these are not incompatible with either health or fertility. They are most likely to be encountered in the transition ages of youth and menopause.

Irregular menstrual periods, that is every five to six weeks or occasionally skipping a month, are of no great significance. In some women, it just takes longer to complete a cycle, which means that the changes occur in orderly sequence, including ovulation, and menstruation is normal. In other cases, hypomenorrhea indicates a depression of endocrine function such as was encountered in Jane, the first case of amenorrhea. Hypomenorrhea in itself is not harmful to the woman and usually requires no therapy other than attention to the woman's general health.

Excessive bleeding, on the other hand, whether prolonged, too profuse, or too frequent, may be a threat to the woman's health and therefore requires careful consideration.

FUNCTIONAL BLEEDING

The pattern of menstruation, as we have seen—the length of the cycle, the amount and duration of the flow—varies so greatly among women that the normal shades into the abnormal. It may therefore sometimes be difficult to say when vaginal bleeding, that is excessive in one or more of its characteristics, ceases to be normal menstruation and becomes functional bleeding. For practical purposes an arbitrary line must be drawn somewhere. Doctors have designated twenty-one days as the shortest cycle and seven days as the longest duration of flow that may still be considered normal. Anything outside these limits we shall call functional bleeding. This will include a host of bleeding patterns, for no two cases of functional bleeding are exactly alike. One case may have periods every two weeks lasting five days; another, every six weeks lasting ten days;

and still another, periods in which there is no regularity as to the time or the duration of the flow.

Mechanism of Functional Bleeding

All cases of functional bleeding have the same general physiologic basis—failure of the ovaries to produce their hormones in a cyclic manner and in the optimum amount. Quite obviously, this allows for great variation, for failure can occur at any time in the cycle and can be of any degree. The ovarian changes which take place in the normal cycle are follicle growth, ovulation, corpus luteum growth, and corpus luteum regression. The mildest degree of functional bleeding results when the luteal phase occurs but is cut short. In such cases, the periods come slightly earlier than every three weeks. The usual condition underlying functional bleeding is that in which there has been no ovulation and therefore no luteal phase at all.

When ovulation fails to occur, the cycle of change in the ovary is reduced to follicle growth and follicle regression. This may be fairly regular, corresponding to the usual ten- to fourteen-day life span of the follicle, and bleeding occurs every two weeks. In more marked degrees of failure, the ovary loses completely its ability to function in a cyclic way and becomes quite erratic. One follicle may last only a week or ten days and is followed by others which last as long as four, six, or eight weeks, so that bleeding recurs at completely irregular intervals and continues a varying length of time. It may be quite profuse, very scanty, or about normal.

What happens to the ability of the ovaries to produce hormones in these varying, abnormal situations? How is bleeding controlled? What causes it to start—and to stop? Why is it sometimes heavy and other times light? The answer to all these questions lies in the ability of the follicle to produce estrogen. In normal menstruation, bleeding occurs when the level of progesterone and estrogen falls—but it is the fall in estrogen that is the deciding factor. The endometrium will bleed on the withdrawal of estrogen even when there has been no progesterone present. This is what happens in cases of functional bleeding.

The follicle continues, past the time ovulation should have occurred, as an unruptured sac lined with secretory cells. It increases in size, and the fluid inside increases in amount. For a while, the secretory cells are able to produce estrogen sometimes even in excessive amounts. But a time comes when they lose this ability either because they are not receiving adequate stimulation from the pituitary or because the fluid inside the follicle exerts such pressure that they become compressed and atrophy. The follicle has now become "cystic" and is no longer able to function. So the estrogen level falls. The length of time the follicle can function varies. It may be one week or six or more weeks. As long as the follicle is producing a steadily increasing amount of estrogen, there is no bleeding. When it falters, and the estrogen level drops, bleeding starts and will continue until other follicular growth produces enough estrogen again. The amount of bleeding will depend on what has been happening in the endometrium.

If the follicle is erratic in the amount of hormones it sends to effect the changes in the endometrium, it follows that the endometrium will be erratic also in its growth and differentiation. It will be recalled that early in the follicular phase, the endometrium consists only of straight tubular glands with many small blood vessels in between. Estrogen causes these to grow, and growth slows down in the luteal phase when the glands are transformed for secretory activity. In functional bleeding, there is only growth because there is only estrogen. The amount of growth depends on the amount of estrogen supplied by the follicle and the length of time it is produced. If the amount is relatively excessive, the endometrium will grow beyond the normal limits. It becomes thick and spongy and, most important, the blood vessels become quite large. When estrogen is withdrawn and the endometrium begins to crumble, the large blood vessels break and profuse bleeding ensues.

Causes of Functional Bleeding

Functional bleeding is a symptom of ovarian failure, but failure that is only partial—a deficiency, but not complete absence of ovarian function. We have learned that amenorrhea is also due to ovarian failure, but more profound. Thus, both too much bleeding and absence of bleeding are the result of the inability of the ovary to produce its hormones in proper amount and cyclic manner. It is understandable, therefore, that the causes of ovarian failure in functional bleeding are practically the same as those of functional amenorrhea. The difference is one of degree rather than of kind.

We might go back to the discussion of functional amenorrhea and insert "functional bleeding" in its place, and we would still be fairly accurate. Failure may be primary in the ovaries or the pituitary, or due to outside factors such as other glandular disturbances, environmental, nutritional, or emotional abnormalities.

Primary ovarian failure, which results in functional bleeding, is most common in the transitional ages of adolescence and menopause. In adolescence, the ovaries have not yet achieved full maturity of function, and in menopause they have grown tired and unable to carry on. It is less common in the Age of Maturity. The nutritional and emotional factors that in the case of Jane caused amenorrhea could just as well have resulted in only partial failure and functional bleeding. Nutritional factors, especially deficiency of the vitamin B complex and vitamin C are believed to be very important causative factors.

Changes in environment or climate may precipitate periods of functional bleeding. Women going from the temperate climate of the United States to the tropics, often experience frequent and profuse periods. Usually this is transitory and corrects itself when the woman becomes adjusted to the climate.

Thyroid failure, on the other hand, is one of the most common causes of ovarian deficiency and functional bleeding in the Age of Maturity. The case history of Edith will illustrate this.

Edith, age twenty, had come from a western state to attend an eastern school. Her problem was irregular and prolonged periods of bleeding. She was having periods that would last from six to fourteen or more days, and they were completely unpredictable. One might occur after two weeks, and the next interval would be five or six weeks. She was finding herself tired to the point of exhaustion and unable to carry on her usual school activities.

Her history indicated the probable cause of her difficulty, which was easily verified by examination and a few tests. She had first menstruated at twelve and was regular and normal until she was eighteen. At that time, she had undergone an operation for goiter—a part of her thyroid gland was removed. She was a well-developed young lady with no physical abnormalities except the tell-tale symptoms of thyroid deficiency—dry skin and hair, brittle nails, low blood pressure and slow pulse. Her BMR was minus twenty-two. The low blood count, which undoubtedly contributed to her fatigue, was the result of the excessive bleeding, not the cause.

The immediate problem was to stop the bleeding. She was given thyroid extract, and response to this treatment was satisfactory. She will, however, have to continue to take thyroid extract for many years to maintain her regularity and fertility.

Edith's case, clear-cut and unequivocal, is an example of thyroid deficiency resulting from surgery. The far more common type of thyroid deficiency is that in which the thyroid is just lazy—does not do its work well. This may be because it is not sufficiently stimulated by the pituitary, or because of its own inadequacy. Sometimes it is unable to function normally—produce a normal amount of its hormone—because of iodine deficiency. Again, the cause of thyroid failure may be a reflection of poor general health, as in the case of Jane's obesity and amenorrhea. Whatever the cause, tablets of thyroid extract or hormone taken by mouth can work wonders. Strange as it may seem, an overactive thyroid may disturb the pituitary-ovarian relationship and also cause functional bleeding; but more frequently hyperthyroidism causes amenorrhea.

Functional bleeding occasionally is the result of an emotional illness. The story of Betty is an unusual and extreme example.

Betty, a girl of twenty-four, had married a service man during the war. When she first sought medical advice she had been married for one year, but had been with her husband only at intervals of several months and then only for a few days. She complained of attacks of extreme nervousness, loss of weight, palpitation, weakness, dizziness, and even fainting. Her menstrual periods, previously normal, had been coming too frequently for several months and were very profuse. Examinations and tests revealed a rapid pulse, elevated blood pressure, tremor of the hands, underweight, a high BMR, and an abnormal blood count and sugar tolerance test. These findings were suggestive of hyperthyroidism.

When she was treated for this, however, there was no improvement. Betty was still ill, with episodes in which all her symptoms became alarmingly severe. It was a baffling case—until months later the truth came out.

Betty had married a boy, whom she liked well enough, to please her aunt who had cared for her since childhood and whom she loved dearly. But Betty was emotionally immature, incapable of accepting, much less of enjoying, a normal adult sex life with her husband. Every time he came to see her, or she thought he was coming to see her, she had one of her violent "attacks." Her mental and emotional conflict was translated into violent physical symptoms of endocrine imbalance. With the help of a psychiatrist, Betty was able to resolve her emotional difficulties, and has been physically well since.

The treatment of functional bleeding has two aims—to stop bleeding and to restore the endocrine mechanism to normal. The measures taken to stop bleeding will depend on its duration and severity.

In earlier days, all a doctor could do was put a woman to bed, elevate the foot of the bed, put an ice bag to her abdomen, and give her ergot. If this did not help and the situation was critical, that is, if the woman was losing too much blood, she was sent to the hospital and the uterus was scraped and perhaps a transfusion given. These measures may work fairly well, and are still sometimes used. But this is treating one symptom only—bleeding; and ignoring the cause—endocrine imbalance. To effect a cure, the doctor must use the basic physiology of bleeding.

In the normal cycle, we saw that menstrual bleeding follows the fall in estrogen level and that menstruation ceases when the follicles that are to participate in the next cycle start producing estrogen. This new supply of estrogen stops the crumbling of the endometrium and initiates growth. It revitalizes the lining of the uterus.

In the disturbed physiology of functional bleeding, we see again that it is the rise and fall of estrogen with follicular cystic activity that accounts for the bleeding. So the key word of bleeding is estrogen. Bleeding can be stopped if enough estrogen is given. We now have extremely potent forms of estrogen that given, either by mouth or injection into a muscle or a vein, will stop bleeding within a matter of hours. But bleeding will recur unless something is done to restore normal endocrine balance.

Occasionally, when the endometrium has been subjected to excessive and prolonged estrogen stimulation, it becomes quite thick and spongy—a condition called cystic hyperplasia. This sort of endometrium has lost its ability to respond normally and bleeding continues in spite of such medication. Then a curettage becomes necessary to remove this excessive tissue and give the endometrium a new start.

To restore the endocrine mechanism to normal, the same measures used in amenorrhea may be employed. Cyclic administration of estrogen and progesterone is used as a pump-priming procedure in the glandular mechanism as well as to restore the normal structure of the endometrium. Thyroid extract is especially helpful in restoring the normal cycle. Frequently, it is given even though the BMR is normal. Iron and liver are usually necessary to correct the anemia.

There still remain the general supportive measures. The things a woman must do for herself are perhaps most important of all. They bear repeating: an adequate well-balanced diet, sufficient rest, a good balance of work and recreation, freedom from emotional stress and strain, and avoidance of overindulgence in alcohol, smoking, coffee, and other stimulants. In this, as in all functional problems of women, teamwork is required, teamwork between the woman, her doctor, and nature. Nature, the wisdom of the body—the complicated mechanism the body possesses for survival, is a marvelous thing. The body has wonderful recuperative powers when given half a chance. If woman affords nature the opportunity and the doctor gives a helping hand, nature will strive to restore the normal balance of good health. Such teamwork is usually successful.

BLEEDING THAT IS NOT FUNCTIONAL

Vaginal bleeding is a recurrent experience that woman accepts as a normal part of her life, and variations in the pattern may not be too disturbing to her. Herein lies a danger. Bleeding from any other part of her body she would instantly recognize as abnormal and probably would immediately seek medical advice as to its significance. Bleeding from the vagina carries no such implication, and she is apt to ignore slight amounts or put up with excessive amounts for some time before seeking medical care.

Although it is true that all menstruation is bleeding and is normal, it does not follow that all vaginal bleeding is menstruation and therefore also normal. Vaginal bleeding may be the signal that something is wrong and should be heeded promptly. Some types of vaginal bleeding are functional, as we have seen, but others indicate the presence of a disease process that may endanger the health or life of the woman. The woman cannot tell the difference—only a doctor can differentiate between the two. But the responsibility lies with the woman to suspect that her vaginal bleeding is no longer normal and to seek medical advice promptly.

The woman must recognize that she has this responsibility of being alert for danger signals and presenting herself for examination. The surest way she can stay on the alert to recognize the first warning that something is wrong, that danger may be lurking, is to make a habit of keeping an accurate written record of the occurrence of all vaginal bleeding. An excellent way is to have a one-page calendar for the whole year, and each month mark the occurrence of menstruation on it. A good picture can be obtained if different signs are used to indicate the character of the flow. A cross may be used to mark each day of average flow. If the flow is more profuse on one or more days, the crosses may be underlined. The days when there is only a little dribbling or spotting, usually at the end of the flow, are marked by dots. After a few months of recording, the variations in the length of the cycle and the pattern of flow will be established, and the woman will then be able to recognize early and slight deviations from normal when they occur.

When a woman has had a light flow as her usual pattern, and it changes to a heavier or longer one, it frequently indicates the presence of an abnormality of the pelvic organs. Fibroids of the uterus are the most common condition. Profuse periods are not the typical symptom of cancer. This change in pattern of flow is one kind of warning signal. Another is spotting.

No amount of spotting is ever too small to be recorded. Spotting, of any kind or degree, should never be ignored. It may be just a tiny bit of spotting after intercourse or in a douche; a slight staining of the clothes or a pinkish discoloration of toilet tissue, but spotting is always important. If it recurs or persists, the woman should report for examination immediately. All spotting should be considered a warning of danger. Spotting may be the earliest sign of cancer of the cervix or body of the uterus. And it is in early detection that chances of cure lie.

The appearance of spotting is not a reason for the woman to become panicky, for not all spotting is due to cancer. There are many other things that can cause it. Raw spots in the vagina or on the cervix may bleed slightly. A little tumor of the cervix called a polyp, is a very common source of vaginal bleeding because it is a soft little mass of tissue consisting mostly of blood vessels. Also, women frequently have a little spotting for one, two, or three days half-way between their periods—at the time of ovulation. But only the doctor can determine the cause of spotting in each instance. This much a woman must know and always observe. It does not matter whether she has just seen her doctor or been to a cancer detection center a week or month previously and has been told that she is in perfect health, she must still consult her doctor immediately when spotting occurs. For cancer can be within the uterus, where the eye cannot see it, nor the hand feel, nor smears reveal the first small changes. Spotting warns that further examination is necessary.

How can a doctor make the diagnosis of cancer? There is only one sure way—to see the cancer cells under the microscope. To have cells to examine, he must take some tissue from the woman's body. If he sees an ulcer on the cervix or a little "piled-up" area, either one of which looks suspicious, he will cut off a small bit for a biopsy and send it to the pathologist for study. But if the bleeding is coming from higher up, he must do a dilatation and curettage (D & C). This merely means that the cervix is dilated or stretched so that an instrument may be introduced high in the uterus and the walls scraped. These scrapings are also biopsy material for study. Curettage is a simple procedure. It requires only a few days hospitalization and entails little discomfort. But it can be life saving if cancer is present or avert a more serious operation, such as hysterectomy, if the bleeding proves to be innocuous. When her doctor recommends a curettage, a woman should have it done as soon as possible and avoid the inevitably anxious waiting.

The importance of early recognition of serious symptoms and prompt attention to them is illustrated in the case of Patricia. Patricia, a lovely young woman in her mid-thirties, had been under my care for a minor condition totally unrelated to bleeding. On the day she was being discharged, she asked how often a woman should have a pelvic examination. As it happened, another case just preceding her illustrated the answer. This woman had very casually come into my office for a physical examination—her first in ten years. Fifty years old, she stated that she had stopped menstruating two years before. But about six months previous to this visit occasional spotting had occurred, which she took to be menstruation, and had continued with slightly increasing severity. On examination, a cancer of the cervix was found, which appeared to be too extensive for hope of cure. I told Patricia about this case saying that if Mrs. X had come in when the spotting was first noticed, certainly her chances would have been better, and perhaps her life might have been saved.

My purpose in telling Patricia was not to make her fearful of cancer but to impress on her the responsibility that she herself must bear in maintaining her health. Regular examinations at six months or yearly intervals are important, but a woman should always report to her doctor no matter how recent her last previous examination, when any unusual symptoms occur, especially spotting.

Patricia expressed surprise that spotting was so significant, stating that she was under the impression that cancer started with a lot of bleeding. This bit of information was to prove very important to her. About three months later she returned and told me, hesitantly, that she had noticed a little spotting for two days.

On examination, the cervix appeared clean and free from any suspicious areas, and the body of the uterus felt normal. Because of the negative findings and the fact that the spotting had appeared only once, which could have been the bleeding of ovulation, Patricia was told to wait another month and watch for the bleeding and note its relation to her menstrual cycle.

The next month she reported that after her period she was clear for three days, then there was just a little discoloration, sometimes pinkish or brown, for three days. This stopped for two days then recurred. She was advised that a biopsy should be made—that she would have to go to the hospital for a curettage. Like most women, she did not like the idea of a hospital or an operation and asked if a "smear test" wouldn't do just as well.

The answer, of course, was emphatically "no." The smear test was never intended to be used as a diagnostic procedure. It is useful only as a "screening device" in women who have no symptoms. Occasionally, suspicious cells are found, which indicate that further investigation is necessary. But the failure to find cancer cells in the vagina does not necessarily mean that there is not a small growth in the uterus, which may not be shedding cells. Suspicious findings or symptoms must always be investigated by adequate biopsy.

Patricia had a curettage. The surgeon reported that the general appearance of the tissue removed was that of simple hyperplasia (overgrowth) of the endometrium but that he could not be sure until it was examined microscopically. We hopefully awaited the pathologist's report that all was well and that would end the problem. Unfortunately, that was not the case. He found cells in the tissue that were abnormal. He described them as "precancerous," that is, cells that would likely become cancerous.

Carefully considering all the factors in Patricia's case, it was decided that a hysterectomy (only the uterus removed) was the best procedure, and this was done promptly. Patricia came through the operation in splendid form and was quite surprised that it was not the harrowing experience that she had been led to believe it would be. Within a few months she was feeling better than she had before the operation. As a matter of fact we all were, because we knew that Patricia had been relieved of the possibility of cancer of the uterus. This happy ending occurred only because Patricia reported the earliest sign, and this was investigated promptly. The lives of thousands of women each year can also be saved if they seek advice and act accordingly at the very earliest sign. Bleeding should always be investigated.

We have reviewed the function of menstruation when it is normal and the abnormalities of amenorrhea, hypomenorrhea, and functional bleeding. These are woman's intimate and personal feminine functions. There are other aspects of her femininity that are also important. The physical aspects of her personality that she presents to the world are apparent in her physical health and beauty. The emotional aspects—how successful she is in achieving happiness within herself and in her relation to the world around her—constitute an important element in her mental health. We shall turn to these in the next three chapters.

VI

HEALTH AND BEAUTY IN MATURITY

WHAT DO WOMEN WANT? What is the ideal toward which they strive? Of course there is no one answer. The wit will say that is because women do not know what they want—or want any one thing for long. But women do know what they want. It is merely in the intensity of their desire, the opportunities they have, and the means they employ in achieving their goal that there is such variation.

Women want most of all to achieve the perfection of their femininity. That is, they want to feel assured within themselves that they are normal women capable of playing well their feminine role. It also means they want the recognition and acknowledgment of their attainment by the world of others—by their own sex as well as the opposite sex. It is in the interpretation of what constitutes the acme of femininity that makes the difference in her aims. We have described it as maturity on all levels of the feminine personality. But this is not the standard that modern society has set for her. Society has not emphasized the many facets of the mature feminine personality that must be attained and maintained by constant effort. Nor is the goal of maturity presented as a dynamic, ever-changing, ever-developing process that makes and keeps her life rich and full.

Society has stressed as ideals of maturity only the physical aspects of her personality. Her physical appearance and physical sex attractiveness are represented as the goals of her existence. Youth and beauty are the attributes to which she must dedicate her energy. She must fight the ravages of time—stay, as long as possible, the horrors of "maturity."

Youth is interpreted to mean the alluring curves of her body as her femininity unfolds, the clearness of her complexion, the gleam of her hair, the sparkle of her eyes. These are the attributes of beauty she is urged to nurture by external means, ignoring the fact that all are the expression of normal body physiology as yet unsubjected to the stress of living and the abuses the woman heaps on herself. Much of the attractiveness of youth is the freshness of good health, which is vitalized by keen enthusiasm for living, with enjoyment for today and high hopes for tomorrow. These are the qualities of youth that are worth striving for. There is nothing wrong in evaluating highly youth and beauty, singly or together. The trouble comes in making a fetish of them and failing to recognize that the basis of each is good health.

Unfortunately, the beauty of youth is not every girl's heritage which she carries with her into maturity. The failure to attain the badges of femininity contributes some of the most trying problems in the Age of Youth. We shall therefore consider them more fully in that age and explore now only the meaning of health.

BASIC INGREDIENTS OF HEALTH

Health is not just the absence of illness or disease. It is a dynamic quality of living. Nor is health our birthright. It is the result of what we do with ourselves and to ourselves in mind and body, a state of well-being that must include all the facets of maturity.

The essential ingredients of health are available to every woman. Her health in maturity will depend on her own efforts to secure it. However poor may be her heritage, whatever crippling may have been inflicted by childhood illness, however lacking her previous history may have been in physical stamina—health can still be hers if she learns its true meaning and diligently seeks to acquire it.

To have health—for the present and in the years ahead—woman should understand what its basic ingredients are and should not be misled by the false promises that are offered on every hand. Subscribing to fads of diet or exercise, or taking pills, tonics, or elixirs will not light the spark of inner well-being, nor will creams and lotions give woman the outer glow of good health. Health culture does not come in easy installments, to be utilized at certain intervals, such as massage, vibratory cushions, shaking tables, or exposure to assorted colors of light or heat rays. In fact the cultists have done a great deal of harm by attaching to the pursuit of health a meaning that is false, either that it is unpleasant, irksome, even repulsive, or that it is the pursuit only of a crank. Nothing could be further from the truth. The pursuit of health is a way of, and an investment in, life that pays dividends in the improved appearance, the increased feeling of well-being, and the increased efficiency and zest for doing, as well as accumulating the capital gains of a strong, healthy body for a long life.

The basic ingredients of health consist of the triad of good health habits: (1) adequate physical exercise, rest, and relaxation; (2) good nutrition; and (3) a healthy attitude toward life. These seem simple and obvious, but few can lay claim to the acquisition of the habits and strict adherence to the rules of good health. In the rush of everyday living all are frequently violated or ignored.

Women do not usually consider exercise a feminine virtue and are therefore not as likely as men to overexert by sporadic indulgence in strenuous exercise with occasional dire results. But every woman needs a certain amount of exercise. It should have become a pleasant habit early in maturity, which woman will continue throughout her life.

Exercise has its primary effect on the musculature of the body, increasing its power, strength, efficiency, and endurance. But it also improves the efficiency of respiration and circulation so that daily activities may be performed with less fatigue. Especially if it is accomplished through out-of-doors activities, it provides not only diversion from work-a-day worries, but also the opportunity to appreciate and enjoy the enduring verities of nature. Exercise will provide an outlet for emotional tensions, worry, and frustration, which have become so great a part of our everyday lives. From such exercise one may return to the tasks of the day with emotional tension lessened and with renewed vigor.

Rest and relaxation, moments of peace and quiet, hours of sleep are too often sacrificed to add a little more time to the active day. A woman should realize that the energy she has to spend has definite limitations, and the demand for resupply is rigid. She must budget her expenditures of energy and maintain a safe balance by redeposits in rest and nutrition. She will pay a fine for overdraft, in fatigue, nervousness, irritability, loss of efficiency, and eventually actual illness.

Good health habits are inseparable and mutually dependent. Exercise is most effective only when the body is well nourished and when the exercise is interspersed with periods of rest; and the body can only be well nourished when it has not only an adequate diet but also periods of rest and active exercise. Physical health enhances the potentiality for mental health, and physical deficiencies are the cause of many psychological disturbances.

Women are living longer, but whether they will live better and be able to enjoy these added years depends to a great extent on the degree of physical and mental health they bring to these years. They should start to build this kind of security, that of health, early in life. Infancy is not too early, but maturity is not too late. Woman's last age will be one of serenity only if she starts early to prepare for it. An important part of this preparation is good nutrition.

In this land of abundance everyone should be well nourished. Although we see little evidence of actual lack of food—starvation—there is plenty of evidence of malnutrition. There are indications that malnutrition is undermining our health in every age of life. Children tested for physical strength and endurance, for example, have not shown the stamina of children of far less privileged countries. The juveniles who present behavior problems, often come from homes where living conditions are poor, not always because of economic conditions, but because there is a lack of a healthy routine of living, including regular and adequate meals in a family group, lack of opportunity for the vigorous and enjoyable physical exercise that youth requires, as well as the much emphasized element of emotional stress. Many of the medical problems of adolescent girls and young women are due in part to faulty nutrition either through ignorance of normal nutrition or by self-imposed restriction of diet. Maternal and infant mortality, which have already been greatly reduced by better medical care, will be reduced still more when women practice good nutrition long before the first pregnancy.

A large percentage of our population is overweight, which is not necessarily hypernutrition or overabundance of all the elements of diet. Many are actually undernourished in some of the essentials of normal nutrition. This is also true of many individuals of normal weight who are not enjoying the health that should and could be their's because of hidden hunger—unrecognized nutritional deficiencies.

The practice of good nutrition affords the opportunity to enjoy good health for a long life. Acute and chronic illnesses due to infections can for the most part now be controlled by the new wonder drugs, but the individual's recovery will be speedier and more complete in proportion to her nutrition. Surgery has been made safe and effective by new drugs and new techniques to correct abnormalities in any part of the body, but only if the individual's body nutrition is adequate to meet the stress of surgery and to make a complete and adequate recovery. Finally, in the problems of aging, many of the so-called degenerative diseases that lead to disability, chronic illness, and deterioration can be stayed by proper nutrition. If a woman wants to delay the signs of aging—and what woman doesn't—if she wants to stay well, feel well, and look well, she must, while she is young, establish the habits that ensure good nutrition.

An understanding of the basic principles of good nutrition and a realization of their importance are elements of physiology that every woman can and should achieve and practice daily. Woman has a double responsibility in learning and daily applying sound knowledge of nutrition. She has not only her own health and long life to provide for, but she usually is responsible for the nutrition of her family, providing a well-balanced diet and establishing good eating habits in her children.

We are apt to think of nutrition solely in terms of what we eat, but this is only one part. Nutrition follows through the processes not only of the supply of food for body needs but also the digestion of foods to simple substances, absorption and transportation to each cell and tissue, and the utilization of these food elements.

Thus nutrition consists of two parts: what nature needs, or diet; and how nature uses it, or metabolism.

NUTRITIONAL NEEDS

We are all interested in the food we eat. For that reason we are deluged with all kinds of diets—some good, some bad—each purporting to contribute in a certain way to our health or happiness. Some are designed to enhance the pleasure of eating and others to ensure good nutrition. Some promise certain weight loss, others weight gain. Some diets, by their restriction, are supposed to protect their adherents from certain illnesses.

All diets, for whatever purpose devised, should provide the essential elements of nutrition in sufficient quantities, and they should be palatable. Every adult should be able to scrutinize a menu for a meal or for the whole day and instantly recognize whether it is adequately nutritious. But just knowing is not enough. They should have established the habit of subscribing to such a diet. It is our responsibility to supply nature with the proper material in the proper amounts at proper timing. If we do so, the reward is good health. If we fail, the deficiencies will show up in changes of appearance, loss of energy, lack of a feeling of well-being, fatigue, loss of mental acuity, nervousness, mental and emotional depression, instability and illness.

There are certain qualities a diet must possess to ensure good nutrition: it will contain the protective and energy-producing foods in adequate and balanced amounts; prepared and served in an attractive and appetizing manner; and apportioned according to a daily schedule that corresponds to the cyclic change of body needs. This is not an impossible order—nor even a difficult one—but it does require knowledge and some effort.

The protective food elements provide the necessary building materials to keep the body as a whole and each cell, each tissue and organ, in the peak of condition for normal function, and allow also for growth and for repair. These are the elements the body cannot manufacture but must be supplied in regular and adequate quantities. The amounts needed are not the same for everyone but vary with age and sex, the size and activity of the person, and in sickness and in health. They are the protein foods, the minerals, and the vitamins.

The energy-giving foods include carbohydrates, fats, and proteins. The carbohydrates are the source of quick energy and are the first to be used for that purpose, because they are quickly broken down to usable form— the simple sugars. When the intake is just sufficient for energy, they are completely used up; when in excess some is stored as a form of sugar, but the larger amount is converted to a more concentrated form of fuel and stored as fat. The fats and proteins of the diet can also provide energy, but they must first be converted to simpler form, which takes more time.

Foods are rarely pure proteins, fats, or carbohydrates but are mixtures to which are added some indigestible material (cellulose) and a considerable amount of water.

Calorie is the unit by which the energy value of proteins, fats, and carbohydrates is measured. Calories therefore are merely a means of measuring quantity, not of evaluating the quality of the diet. When used as the only standard of measuring a diet, which is too often the case, the result is likely to be a poor diet. To select a diet by calories alone is like buying a sealed box by its weight without knowing its contents. It might be a pound of sand or a pound of gold. Usually when the diet contains the necessary protective food elements, some energy producing foods, and some bulk in every meal the calories fall into place.

There must be a schedule by which these elements are supplied corresponding to the needs of the body. Food should be taken at regular intervals throughout the day, and each meal should have a proportionate amount of each kind of food. This means a good breakfast high in protein, a comparable well-balanced lunch, and a moderate dinner. Besides the proper chemical values and timing, the diet should be both appetizing and satisfying. These qualities provide the control mechanism of amount of food eaten.

THE CELL AND THE ELEMENTS OF NUTRITION

The atom bomb and the food we eat would seem to be worlds apart— one the threat of death and the other the source of life—but that is not entirely true. We are living in an age when scientists are delving into nature's innermost secrets—the chemistry and physics of her tiniest particles. Nuclear physicists have pursued the atom, while biochemists have sought out the mysteries of the living cell. Both are seeking to understand the same thing—the physico-chemical forces of these tiniest particles, and the laws that govern them. The physical laws that explain why chemical substances behave as they do, according to their physical structure and the energy bound within, explain not only the nature of the atom but also the chemical processes in our own bodies, our own cells, and in turn the food we eat.

The cell is the basic unit of living tissue and although minute in size is exceedingly complex as to its function, for it is within the cell that life processes take place. The activity of all cells is accomplished through chemical reactions and the accompanying exchange of energy. Each cell is thus a minute chemical laboratory, which is set up (structure) to perform certain chemical processes (functions). There are, of course, many types of cells that have different structures and perform different functions for the welfare of the body as a whole, as is obvious in the difference between the muscle cells, whose main function is the transformation of chemical energy to physical energy, and the gland cells, which manufacture special chemical products for the body needs.

All living cells contain the three basic organic substances—proteins, carbohydrates, and fats—and some inorganic or mineral elements. These are not present in the same amount or used in the same way by all cells, which accounts for the differences in the structure and function of the many thousands of kinds of cells that make up the body.

Each cell in order to maintain its identity, its integrity of structure, and to perform its various chemical functions must have its basic elements of nutrition and oxygen brought to it by the blood stream. The various groups of foods in the diet consist of complex molecules that must be reduced to simple blocks before they can be brought to and used by the cells. This is accomplished in the digestive tract. Foods are broken down to their typical kind of block—proteins to amino acids, carbohydrates to simple sugars, and fats to fatty acids (in part).

Proteins are exceedingly complex organic substances made up of a specific kind of block, the amino acid, linked together in a specific way. An amino acid is not a hypothetical substance or transitory, but is a true organic chemical compound.

It is the composition of the protein molecule—the kind of amino acids contained and how they are arranged—that is most important, because this determines its chemical properties and in turn the physiological potentialities. There are some nineteen to twenty-three amino acids in body proteins. With this number of building blocks that may be put together in any arrangement and combination, an infinite variety of proteins is possible, just as all the astronomical numbers which measure outer space are made of only ten digits. Most body proteins consist of long chains of many kinds of amino acids, usually as many as fifteen to eighteen. To this basic structure may be linked any other type of organic compound or mineral. Globulin, for example, is one of the most versatile of the body proteins. In the blood one fraction of the total globulin has a pigment-bearing (iron) complex—hematin—attached to form the hemoglobin of the red blood cell, while the gamma globulin is the agent of immunity. In another compound, the thyroid hormone, thyroxine, is attached to form thyreoglobulin.

All these amino acids are necessary to make up the different kinds of proteins of the body. Some cells of the body can synthesize some of these amino acids from other substances. There are some amino acids, however, that the cells do not have a facility to manufacture. These are the seven to nine essential or indispensable amino acids that must be provided as finished products in the food.

The "complete proteins" of the food will contain all of these essential amino acids, as well as others, and they are found in generous amounts in the proteins of meats, milk, and eggs. The "incomplete proteins" are lacking in one or more of the essential amino acids. As examples, casein, the typical protein of milk, is a complete protein that will maintain life and good health. Gelatin, on the other hand, is an incomplete protein, deficient in some of the essential amino acids. Its use as the only source of protein in the diet would lead to malnutrition.

The cells of the body take the amino acids and build them into an assortment of products. They are essential elements of cell structure—the cell wall, the nucleus—and many of the products of cell metabolism contained in the cytoplasm such as some hormones and enzymes.

Every physiological function of the body (and this includes the psyche as well as the soma) has some specific physical structure, some necessary chemical basis. Proteins enter, in one way or another, into all of these. The genes, which provide the life-giving function to the cell, are nuclear proteins. Many of the hormones are protein in nature, including the important tropic hormones of the pituitary. Enzyme activity, the acquisition of immunity to infectious agents, allergy, cell growth and repair, maintenance of fluid balance, to name only a few, are other functions of the cells that require proteins.

The cell cannot store amino acids or hold them in reserve, even for a short time, until other amino acids come along that are needed to synthesize some specific protein. The cell must have all the necessary amino acids simultaneously. Amino acids that are not needed or cannot be used for protein synthesis are broken down further. The amino group is excreted in the urine as ammonia. The other portion may be synthesized into appropriate form for storage as fat or converted to sugar for energy. The cell does not ordinarily use proteins as a source of energy for its chemical processes. However, if the fuel supply is low or inadequate, proteins can be used for this purpose.

The carbohydrate foods (starches and sugars) are complex molecules made up of carbon, hydrogen, and oxygen. In the process of digestion these are readily and rapidly broken down into the simple sugar—glucose (also called dextrose)—and absorbed into the blood stream for quick delivery to all parts of the body. Its primary function is to produce the necessary energy for the chemical functions of the cells. Not all of the particles are completely used for energy all the time. Some are used in the synthesis of proteins, and others are combined with a phosphate radical by which energy is concentrated to a far greater degree and stored for use at another time. Sugar is also necessary for the proper metabolism of fats. When there is an excess of glucose or sugar, it must be converted into some other form because the body cannot store glucose as such. A certain amount is converted to glycogen, primarily in the liver and the muscles, which is readily available as a source of glucose when needed. This is the source of steady supply. Glucose in excess of this is converted and stored as fat, which is not available for reconversion to glucose but can be used by the body as a source of energy.

Not all the sugar provided the cell is derived from pure carbohydrates of foods. Some comes from the breakdown of certain amino acids and fats. They are used, however, in the same way as the ingested sugars.

The fats or lipids are a group of substances that are insoluble in water but are soluble in such solvents as alcohols, ether, or benzene. There are two main groups of lipids: the oils and fats, which have the fatty acids as the characteristic block; and the steroids, which include cholesterol, certain hormones, and the fat soluble vitamins. While grouped together, they really have little in common from the standpoint of molecular structure or physiological function.

Lipids are complex organic substances in which a fatty acid is the typical constituent or block. There are many fatty acids in the fats of food. Most of these the body can synthesize, but there are three that it cannot. The fatty acids the body needs but cannot synthesize are the essential fatty acids. They are all unsaturated fatty acids and are found in small quantities in animal fat but quite abundantly in the natural plant oils.

In this day of weight-consciousness, we are apt to think of fat as a superfluous and undesirable constituent of the body. Actually, fat is both useful and unique in the role that it plays in total body economy. In the first place, fat is the way the body stores fuel for energy in a concentrated form. It cannot store protein or carbohydrates except to a very limited degree. But it can and does store fat in almost unlimited amounts (some times to our sorrow). It is particularly suitable for storage because each unit weight of fat carries twice the energy or calorie value of either proteins or carbohydrates. Ten per cent of normal body weight consists of fat—enough calories to supply energy to the body for one month. The body has special storage places for this fat—in adipose tissue, distributed throughout the body but concentrated in fat depots, which also serve the useful purpose of padding vital organs, furnishing support and even beauty to the body in the feminine curves and the soft smooth surface of the skin.

The cells of adipose tissue are highly specialized, taking up fats when they are in excess and delivering them on call when there is need for them as fuel for energy, to spare the more necessary sugar or the vital proteins. Very little is known as to the regulatory mechanism involved, but it is presumed to be hormonal in nature.

The storage fat in adipose tissue comes not only from the excessive ingestion of fat but is the means whereby fragments of carbohydrate and protein, in excess, may also be stored.

Fats are important for other reasons. Some are essential in cell architecture. This is especially true in nerve tissue, where they serve as insulation. The fatty acids that are used in cell structure become an integral part of the cell structure, and are not available for use even in starvation.

Fats are an important constituent of the diet because they occur in almost pure form and have a relatively higher caloric value than other constituents. It would be difficult to eat enough low-caloried food—such as vegetables and fruit—which contain large amounts of unusable bulk and water. And it would be difficult to have a completely fat-free diet. Most meats are high in fats, as are eggs, cheese, milk, and nuts, and even vegetables such as string beans have some fat. Also fats carry the fat soluble vitamins A and D.

Minerals are important to normal cell function. We may think of iron as the most important mineral, but sodium, potassium, calcium, phosphorus, iodine, and the trace elements are also necessary minerals provided by foods. These mineral elements are so interrelated and balanced one against the other in body metabolism that we do not speak of a specific function of each. The equilibrium of certain pairs of minerals is exceedingly important in regulatory mechanisms—sodium and potassium in the maintenance of fluid balance, or calcium and phosphorus in normal bone structure. However, different kinds of cells use some of the minerals in different amounts. For example, 90 per cent of the iodine of the body is found in the thyroid cells, and the greater proportion of iron in the red blood cells.

The organic compounds—amino acids, glucose, and fatty acids—supplied to the cells are rather stable units, and the complicated chemical processes that take place would therefore be very slow if they were unaided. Ordinary table sugar, sucrose, which is two molecules of simple sugar, can be dissolved in water, exposed to oxygen of the air, or heated, yet it retains its chemical identity. Pure oils and fats change very slowly in character, and even protein when protected from bacterial action and heat, remains intact. Yet the cells perform their complex cycles of chemical reaction readily and exactly because of the presence of substances that speed up these reactions. These chemical expediters are called enzymes.

An enzyme is a complex chemical substance, protein in nature, which acts as a catalyst. That is, it speeds or facilitates a chemical reaction without contributing any fraction of itself to the end product. It is biosynthesized (manufactured) in the cell. It may be used either in the cell or poured into one of the body fluids (such as digestive juices).

An enzyme alters only the rate of chemical change. Each enzyme (there are thousands that contribute to the body's chemical processes) is specific for one type of reaction that it will expedite. The specific reactions are of many types. Enzyme action is necessary for each step in the synthesis (which consists of many steps) of organic compounds— amino acids to proteins, fatty acids to fat, sugar to glycogen. And enzyme action is essential to the breakdown of the complex molecules to simple structure with the resultant release of energy.

Some of the enzymes have been known for a long time, but the knowledge of their identity, their distribution, and their role in cell metabolism belongs to the atomic age.

Vitamins are called "accessory" food factors because they do not contribute material to the final product of cell metabolism. Rather they are organic catalysts that the body needs but cannot manufacture. They either influence certain phases of cell metabolism directly or serve as an integral part of an enzyme system.

We have spoken of the cell as the smallest independent unit of life and stressed that it is a chemical laboratory in which activity is ceaseless. There are two other concepts of the cell that also must be emphasized. Cells are not independent but are minute entities specialized in various ways and effectively integrated to maintain the vitality of the body. Cells have a definite life span, which does not correspond to that of the body as a whole. They are constantly being replaced by like ones—as far as possible—to maintain the integrity of body structure and function—the personality.

Vitality

In speaking of the wonderful mechanism of the body, we compared it to a machine. This was apt (with certain reservations) when we were considering the various levels of control and how they succeeded in integrating the general functions of the body into a smoothly functioning whole. But when we come to consider the biochemical processes, it is a mistake to think of the body as one large machine.

A machine we visualize as a solid structure, rigid and permanent, which requires one kind of fuel for production of energy to run the machine and one or several raw materials that the machine converts into finished products. The body is not like this. Rather it is an aggregate of millions of cells, grouped together into tissues and organs to perform specific types of chemical procedures. Each is dependent on the others, each contributes to the welfare of the whole, and each requires for normal function all the elements of nutrition. And they perform functions that no machine can, such as growth, repair, and reproduction. The sum total of these functions is vitality—life.

We may think that because the body has a fixed size and form and a definite weight that it is also solid. Actually the body is not solid at all. The body as a whole must exist in an external environment of air. But each of the living cells must have an environment of fluid to exist and carry on its chemical processes. Dry cells are dead cells, such as the outer layers of the skin. This accounts for the fact that 65 to 75 per cent of the total body weight is due to water. Most of the tissues are made up of 70 to 80 per cent water; even bone, which seems hard and dry, is 20 per cent water.

Body function is not rigid and mechanical. We might get the idea that nutrition is on a production-line basis: that raw products are poured in; that proteins, carbohydrates, and fats are refined and together with minerals and water are passed along, each retaining its identity, to the cells of fixed structure; and that each cell takes what it needs and discards the unused elements as waste products. This is a static, rigid state which is not the true picture. Body function is dynamic, because ceaseless change is the life quality of all cells.

Each cell of the body is constantly receiving a supply of chemical material from the blood stream, some of which it uses as fuel, some to build up its own specific substance to maintain its integrity of structure and function, and it is constantly returning chemical material to the blood stream. Different kinds of cells need, besides the basic elements of nutrition, specific chemicals for their particular kind of function—the thyroid gland needs iodine, the bones need calcium. This readily available supply of chemical material distributed in the fluids throughout the body is called the common metabolic pool.

Personality

We may think of the body as a permanent structure with individual characteristics which are lost only after life has ceased. We see ourselves looking much the same day after day. We identify our friends by their external characteristics, even after years, and attribute the changes we see to aging—a little fatter or a little thinner perhaps, a few more gray hairs, a few more lines in the face, but they are in truth not the same individuals as far as their physical structures are concerned. It has been estimated that every seven years marks a cycle in which the body has completed the replacement of all its chemical substances. This is accomplished in part by the continuous turnover of all the chemical substances, as we have seen in the metabolic pool. The rate of change, the time required for complete replacement varies. As for protein, an indispensable unit of cell architecture, it is said to be about two years, while iodine, which is used almost exclusively in the rapidly expended thyroid hormone, it is a matter of days. But there is also another way in which changes occur, and that is the constant replacement of old cells by new in every tissue and organ of the body except one. Nerve cells of the brain and spinal cord do not have the power of reproduction—replication. But even in these there can be regeneration of fibers (the connecting element of the cell) after injury, even formation of new fibers as experience dictates the need for them. And nerve cells experience turnover of their chemical substance.

Each cell has a limited and characteristic life span—some longer than others. In any tissue, new cells are constantly being formed and growing to maturity, while old cells are constantly being broken down and discarded. When tissues are injured or damaged, sometimes the injured cells are replaced, but most often the damage is repaired by a simpler structure, and the debris is returned to the metabolic pool as usable material or as a useless waste product to be discarded. Each of the new cells looks like and functions like its predecessor.

Individual "personality" is based on body structure and the particular characteristics of function of the whole and each of its parts—psyche and soma, cell, tissues, and organs. The integrity or individuality of physical personality is not maintained by inactivity and rigidity of structure but by constant change as the result of replication, growth, and repair, which is in turn dependent on nutrition. Thus, because a woman has reached maturity does not mean that growth has ceased. She will not increase in height, her structural proportions will not change greatly, but growth will continue as long as she lives.

The skin affords a good example of the continuity of growth. Every day old cells on the surface are dying and being discarded—rubbed off as a flaky material—because deep in the vital basal layer of the skin new cells are constantly being formed, grow to their mature form, and are pushed upward. When the skin is injured by a pin prick, a cut, a burn, or an infection, it heals or repairs itself by growth of new cells. This process of growth is happening every day in every tissue of the body, even the bones. Repair is constantly needed to offset the effects of the wear and tear of daily use.

The beauty of this organ, which we so highly prize for its attributes of soft and smooth texture, delicate and subtle coloring, luxuriant and lustrous hair, firm, smooth, and well-formed nails comes as a result of the dynamic processes of nutrition, growth, and repair, which reside deep within its structure.

The skin, to be healthy, to grow, and to be repaired, must have the same elements of nutrition as the cells of any other organ of the body, and it receives this nutrition in the same manner—from within, by the blood stream. It must have the right kinds of proteins for growth and repair and sufficient energy producing foods and vitamins to accomplish these chemical processes. Deficiencies produce changes we can see, which mar the beauty and undermine the health of the skin.

This process of continuous growth of the skin is directed by the growth hormone of the pituitary assisted by the thyroid hormone and the sex and adrenal steroids. The importance of each of these becomes apparent when one is deficient. For instance, when the thyroid is deficient, the skin is thick and dry and the nails brittle. In adrenal deficiency the skin has a peculiarly distributed increased pigmentation. In women, when the adrenals become overactive and produce an excess of the male hormone, the result is overactivity of the sebaceous (oil) glands leading to acne and male distribution of body and facial hair.

The endometrium is another tissue that demonstrates even more markedly the ever-active processes of growth and repair and their regulation, for here these occur rapidly in recurring cycles that constitute the most characteristic badge of femininity—menstruation. The endometrium requires for its functional cycle the same nutritive factors and the same general regulatory mechanism of growth as any other tissue. But here there is greater loss of tissue proteins and blood elements, which must be replaced. And the changes that occur are more than mere growth, they are differentiative changes, changes in the pattern of structure, which require their own growth hormones—estrogen and progesterone. Thus, failure of growth may be due to the deficient supply of the nutrients, or it may result from the lack of its own specific growth hormones from the ovaries.

NUTRITION AND THE ENDOCRINE GLANDS

It is the wisdom of the body that keeps the two phases of metabolism in harmonious balance. Health is the accurate and optimum balance between tissue destruction and tissue repair, which is achieved through the regulatory mechanism of nutrition, endocrine function, and nervous control. Good nutrition is mandatory for normal function of the body, which includes normal function of the endocrine glands; and the endocrine glands play an indispensable part in the body's utilization of every element of nutrition—not only proteins, carbohydrates, and fats but minerals and water as well. We cannot say that any one hormone controls exclusively a specific phase of metabolism, for each is quite complex. For instance, insulin from the pancreas is essential in the metabolism of carbohydrates, but it requires assistance from the thyroid, pituitary, and adrenal glands. Protein metabolism involves the corticoids of the adrenals, the pituitary, and thyroid hormones, and the sex steroids. And the thyroid sets the pace for all metabolism.

When glandular function is abnormal, nutrition suffers. This is quite obvious in certain serious, but fortunately rare, conditions. Obesity of a peculiar type is one of the cardinal symptoms of Cushing's Disease, which is due to a hormone-producing tumor of the pituitary gland. Emaciation is characteristic of several endocrine abnormalities such as adrenal insufficiency (Addison's Disease), pan-pituitary failure (Simmond's Disease), and thyroid hyperactivity or thyrotoxicosis. More subtle forms of malnutrition occur as part of less severe degrees of endocrine imbalance.

Malnutrition, on the other hand, results in glandular deficiency. The endocrine glands must have the proper nutrition to perform efficiently. They need specific elements of nutrition to maintain the integrity of their structure and function, just as all other tissues need material to grow, replace, and repair. They also have another need, that is, specific material that is used to elaborate their hormones. Since hormones have different chemical structures, the building blocks needed by each gland will vary, although not very much is known about the actual process involved in the elaboration of hormones. The pituitary hormones are protein, requiring specific amino acids. The thyroid must have, in addition to protein, the specific element, iodine. The sex hormones and other steroids are derived from cholesterol.

The ovarian cycle is a significant example of the need of proper nutrition for woman and her normal glandular functions and personality. In the ovary, the follicle grows from a few cells to many cells, elaborates the ovarian hormone estrogen, and is then transformed into the corpus luteum, which serves its purpose and then disappears. The follicle must have the general nutritive factors and its own specific growth hormones—the gonadotropic hormones of the pituitary gland. It needs nutritive factors and withdraws them from the metabolic pool, but it does not waste them as does the endometrium. The products are returned to the blood stream.

There is one other facet of metabolism that it is important to mention; that is, the metabolism of the hormones themselves. We have seen the wisdom of the body in maintaining balance of hormone production such as the ovarian-pituitary balance and the thyro-pituitary balance. But what happens to the hormones? They are chemical messengers. They tell the cells what to do, but do not themselves enter into the chemical process. Since they are being produced constantly by the glands, how does the body keep them at the optimum level and not allow any excess to pile up? For the most part a hormone maintains its identity and activity for a very short period of time. It is broken down and some of the fragments are returned to the metabolic pool, others are discarded. How and when this happens varies for each hormone. As an example, the liver plays an important part in the metabolism of the ovarian hormones where they are broken down into inactive fragments, and here again nutrition enters. The liver must have, among other things, sufficient vitamins, especially of the vitamin-B complex, to do the job properly. When the liver cannot perform this, excessive estrogen may accumulate in the blood stream. Excessive estrogen causes extreme growth of the endometrium, which results in excessive menstruation. In treating profuse, excessive menstrual bleeding, we try to restore liver metabolism by the administration of the vitamin-B complex and also to restore the protein and iron lost in the excessive flow, as well as to correct the cause of the endocrine imbalance.

THE MECHANISM OF CONTROL

Long before the meaning of calories was known or the necessity of various essential food elements was understood, man knew when to eat and when to stop eating and for the most part felt the necessity of obtaining a varied diet. The faculty of eating—the desire for food—is inborn. It is a part of the wisdom of the body not only that the urge to eat is present, and a powerful drive in everyone, but also that under the right environmental conditions a person will naturally select the right kinds of foods and be satisfied with what is the required amount. Primitive people today eat a nutritious diet, as far as the environment affords the various foodstuffs, and in some instances show a higher standard of nutrition than those of more civilized or cultured areas. Experiments in our own country demonstrated that babies and children under optimum conditions when allowed to select their own foods will choose a good variety of foods and do not eat excessively. Experiments in natural selection of food, using young men in the services, revealed that while at first they ate excessively, they too settled down to a good diet.

What is this wisdom of the body that controls the supply for nutrition? What is the physiological mechanism that controls eating?

The process of eating is directed by three types of sensation—hunger, appetite, and satiety. Hunger is a physiological reaction, the body's way of announcing that food is needed. It is recognized as a "rumbling in the tummy," a feeling of emptiness, which is caused by increased muscular contraction of the stomach when it is empty which disappears when the stomach is filled. Under the conditions in which we live today, food is abundant, and hunger as a condition is a pleasant sensation because it is easily satisfied. But in the situation where there is not enough food, hunger becomes a dominant force that sweeps aside all other drives, and with them ideals, hopes, and ambitions. Intellectual people of highest culture who experienced the hunger in concentration camps, which was both extreme and chronic, tell us that food was incessantly uppermost in their minds, and dominated their conversations, their thoughts, and their actions. Cannabalism, horrible as it may seem to us, has been acceptable to isolated groups of civilized people cut off too long from all other food supply.

Appetite, on the other hand, is the desire for food. It is a psychological reaction and does not always reflect the needs of the body. As in all other desires, it is conditioned by past experience and may be exercised to satisfy needs other than hunger. To a certain extent a normal appetite reflects a normal balancing of emotional drives, self-satisfaction, and application of good habits. Abnormal appetite (too little or too much) can result from a disturbance of any one of these factors. Some people have an excessive appetite that may be satisfied with any food as long as it is supplied in large amounts; while in others the excessive appetite is a craving for a particular type of food. In most instances these are the results of bad habits. In the opposite situation—loss of appetite—the person has no desire to eat, although the needs of the body may be great.

Satiety is the appeasement of appetite. Hunger and appetite normally occur simultaneously, but even after hunger is appeased by a hearty meal most people still have appetite for the dessert. Appetite and satiety then are the deciding factors in why and how much we eat.

What is the mechanism that blunts the appetite, tells the person she has had enough? Where does the appetite originate in the first place?

There is a part of the brain, the hypothalamus or old brain, which is the control center for important self-regulatory functions of the body such as temperature control, water balance, breathing, heart action, and sleep. Here also is a control center for appetite. When that center is stimulated, it transmits messages to the conscious brain and makes the person want to eat. When the appetite center is depressed or satisfied, no such messages go out. Appetite is not appeased by the bulk of the food ingested or the conscious recognition that one has eaten enough. It is the result of a chemical communication to the appetite center, which relays the message to the conscious brain. This chemical messenger of appeasement is blood sugar, and it works something like this: The carbohydrates (sugars and starches) of food are converted in the intestines to glucose, which is absorbed into the blood stream and carried to all parts of the body. Some of it is used by the muscles for energy, some is stored in the liver as glycogen, and the excess, if any, is deposited as fat. When a situation arises that more glucose is needed by physical activity, the glycogen can be reconverted back to sugar. The storage and delivery-on-call of glucose is accomplished by means of hormones from the pancreas, the pituitary, and adrenals. This glucose is the fuel of the body and is constantly being used up. Therefore, it must be regularly replaced by the ingestion of more glucose-producing foods. The appetite center in the hypothalamus is very sensitive to these changes of blood-sugar levels. When the level is high, it is soothed and remains quiet, but when the level is low, it sends out the alarm to the conscious brain that more food is needed.

This is an oversimplification of a complex mechanism, but it gives an idea of the basis of normal appetite. And from it we can see possibilities that would reduce the efficiency of the appetite center. When the glands cause the sugar to be stored too fast, an excessive amount of food may be ingested before the blood level of sugar has increased enough to appease the appetite center. The same condition would result if the appetite center had suffered some injury, an acute illness or infection that actually reduced its efficiency. In persons who constantly overeat—the appetite center is constantly flooded with high glucose. It comes to expect a high level as normal.

THE MEASURE OF NUTRITION

How do we measure nutrition? How can we say that one person is well nourished, another undernourished, and still another malnourished?

It used to be generally believed that nutrition was measured by weight, that a person who was well nourished was of normal weight; therefore a person of normal weight was well nourished. This we now know is not true, and doctors have learned to look for signs and symptoms of malnutrition in persons of normal weight and in obesity as well as in underweight. Nonspecific symptoms such as fatigue, irritability, nervousness, insomnia, pain in the legs or headaches may be indicative of deficiencies of some essential food elements. Sore swollen tongue, cracks at the corner of the mouth, skin changes, high blood pressure or low blood pressure, low blood count—these symptoms may be physical manifestations of nutritional deficiencies.

The search for nutritional deficiencies can be carried further by chemical analyses of body fluids. But the most important part of detection is, first, to suspect that deficiency may be present and, second, to analyze the patient's eating habits by a detailed nutritional history. Perhaps someday a physical checkup will no longer be only a search for disease but will be a profile of the health of the individual with the characteristic features contributed by nutrition, degree of physical fitness, and emotional attitudes.

Weight, however, always has been and always will be an important measure of nutrition if for no other reason than that it is so obvious and easily measured and also because abnormal weight is always the sign of malnutrition in one form or another.

"Ideal weight" is defined as the weight at which the person can be expected to live longer and live better. A woman's ideal weight depends not only on her height but also on her type of body build or bone structure. She should attain this ideal weight as she achieves physical maturity— about age twenty-five—and maintain it thereafter. It is not healthy to put on weight with the added years of life. A longer span of life may be expected if she does not gain. As a matter of fact, there is a definite health advantage in being slightly underweight after the age of forty.

We have tables of "normal" or "ideal" weight because so many people have tended to have the same weight for a particular height, age, sex, and build. Does it follow that all these people always eat just the amount of food their bodies need day in and day out? Not at all. Their weight may be normal because of their superior self-control, but more frequently they are just lucky that they have a body that functions efficiently but not rigidly.

"Ideal" or "normal" weight is another manifestation of the wisdom of the body. There is a "normal" weight because the body possesses and uses an efficient weight-regulating mechanism. For proof that the body possesses an efficient weight-regulating mechanism we may go to statistics on overweight. We find that only one person in four or six is moderately overweight; only one in thirty becomes seriously obese; and one in a million reaches the proportions of the fat lady in the circus. Stated another way, we find that five out of every six people maintain a normal weight, twenty-nine of every thirty never become truly obese, and there is only one chance in a million that a person will be monstrous. We would be unrealistic to suppose that all these people of normal weight always eat just the right amount of food.

Another bit of evidence of the weight-regulating mechanism is to examine the eating habits of any one person. The amount of food required for a person's physical needs can be accurately measured. If the amount of food eaten is just sufficient to supply the needs of the body, the weight will remain the same. We would expect therefore that if an excess is eaten, it would invariably be stored as fat causing a gain in weight. But this does not always happen.

When we consider the amount of food most of us eat, it is a wonder we are not all exceedingly obese, for we are all guilty of consuming, at one time or another, considerably more food than is needed. Think of the holiday dinners, picnics, parties, and TV snacks when goodly amounts of high caloric foods are eaten. It has been estimated that eating a single slice of bread or drinking one glass of milk a day in excess of the needs of the body, is sufficient to lead to the storage of twenty-four pounds of fat, or gain in weight, within a year. But this does not occur in the normal individual. The body is able to regulate weight by some mechanism that is not completely understood.

The weight-regulating mechanism has its limitations, however. There is no "perfect animal" whose habits of animal functions such as eating, sleeping, and sex activity, conform strictly to body needs. We eat for many reasons besides body needs, and we all overeat at times. This overeating is a stress to which the body can adjust for a while, but if continued and excessive, the weight-regulatory mechanism breaks down and obesity is the result.

VII

WOMAN'S PERENNIAL PROBLEM

IT IS A FAIR ESTIMATE that every woman at some time in her life will be dissatisfied with, and concerned about, her weight. Some are disturbed because they are gaining or are already overweight. Others are concerned because their figures do not conform to their concept of ideal measurements. There are a few who will want to gain weight.

Normal body weight is exceedingly important to woman, not only as a measure of health but as an attribute of her attractiveness. Weight, as identified with a good figure, is the most dominant and fundamental of all characteristics of beauty. A pretty face loses its appeal when coupled with a body distorted by excessive fat. Woman can change the color of her hair or hide the flaws of a poor complexion, but any degree of overweight she cannot conceal; she must do something to correct it. It has recently been estimated that 26 million American women think that they should lose weight; 8 million have tried, with a varying degree of success; and of those who lost weight, half regained what they had lost very quickly. These women, and perhaps many more, are plagued by the problem of obesity, the greatest stumbling block to both health and beauty and woman's perennial problem.

The word "obesity" may be distasteful, suggesting a person bulging at the seams, with triple chins and a waddling gait, a woman who cannot see her own feet for the shelves of fat except when she looks in the mirror. But it may be applied to someone who is "too fat" or more politely "overweight." The true significance of obesity, however, which should be clearly understood, is that it is one of the greatest health hazards today and is almost completely within the power of each of us to avoid or control.

"Obesity is a condition in which the body weight is in excess of body needs due to excessive deposition of fat." Obesity thus defined may seem to say simply "overweight" due to "too much fat." But note that it specifies not just too much weight, but weight that is in excess of body needs, which implies that there is an optimum weight at which the body will function most efficiently. This eliminates other factors in excessive weight such as heavy bone structure, unusual muscular development, and abnormal fluid retention. A certain amount of fat storage is necessary for normal body function and serves many useful purposes. It is only when the reservoirs are overfilled that obesity is present.

ORIGIN OF THE PROBLEM

In every case of obesity, the gain in weight is due to eating too much. This is an unassailable fact that must be faced. The body cannot make fat from fresh air; it must have food in excess of what it needs. It should be pointed out that obesity refers to an accomplished fact, the person has already stored excessive fat. She may still be gaining, or she may have reached the state of obesity years before and maintained a constant weight since. If she is still gaining, she is still eating too much. If her weight is constant, she has achieved the balance of eating just the amount her body needs at the present time, which may be the same as that of a person of normal weight or even less. This accounts for the fact that some obese persons do not seem to eat excessively. To find the cause in any particular case, one must examine that person's way of life at the period of actual weight gain. But this does not answer the many important questions. What is too much? Why is it too much? Why does a person eat too much?

We are all acquainted with a few persons who seem to ingest a terrific amount of food and never gain weight and with others who complain that even though they restrict their diets, everything "turns to fat," and they gain weight. Here are contradictions and exaggerations, but each has an element of truth that emphasizes the fact that "too much" is a very individual thing. It must be measured in terms of the person, and both the amount and the kind of food that she eats.

We have tables that state the approximate number of calories a woman should eat, with variations allowed for her physical activity as sedentary, moderate, or strenuous. The difficulty comes in trying to classify her activity because it is not only what she does, but how long she does it and how she does it. One woman who works in an office may sit placidly typing all day, while another may be constantly on the move, harried by the stress of getting work done, with interruptions and deadlines, and there are few moments in her day when her body is not in high gear and using more calories than the woman who sits all day. They would not maintain the same weight even though their diets were identical.

How much a person should eat is not measured in terms of volume of food consumed but of the kinds of foods included and their distribution in the day's menu. There is considerable misunderstanding that women bring to their problem of weight control about the quality of foods. Some believe that a person must eat certain kinds of foods to lose weight and other kinds to gain. There is no such thing as "slimming food" or "fattening food." A person will lose weight on high calorie foods if the amount is sufficiently limited and gain weight on low calorie foods if enough is consumed. Similarly, no particular combination of foods renders them more fattening. Nor are nourishing foods such as meat, eggs, and milk to be avoided as fattening just because they are essential to a substantial diet. All foods have some caloric value, some more than others. It is the total number of calories consumed each day, from whatever kind of food, that counts.

Another error occurs in evaluating foods by the class to which they belong. Many of our foods have "concealed" (more properly—"ignored") calories. Cheese is a high protein food, but most cheeses contain a large amount of fat. An apple is a fruit—but a fresh apple is not the same as a baked apple to which butter and sugar have been added. These and other pitfalls can be avoided by using one of the many excellent books on diet that are available.

There is also the mistaken idea that skipping a meal or two and having one large meal a day is a good way to lose weight (or sufficient safeguard against gaining). Actually, the body will burn up more food, use more calories for energy, if the day's allowance is distributed among three meals with a snack in between. A good breakfast speeds up body metabolism (and the use of calories), and frequent refueling keeps it going at this higher speed and also renders the very important service of keeping the appetite in check. On the other hand, if little food is taken during the day, metabolism may remain in low gear, but by evening the appetite is ravenous. The result is an excessively large meal is taken, which the body has little need for and cannot use completely when the day's work is over, particularly if one settles down to a few hours of relaxation, reading or watching television before going to bed. There is but one solution for the body's dilemma and that is to store the excess as fat.

Moreover, there is a difference in the degree that different foods influence the rate of metabolism. Proteins have the power to stimulate cells to more intense or rapid activity. Thus proteins have a "pepping up" quality that speeds up body metabolism so that more fuel is needed, more calories expended. There is also an extra bonus in a high protein diet in that it has a higher satiety value and the appetite is more easily controlled.

Why do some people have excessive appetites, eat more than they need, and eat when they are not hungry? There are two answers, one based on the psychological aspects, the other on the physiological or chemical. They are poles apart.

The psychosomatic school of thought interprets excessive appetite on an emotional basis. They view overeating as an escape mechanism, similar to addiction to alcohol, whereby the individual seeks solace in food to make up for other needs, disappointments, or frustrations. All people who drink even excessively are not alcoholics or mentally ill. And all over-eating cannot be attributed to emotional conflict alone. In this land of plenty, the opportunity to eat is excessive, and most of our social and many business activities are accompanied by eating—morning coffee (with a bun), afternoon tea (with cake), bridge luncheons, dinner parties, and TV snacks. Such overeating is just a bad habit, not evidence of emotional conflict. While it is true that some obese persons are emotionally disturbed, it does not follow that they are obese because they are neurotic. Obesity may just as well be the reason for the emotional disturbance.

Those who would explain obesity on the basis of disturbed body function attribute it to "physiologic overeating," which is not necessarily deliberate gluttony. An obese woman eats only enough to satisfy her appetite, but the trouble comes because her appetite is not satisfied until an unphysiological amount of food (more than the body needs) has been eaten. This person is obese because her weight regulating mechanism is out of gear. This is not meant to be an alibi for the person who is obese nor to brand appetite as a culprit. It is to point out that her appetite is playing a trick on her; but she is not helpless to do anything about it. She may have been guilty of doing things that threw the mechanism out of gear. It is up to her to reprimand and control this faulty appetite. She will be rewarded for her efforts not only by loss of weight, but with a return to normal weight the appetite control mechanism may also regain its sensitivity and work more efficiently.

To have a good appetite is healthy. To have an appetite for the right kinds and right amounts of food is much more—it is the best insurance for a long and healthy life.

AN ALIBI FOR HER PLIGHT

Whatever may be the causative mechanism in any case of obesity, the fact is that the individual has eaten and may still be eating too much. Eating is a pleasant pastime, and most of us overindulge in varying degrees. Human nature being what it is, we do not always admit to our shortcomings, and we look around for alibis. The alibis that women give for obesity are familiar enough, but they should not be accepted at face value. They rarely will hold up under close scrutiny. We may examine a few.

"I can't help being fat, it runs in my family." It is true that fat parents frequently have fat children, and fat children are more frequently found in a family in which one or both parents are obese. But this does not mean that the child has inherited a tendency to obesity, as she inherited the color of her eyes and hair. She may have acquired, not inherited, the food habits of her parents. She learned from them to like to eat, to like the foods rich in calories, and to like an abundance three times a day, and snacks between.

"I gained weight when I had my baby." "I gained weight after my operation." These are common variations on the theme that women gain weight more easily than men and are especially prone to obesity in the passing from one age to another. It is true that more women are obese than men. It is also true that they started in many instances to gain at such specific physiologic epochs in their lives as puberty, pregnancy, or menopause. These are periods when the balance of endocrine gland function is changing and less stable and when imbalance or abnormalities of glandular function are more likely to occur. But there are other factors that are probably more important. In adolescence, there is also a change in physical activity, an abrupt and marked decrease from boisterous activity of childhood to the more circumspect behavior of the young lady. In pregnancy, there is often decreased physical activity with the added psychological factor of "eating for two." For women in general, as contrasted with men, physical activities are less extreme, they need less food, and because they work with food the opportunity for excessive eating, especially nibbling and tasting between meals, is greater. So sex is not an alibi for obesity.

"I don't eat much." "Everything I eat turns to fat." "I eat like a bird." These alibis needn't be taken very seriously, even though the defendant is quite honest in her reliance on them. Of course, a bird only pecks at its food, but it does so all day long.

"I have gland trouble, which makes me gain weight." This alibi will be sustained only in rare cases. Glands are rarely at fault in an obese person who is otherwise normal. When a person is obese due to faulty glandular function, there are usually other physical evidences of glandular dysfunction.

WHEN IS A WOMAN OBESE?

A vast number of women, as we have said, think that they should lose weight. Does this necessarily mean that all are obese? Likely not, but it would be difficult to separate them into clear-cut groups of obese and non-obese. As there is no such thing as an average woman, there is no such thing as an average ideal weight even when we allow for differences in height and body build. When a woman's weight is obviously excessive, say 150 pounds for a height of five feet, or 200 pounds for five and one half feet, there is no question. But suppose she weighs 140 pounds and is five feet five inches; is that obesity? It may or may not be.

The normal body consists of 10 per cent stored fat, and obesity is stored fat in excess of this amount. The 90 per cent is made up of muscles, bones, vital organs, and fluids and stays fairly constant in the healthy individual. With weight changes, it is usually the fat that is variable. The difficulty comes in determining what the actual total weight should be, and the fact that we have no convenient method by which to measure the fat storage.

This may seem to be belaboring an unimportant point, but if 26 million women think they should lose weight, there are undoubtedly many of those who do not and should not, and others who have not admitted to their obesity. And if 26 million people want something in this country, you can rest assured there will be many who will try to meet this want in some way—at a profit to themselves.

Before a woman tries to reduce, she should determine whether she is overweight. This is not done by comparing herself to the women whose figures are their livelihood. Their weight and measurements may be optimum for them (usually they are below normal) but certainly cannot be the criterion for all women. And she should know how much she should reduce. This can be measured only in pounds not inches. (She has only one weight, but she can be measured in a thousand ways. Each measurement may be a little excessive, and the total may be greatly so.)

We have tables of normal or ideal weights compiled from large series of women that allow for variation according to the three types of body build—the small, the average, and the large. But how is one to determine the body build, and establish the fact that a particular woman is over-weight? The simplest way is not to try to fit her to a table of numbers but to evaluate her own body proportions. There are two practical ways of doing this: one seeks evidence of excessive padding of fat; and the other estimates her bone structure.

Does she have extra padding of fat? All women have a way of storing fat in special places to give them the normal feminine curves—throughout the breasts, a little pad on the lower abdominal wall, a generous layer on the hips, and a moderate layer on the neck, shoulders, and arms. The tell-tale pads of fat are on her chest wall and upper abdomen. If she can pick up a roll of fat on the ribs below the arms that is thicker than her finger, or a roll of fat around her abdomen between her ribs and waist line she has too much fat. These same pads of fat show up as bulges above and below a snug fitting bra or over the top of her girdle. Women will vary in amount of fat in other locations and are made quite unhappy about their proportions. Body proportions are an inherited character, which they cannot do anything about. What is her body build? We may estimate body build from the size of glove that she wears—7–7½ indicates average, 6–6½ small, and 8–8½ large, but this is not infallible. Even with these devices we still have to rely on a modicum of common sense, which is based on how the woman looks, how she feels, and how she is able to perform physically.

THE SERIOUSNESS OF HER PROBLEM

Overweight is always a serious problem, and a woman should be encouraged to correct it for her own happiness as well as for her health's sake. Obesity is a stumbling block on the pathway to maturity on all levels of her personality. First of all she is not happy with herself. She is ashamed of her appearance, although she may seek to hide her true feelings with aggressiveness and heartiness. More often she retreats to self-conscious loneliness. She does not achieve the status she would like to have in the world of others. She finds it harder to get a job and may be passed over for advancement. Her social life may be limited, and she does not have her choice for a husband.

On the physical level, obesity is a burden and a hazard. Avoiding or correcting it affords her an important way to avoid many future illnesses and to lengthen her life. Obesity reduces her chances for a normal pregnancy. The likelihood of complications such as toxemia, difficult labor, fetal mortality, etc., is greater for the obese woman. Even her ability to become pregnant is threatened, for obesity may be the cause of menstrual irregularities and lowered fertility.

Surgery and many acute infections are more dangerous in overweight persons. Degenerative diseases develop earlier and are more severe in obese persons. These include heart disease, hardening of the arteries, kidney disease, arthritis, diabetes, varicose veins, and many others. For most of these conditions there is no known cure, but they can be delayed or prevented, and their severity can be mitigated by maintaining a normal weight.

SOLUTION TO THE PROBLEM

Obesity as we have seen has many contributing causes. The correction therefore must take all these into account. It will not be a simple matter, but it is not an impossible one. The following plan of attack on the problem has been assembled with sympathy for the woman's difficulties and the intent to be helpful, not critical or dictatorial. If you are over-weight and truly want to reduce, read the following over carefully. When you can accept the facts as applying directly to you, you are ready to start. If you seek an easier way, you are destined to failure. Remember that losing weight is something that you have to do for yourself; no one can do it for you.

1. Have a heart-to-heart talk with yourself and face the facts: Your weight is too much. It is too much because you have eaten too much. To lose weight, you will have to diet. It is useless to try to excuse yourself.

2. Examine your reasons for wanting to lose weight.

3. Lay out a specific plan of action. It is a strictly do-it-yourself project. Get a well-balanced diet to follow. Do not rely on calorie counting. Set a goal for yourself, the date by which you will be at your ideal weight, allowing a weight loss of one and a half to two pounds a week. Have a regular time to weigh—once a week in the morning, and keep a written record. Restrain yourself from getting on every pair of scales that you see. If you have a chubby friend, invite her to join you. Misery loves company, and competition adds zest. Promise yourself a reward (other than food), at specified intervals if you have lost as per schedule, and deny yourself something if you have failed. Be sure that you have diverting interests, so that you won't have time to be sorry for yourself. Keep busy doing something that brings you pleasure and satisfaction. Allow time each day for a moderate amount of moderate exercise. You are exercising for your health, but it will also help you to lose weight.

4. Go to a doctor if you are unsure of yourself and want help.

What are the chances that you will lose weight and will maintain a normal weight thereafter? The statistics say that you have only a 15 per cent chance of losing weight and only half of that not to regain once you have lost. This need not be disturbing. Your success depends not on probabilities and chance but on your own personal situation—the reason you are overweight, your incentives for losing weight, and how you go about your objective.

The reason for overweight, as we have pointed out, is overeating. It is up to you to learn enough about nutrition to understand where your errors of diet have been, and about yourself for the reasons that you have overindulged.

To think that you would like to lose weight is not enough. There must be determination and motivation strong enough to start you on a definite program and see you through. Moreover, in order to reduce and stay reduced, the incentive and determination must be long lasting, because the world of food about you is not going to change. The opportunity to eat excessively will always be present and tempting. Your determination will be bolstered, your ability to carry through strengthened, if you choose the only correct method, which is knowing and appreciating the truth and importance of nutrition and accepting this as a new way of life.

You will meet with many "get thin quick" schemes. They are enticing, they promise quick results with the minimum of effort on your part, but they are deceptive. They all play up one particular means of losing weight, as by special foods, a particular medication, exercise or massage, but they always contain (in fine print, or a footnote) a restricted diet. We might profitably examine some of these short cuts for which women spend millions of dollars each year in vain.

There are many forms of food advertised as conducive to weight loss such as high-protein bread, fat-free bread, a particular kind of cracker, fruit juice, and candy and the specially prepared fruits and vegetables low in calories. All of these may serve a useful purpose as a part of the diet. The fault lies in the implication that they have some hidden ingredient, some magic property, which induces loss of weight.

High-protein bread or cereals or fat-free breads may be good and wholesome, but the fact remains that they are food, they have calories. They are effective only if they are taken in place of other higher calorie foods and not along with a regular diet. They have a valid physiologic basis in that they have a high satiety value, and if they are taken before a meal may make you satisfied with less. But if you like to eat, they will do little to stop you; only your own determination can do that.

There are crackers that are made up largely of some form of cellulose that the body cannot use, and which expands when ingested with a glass of water to form a much larger mass—to deceive the stomach into believing that it has had a meal. But these crackers have twenty-five calories and as few as six a day will add up to a large percentage of the daily calorie allotment, yet they have no protective nutritional value.

Fruit juices, before meals or between meals, have a valid basis in that sugar is the body's tool for satisfying the appetite. But this kind of appeasement is short lasting, and the appetite soon returns with full vigor.

Medication of one kind or another has long been one of the most tempting short cuts, promising weight reduction without effort. It always has been and always will be the most futile. There is one indisputable fact—there is no safe medication that you can buy or that your doctor can give you that by its action alone will reduce weight.

Before the days of the pure food and drug laws some of the preparations sold for self-medication were harmful, even dangerous. Today they are harmless but also useless. Yet you will find advertised a pill that promises that you will "lose that ugly fat yet eat what you want. Full stomach plan never allows you to go hungry—lets you eat, feel pleasantly full while ugly fat just seems to melt away. Pleasant tasting, safe, no dangerous drugs, no hormones." In fine print it adds: "to be used with reducing diets." The ingredients are dry skimmed milk, sugar, and vitamin C, which are normal elements of diet.

Other medications widely advertised go much further in their claims and are more secretive as to their formulas. They usually claim for their product some special medical background. Some mythical doctor or clinic has devoted "years of research according to the methods of modern science" and come up with "another wonder drug that makes losing weight effortless, positively pleasant. It is like a doctor's prescription." Yet you may have it by signing a coupon and enclosing cash. The analysis of one such product is typical for all.

"Slimdown," the ad says, "guarantees a loss of thirty pounds in thirty days safely without discomfort, without hunger pangs, without frustration, and makes it so calm, so peaceful to lose weight." It then goes on to tell of the doctor who was dissatisfied with the old methods of losing weight, began to search for the ideal medication. He discredits the appetite-depressing drugs because they make the patient feel lost, vaguely dissatisfied, jittery. His devotion to science and his patience are rewarded by the discovery of a secret formula, of medically known ingredients, which works like magic. He gives to these mysterious ingredients suggestive and scientific-sounding names.

"Pacifier," it is claimed, "is the peaceful wonder drug that calms and soothes, keeps you happy, helps you sleep healthfully and calmly."

"Antipater works on the centers concerned with hunger, but allows you to enjoy your favorite foods."

"Gastrofiller" is a remarkable no-calories ingredient "that fools the stomach, makes it feel half full before you sit down to eat."

Behind the mysterious titles we find a mild sedative, which you can buy over the counter, sugar, which is the normal appetite appeaser, and cellulose, which is the bulk producer. It is true that these are medically known, harmless ingredients. But their combination has no magic power to induce weight loss. You still have to diet, although the ad does not say this in so many words.

Sometimes medication is presented, not by advertisers but in popular articles and as news of scientific discovery. As an example, recently newspapers and a very reputable magazine reported that a foreign doctor had found that the chorionic gonadotropic hormone given by injections daily resulted in the loss of fifteen pounds in one month for a few patients. It frankly stated that the patients were also placed on a 500 calorie per day diet, but this was given little significance. The patients would have lost the same amount of weight even if the doctor had used sterile water for injections. There is no scientific support that the chorionic gonadotropic hormone has anything to do with fat metabolism, and no reason has been found in its known physiologic activities to suggest that it could.

By far the most lucrative field for those who would exploit woman's desire to lose weight, and acquire a good figure, is that which depends on passive exercise. This includes manual massage, and any number of mechanical devices from a simple hand vibrator or cushions to elaborate tables. There is nothing wrong with passive exercise—doctors recommend it for certain conditions for its soothing, relaxing, and beneficial effects, or to exercise muscles that a patient can't exercise herself (such as polio victims). Many of these package plans include harmless tablets (consisting of sugar and vitamins) and a diet. What is wrong is the implication that passive exercise is the important and effective element of the regime and that it is the only way to "spot reduce."

Some of these go so far as to explain that massage loosens the fat that causes the unwanted bulges, makes it more readily available for the body to burn or even actually moves it or causes it to vanish. This of course is nonsense. Storage fat is not an accumulation under the skin or even between the cells of tissues or organs. Storage fat is contained in cells specialized for that one purpose in adipose tissue found throughout the body, with few exceptions, as the soles of the feet and the contents of the head! These cells take up the excess of fats supplied and hold on to it until the wisdom of the body calls for it as a source of energy. It cannot be rubbed out, pounded out, or wished away. There is no such thing as "bound fat," as is sometimes claimed, that is tucked away in a form that the body is helpless to use except when broken loose by massage. There is "bound fat" in the sense that certain lipids are essential for normal cell structure, as in all cell walls, and for insulating material in the central nervous system. The wisdom of the body holds these lipids inviolate—for the welfare of the body as a whole.

The only reason that these methods are ever effective is the one that is rarely admitted. They offer the woman a definite regime that she must follow. She must diet, she takes pills (and even sugar pills may give her a psychological lift), and she is checked regularly for her progress, praised, and encouraged. All of these are proper and helpful. And she takes "treatments" for which she must pay—and if she has to pay she is more likely to do what she is told.

The saddest aspect of woman's addiction to these reducing schemes is their wastefulness. This includes not only the monetary expense, which amounts to millions of dollars a year, but expense of one of the most precious things we all have—time. Hours are wasted that could be used to enrich her own life and the lives of those about her.

Although there is no easier way than to diet if you are to lose weight, it is not a sentence to weeks of misery. Rather it should be the entrance to a new way of life, which leads to health and happiness.

What diet shall you choose? Certainly there is no lack of diets available. But you must not choose one by what it promises in pounds lost. You must choose a diet that promises good health and a feeling of well being both during the dieting period and thereafter. You must know what constitutes a well-balanced diet, that is, one that will supply all the body's essential needs, not just one that reduces the calories. In other words, you will have to learn what to eat, a new way of selecting your food, and you will have to acquire new habits of eating, which you will follow the rest of your life. This well-balanced diet is not necessarily a rigid uninteresting one that leaves you hungry. As a matter of fact, once you have acquired the habit of subscribing to it, it becomes the most satisfying and easiest to follow. It is one that supplies an adequate amount of the protective foods—the proteins, minerals, and vitamins—and cuts down on the high-energy foods, fats and carbohydrates, so that the body must use its stored fat. In other words, a high-protein, low-calorie regime.

Calorie counting alone is a poor way to try to lose weight for several reasons. In the first place, we are apt to be too generous with ourselves in estimating the value of a serving. An example is the girl who shopped around for the large apples found only in specialty food stores. They probably weighed two to three times as much as an average apple. She wasn't fooling anybody including herself when she said "an apple is an apple, therefore it contains sixty-four calories." As for other foods, you can only be certain of the calories if you weigh the food, which is not practical. Furthermore, when we select foods according to calories, we are more likely to follow our appetite than our good judgment, indulging in a piece of pie a la mode and a cup of coffee in preference to a meat ball, spinach, and half a grapefruit.

Dieting should serve two purposes, to lose weight and to establish new habits of eating that will abide after the necessity for reducing has passed. Therefore the diet must appeal to and satisfy your appetite. Of course, your appetite may require a little disciplining at first. Sufficient bulk is necessary to give a feeling of satisfaction, and this is supplied by the leafy vegetables. You probably will require some sweets to be completely happy, so you will have to learn to rely on fruits for this, and you will be surprised how you will come to look forward to and relish an orange for dessert after you have accepted the fact that pies and cakes are not for you. Lastly, there must be variety. However much you like eggs, if you are directed by a diet to eat two eggs three times a day, you will soon come to the point where you would rather not eat at all. So it is with any other rigid regime. You will soon tire of it, go off your diet completely, and return to your old habits of eating. The result will be that you will quickly gain back all you have lost, and you will be oppressed by the feeling of failure, and the futility of trying to lose weight.

When the calories are counted, and adequate protection foods of agreeable variety are assured, the next step in making a good diet is to divide the food into three meals a day with perhaps something between. Remember this is not a marathon to see how long you can go without food. Rather it is learning to eat within your means to take care of food, just as you budget to live within your income.

You cannot skip breakfast or lunch so that you can have a big dinner and expect to lose weight. There are several reasons for this, as we have already seen. First, it is not as hard to diet all day if you have had food in the morning. Second, breakfast is the most important meal of the day. You need the food not only to start the engine running but to keep it going at top speed of efficiency all day. A cup of black coffee with a cigarette is no substitute. Neither can you sleep through breakfast time and consider that you have saved on calories. Your body is using very few calories during the early morning hours of sleep.

Three meals a day does two helpful things. It makes dieting easier because it reduces the consciousness of the fact that you are denying yourself some food, and you feel better because your body has a continuous supply of fuel for energy. There is an extra bonus the body gives you: it will burn up more calories when given food in divided amounts throughout the day than it will in one large meal a day. We have compared the body to an engine that requires a certain amount of fuel, as a car that gets so many miles per gallon of gas. But this is not quite accurate. The body can adjust (within limits); a car cannot. When you overeat, as we saw in the discussion of normal, the body can adjust and burn up more fuel, and when your intake is less, it slows down and burns less. So if you deny it food for twenty-four hours, it slows down and is less able to use what you supply in one large meal.

Exercise alone is of little value in the quest for weight loss. A person must walk thirty-six miles at a good pace to burn up one pound of fat. It may defeat its own purpose, for it increases the appetite so that many more calories are ingested. If your excess weight is only a few pounds, you will benefit by exercise in a general increase of well being. But if weight is greatly in excess, exercise can be dangerous. With marked obesity, the heart is already overburdened, and exercise may be too great a strain. Obese persons are more apt to injure themselves or fall.

Alcohol is out while you are on a diet. First, all alcoholic drinks have a caloric value, some greater than others; second, alcohol increases the appetite and decreases the will power; and in some persons alcohol leads to the retention of fluids, obscuring any weight loss you might have accomplished.

THE DOCTOR'S PART

First of all, you must choose a doctor who is really interested and experienced in the problem of obesity. It is helpful to have someone to whom you report each week, who is genuinely pleased when you lose, and who will sit down and help you discover the reasons for failure when you don't lose or when you gain. You will be examined on your first visit and checked from time to time to see that you are maintaining good health.

Your doctor will use whatever means are necessary to determine why you are overweight. He will investigate to see if your glands are in any way responsible. He may discover nervous tensions, the importance of which you have been unaware, which cause you to overeat.

A BMR may be done, but the chances are that it will be normal. Most overweight people do not have a low BMR, and thyroid or any other glandular deficiency is rarely the cause of obesity.

Will you be given thyroid? That will depend on several things, mostly your doctor's attitude toward thyroid medication. Some doctors are rigidly opposed to giving thyroid in any circumstance. Others are not afraid of thyroid medication and explain its usefulness in this way. The body does not use a fixed amount of energy all the time. Rather when the supply is limited, it tries to adjust to a lower level of need by decreasing the rate of metabolism.

Will you get one of the appetite killing drugs? That too depends on your doctor. Most feel that they are not harmful if properly administered, and may be very helpful especially in the first few weeks when you are breaking away from your old habits of eating.

Constipation is likely to result from the reduction in the bulk and carbohydrates in your diet. Laxatives, mineral oil or enemas should not be resorted to. Rather, the bulk should be increased. There are many products on the market which have psyllium seed, agar, and other forms of bulk, which the body cannot digest. As a matter of fact these products are the bases of some of the patent medicines advertised for obesity, on the theory that taken before meals, they gain bulk in the stomach, relieve hunger, so that the appetite is satisfied on less food.

When your weight is down, what then? You should congratulate yourself for you have accomplished a difficult job. You have proved that you are mistress of yourself. You will live longer, and you will live better. You have established normal habits of eating, and are going to keep them, to maintain your normal weight.

Will you have to diet the rest of your life? That only time will tell. This much is certain. You must live on a restricted diet and watch your weight for many months. If you suddenly go off your diet, and eat all you can, you will regain your previous weight much faster than you lost it. Happily when the excessive burden of obesity is lifted and the body becomes adjusted to less weight, there is an increase in efficiency of the weight regulating mechanism, so that a person can again eat more and not gain weight. But most will always have to be careful of their food intake.

VIII

EQUANIMITY

"AM I NEUROTIC?"

"Do you think all my symptoms are psychosomatic?"

These are questions that women are frequently asking doctors when they find themselves depressed, nervous, irritable, or beset with unaccountable aches and pains. Many times they hesitate to go to a doctor for fear of being brushed aside with the comment that there is nothing wrong with them, patted on the back and told "just forget it, it is only your nerves," or that they are mentally sick and should see a psychiatrist.

Why does modern woman ask these questions? Why should she be fearful that her illnesses may be of the mind rather than the body? Her grandmother had no such thoughts. The answer is not to be found in woman's being different. It is the world in which she lives that disturbs her equanimity.

Modern woman is a part of a new era. Depending on the vantage point of interest from which one views it, this atomic age has many meanings. In the field of human health it could be characterized as the new era in surgery, endocrinology, antibiotics, or nutrition because of the advances made in knowledge and its application in these fields. It could also be called the new era of psychology. The sciences of psychology and psychiatry are products almost exclusively of modern times and have in turn had a tremendous impact on modern culture and on each of us as individuals.

126

THE ERA OF PSYCHOLOGY

"Psychology" is a broad term that encompasses the search for knowledge of how man behaves: that is, how he perceives, thinks, feels, and reacts in relation to himself, his fellow man, and the world about him. This search, of course, is age old, but it is only within this century that it has become a true science—knowledge based on facts obtained by scientific methods of investigation. Previously, there were only theories, which often were only figments of someone's imagination.

The science of psychology has given us much information on what constitutes normal behavior. These concepts are the basis of our definition of maturity—the ability of a person to live, with a reasonable degree of success, comfortably, purposefully, and productively both within one's self and among people. But psychology has not yet arrived at the answer of how best to achieve maturity, or what makes us falter along the way.

The application of these advances in the understanding of how the human mind functions in health and disease adds to mankind's potentiality for a rich, purposeful, and productive life. It can, however, be misapplied and become a detriment to his growth to maturity. This is being done day after day through the vast media of communication. There is a constant bombardment of pronouncements on all the facets of the world about us—political, social, sexual, and health. Frequently they are half-truths, misinterpretations, biased and slanted or even false. These may serve to obscure man's true goals, establish false standards for achievement, and generate confusion, anxiety, and fear. The broader implications as applied to society as a whole are far beyond the scope of this book. We are concerned with the effect on the individual—particularly woman.

Woman has felt the impact of the new era of psychology in every aspect of her life. As a housewife the choice of everything she buys, from a lipstick to the family car, is influenced by the effective use sellers have made of the psychology of advertising and merchandising. Such advertising frequently makes her want to buy things she does not need. In industry, she has found certain jobs previously restricted to men open to her because psychology with its new methods of testing aptitudes has proved that there are things women can do better than men. She has a shorter working day, with coffee breaks because their importance in diminishing fatigue and increasing efficiency has been demonstrated. As a mother she is told that it is no longer enough to care for a child's physical needs, but she must also understand child psychology. When the child enters school, the mother is introduced to the psychology of modern education.

It is to woman, as a person, however, that the greatest impact is delivered by the forces of psychology. The composite ideal of womanhood that the propaganda of advertising has prompted is false, and it is detrimental to her maturity, because it stresses physical appearance to the exclusion of all else. She cannot avoid the constant attempts at indoctrination on the vital necessity of various items of cosmetics for the attainment of beauty; of garments that will mould her figure; of machines that will reduce her; of services of salons that will improve her appearance. Such indoctrination seeks to brainwash woman to complete conformity. That she is vulnerable is due to the fact that within every woman there is a strong and positive drive to be attractive, to be pleasing in appearance, and to have her femininity recognized and appreciated. This drive is both worthy and realistic. But it is being subverted for ulterior purposes. That such propaganda is successful from the advertiser's viewpoint is attested by the fact that the money spent in the purchase of these products and services amounts to millions of dollars each year. The real cost to woman, however, is in the time and effort wasted and the false standard of feminine maturity, which can never bring her fulfillment and happiness.

The psychology of advertising exploits woman herself as a selling device. The feminine form, usually scantily clad and provocative, is used to draw attention to anything and everything. And her feminine ideals of wife and mother are made the basis of proclaiming the virtue of anything from automobiles to washing powder.

MENTAL HEALTH

We have been concerned in the preceding chapters with the components of physical health, the characteristics of woman's body structure and function in maturity. In every phase we have had to include the nervous factors, for the story would have been meaningless without them. We have already outlined the attributes of health as the ideal of maturity. They include woman's psychological, physical, and sexual well-being, all of which are important and interrelated.

Health, however, is usually considered as having only two components—the physical and mental. What is the meaning of "mental health"?

We have used the term "psychological" in the same sense that "mental" is usually applied; and for a reason. It is necessary to differentiate woman's mental capacity to learn, to think, and to apply knowledge, from her purely emotional reactions. Whether we use psychological or mental as the inclusive term applied to the total function of the mind, neither is synonymous with emotional.

Too often mental health is considered from the emotional aspect alone. By this standard a person is mentally healthy who is happy-go-lucky (free from anxiety, guilt-feeling, and fear), doing routinely what is expected of her (free from frustrations and conflicts), bearing her burdens with complacency, self-satisfaction, and self-respect. Mental health is far more than this ability to accept, adjust, and be happy in what life has to offer. It must also have a dynamic quality, which contributes purpose and meaning to life.

There is no hard and fast definition of mental health, and there are no specific rules for its attainment. We are only beginning to understand the basis of mental health and its expression in man's behavior—how he thinks, feels, and acts in relation to himself and the world about him. This understanding is derived from sound scientific study dealing with facts that can be observed, tested, and measured in the behavior of individuals of all ages.

These truths—facts of behavior and their significance to mental health—have been contributed by investigators following many disciplines of science such as genetics, physiology, pharmacology, anthropology, and sociology as well as psychology. No one of them started with the purpose of collecting only facts that would prove some particular theory he might have devised. Rather, according to the dictates of true scientific research, he collected all available facts, tested them, verified them, and allowed the facts to speak for themselves. Researchers in these various fields have been interested in different aspects of behavior and therefore followed different lines of study. But as their findings are being brought together, they are like the parts of a jig-saw puzzle, from which a picture begins to emerge that depicts the true pathway to maturity and mental health. Not all the parts are available, not all fit perfectly, but the picture is definitive enough to give us hope that we will some day know how to assure the achievements of maturity on a large scale.

The foundation of the concept of mental health is knowledge of the structure and function of the organ that controls behavior—the brain—which is where mental health resides.

The Brain

The mind—the psychological personality—is the function of the brain, an organ of flesh and blood. This brain of ours is wonderful, complex, and mysterious. In its millions of cells and connecting fibers resides our ability to remember, to forget, to have aims and ambitions, determination and self-control, to love, to hate, to care, to be indifferent, and to fear. In it resides also our ability to appraise realistically our talents and the capacity to face the realities of life. The brain directs and co-ordinates all the physical activities of the body. When it is destroyed, life goes. When parts of it are destroyed or injured, some nervous function is lost. There is no thought, no emotion, no element of nervous control of the body that does not have a physical basis somewhere in the brain. Because we do not know where all these functions reside or how they are achieved does not mean that there is no physical basis for their existence.

We have already seen that health in any organ (or the body as a whole) is measured in terms of the efficiency of its behavior, its ability to perform its own particular functions. Normal function requires normal structure and has a specific physiologic basis, which includes chemical as well as physical changes. This is true also of the brain, although we have only recently acquired the facts of structure and function to prove it.

The human brain has been inaccessible for exploration until the present era. Long ago scientists found where certain functions of the brain were localized—sensation (sight, smell, touch), motor activity (speech, muscular function), and the higher mental processes (reason and judgment), as well as the regulatory functions (breathing and heart action). But little could be determined about the pathways of mental activity that made this organ function as a whole. Now scientists are delving into and finding answers to the physical basis of mental processes, such as memory, imagination, and emotions, and the nervous pathways involved in mental activity. The brain is being explored along many trails. The starting point for these ventures into the unknown realm of physiology was established by the accumulation of knowledge in many fields such as endocrinology, nutrition, pharmacology, and surgery. The tools are provided by the modern advances in chemistry and physics. Much progress has already been made, much new information has been gained, and there is promise of a great deal more to come.

One interesting method of exploration is the electrical stimulation of areas of the brain. This is usually done during surgery but may also be accomplished by the implantation of electrodes. Both are harmless and painless to the subject. Moreover, the subject is conscious (not anesthetized) and can relate his mental experiences. By such stimulation or delivery of a minute electric shock to a tiny area of the brain, specific mental experiences are induced. Some produce pleasure, some fear. Some bring into vivid focus events long past and forgotten. Some are silent.

The electroencephalogram is a means of recording activity of the brain just as the electrocardiogram does for the heart. The patterns of normality have been established and the significance of deviations is being recognized.

Many pathways of chemical exploration are also being followed. There is revealing evidence that chemical changes play an important, perhaps dominant, part in the function of the brain. The appetite or affinity of certain cells for certain chemicals and their vulnerability to others has been used to localize and clarify the mechanisms of mental processes. The mind can be poisoned by the administration of certain drugs and will produce typical symptoms of certain mental illnesses. These disappear when the body has metabolized (got rid of) the poison. On the other hand, there are drugs that accentuate healthy qualities of the mind. Some induce tranquility. Some increase awareness and energy and erase fatigue. There are some that increase our energy and willingness to do a job and make it seem less difficult, although they do not increase our competence to do it. Radioactive tracer substances are used to reveal which cells use certain chemicals and at what rate. This has been extended to the identification of overactive areas such as occur in certain types of brain tumors.

These are but a few examples of the explorations that are revealing the physiology of the brain.

The brain, as an organ of the body, requires the same basic ingredients of physical health as any other organ or tissue, or it will falter in its function. There must be adequate nutrition, an abundant and continuous supply of oxygen, rest and relaxation, and exercise.

The brain being the most highly specialized organ has special protective devices. The most obvious are the anatomical—the heavy casing of bone and the layers of membrane that shield it from external injury. But it has an internal security system also by which its internal environment is kept in even more perfect equilibrium than that of other organs of the body. The proteins and lipids that are incorporated in the structure of brain tissue, unlike those of the other organs, are not subjected to call to the general metabolic pool. As an example, the brain structure is not subject to wasting as are the muscles in illness and starvation. Furthermore, this internal security system provides a barrier that monitors the entrance of chemicals brought by the blood stream. It allows only slow entrance to most chemicals except glucose and bars to a certain extent those detrimental to the structure and function of the brain. It is conceivable, and there are some facts to prove it, that a break in this internal security system would seriously affect the function of the brain and, in turn, mental health.

It is not happenstance that one-fourth of the body's blood supply goes to the head—the brain. The brain needs an abundant and steady supply of oxygen. When the supply is only slightly decreased below normal, consciousness is lost temporarily. When the blood supply, and oxygen, is cut off completely for even a short period, nerve cells are injured or die. The familiar examples are: "large strokes," which involve either vessels supplying large areas of the brain and result in loss of specific functions or small vessels that supply vital structures and result in sudden death. The "small strokes" are due to damage to small areas and cause personality changes and mental deterioration.

This abundant blood supply also brings glucose, the basic fuel for energy that is necessary for normal function of the brain cells, even as it is for other cells of the body. Mild hypoglycemia (low blood sugar) leads to nervous irritability and other symptoms of decreased mental efficiency, while marked hypoglycemia, such as may occur after an overdose of insulin, may produce convulsions and shock and, unless relieved, death.

The brain as an organ is made up of cells that are involved in the same processes of dynamic metabolism as any other cell of the body. They are carrying on physio-chemical processes that require oxygen and other chemical components from the general metabolic pool. They, too, have enzymes that expedite these physio-chemical changes. Enzymes have been isolated from nerve cells that are specific for those cells and essential to their normal function. There is well-founded evidence that suggests that certain mental illnesses may be due to toxins, possibly derived from faulty metabolism, which interfere with the enzyme systems of certain brain cells. Furthermore, brain cells are subject to the regulatory mechanisms of hormone function. We shall have many examples of this in each of the ages.

The brain must have rest, which it normally gets in the hours of sleep. It is limited as to the time it can function normally without rest. Experiments have demonstrated that four days without sleep is about the maximum that can be endured without damage to brain function and various temporary manifestations of mental illness.

The brain needs exercise, which is stimulation by contact with a changing environment of ideas, people, places, or things. It is a strong mind with deep inner resources that can withstand solitary confinement with nothing to occupy it for any length of time. "Brain-washing" is a familiar example of how the factors of mental rest, mental exercise, and mental nourishment may be used and abused to distort, weaken, and deprive of its function a mind once healthy and vigorous.

The exploration of the brain is being accomplished by the collaboration of specialists in many fields—neurologists, neurosurgeons, biochemists, physicists, psychiatrists, as well as physiologists interested in nutrition and endocrinology, and pharmacologists concerned with the effect of drugs. This type of scientific research is just beginning to yield results, but it promises rapid progress with further explanation of the physical basis of mind and behavior, and will relegate to the museum of medical anachronisms the paper-pencil-couch technique of "research" and "therapy."

Achieving Psychological Maturity

To achieve maturity on the physical level, there are patterns of growth and maturation that start at the moment of conception and continue through the different ages. How these patterns are laid out, what they are, and how they evolve are dependent on two governing forces: the genetic or inherited patterns of growth; and environmental factors, which include not only the presence of certain needed elements but also a minimum, if not complete absence, of harmful or detrimental experiences.

The achievement of psychological maturity is subject to the same forces. The part these forces play may be broadly summarized in the following principles, recognizing that there are some duplications as well as omissions.

1. The Seeds of Maturity Are Present at Birth.

The future of our physical personality is laid out in the genes of the original germ cells. First of all we are human beings because of the genes, which carry the pattern of growth and development to human form, including the human type of nervous system and our most precious endowment, a human brain. The pattern is the same for all of us, but the results are never quite duplicated, for no two people, not even identical twins, are ever exactly alike. Individual variations do not apply to physical characteristics alone, such as body size and color of hair, but also to mental capacity—the ability to learn and apply knowledge and aptitudes for particular types of learning.

Furthermore, the genes carry a pattern of growth to maturity on the psychological level as well as the physical. That is, there is a timetable for the development of the brain and its functions just as for any other part of the body.

Geneticists have demonstrated that normal development depends on normal genes and that some forms of mental deficiency are transmitted by faulty genes from one generation to another. This represents a massive insult visited on germ plasm. We know very little of what the effect of minimal insults to the germ plasm of one individual may be in succeeding generations, but the dangers of irradiation have brought this into focus as a real problem in future health, mental as well as physical.

The environmental factors in physical growth and development begin to exert their influence long before birth, indeed at the moment of conception, and they determine whether survival is possible and whether development shall proceed along normal patterns. The body can be stunted or malformed by too little of what it needs or too much of harmful experience. We know a great deal of what the needs are during this period before birth, but we are just beginning to learn the identity of harmful factors and have only a glimmer of what may be too much or too little.

2. There Is a Pattern of Growth to Psychological Maturity.

The seed germinates, and the organism grows to maturity according to a definite pattern. Just as there is a definite pattern in which the individual learns to use and control the physical powers and gain proficiency, there is also a pattern to her psychological development. The two are interrelated and mutually supportive. The individual's ability to comprehend, use reason and judgment, to learn and apply knowledge, as well as his emotional development—all follow a definite sequence. The recognition of these changing mental and emotional facets in the personality has become important in understanding behavior during the formative years.

These patterns, mental and emotional, are not rigid. Psychologists have pointed out that the rate or time element is an individual characteristic. Some children are slow, some accelerated. Thus mental age and emotional age do not necessarily correspond to the chronological age. There is also individual variation in content, in aptitude to learn, as well as in intensity of the emotional aspect.

3. The Forces of Growth Originate Within and Without.

The ability to grow and mature is an inherent property of all living things—plants and animals. A seed germinates and grows to a specific kind of mature plant within a specific time period. To do so, it needs a favorable environment of moisture, heat, light, and adequate nutrition. It also needs an environment in which impeding or destructive elements are absent. We have already discussed the relation of internal environment in physical health to normal brain function. Little is known of the external physical—the climatic—effects on development. But the study that is being devoted to the effect of space travel—weightlessness, rays, etc.—

suggests the importance that the physical elements of the environment may have on mental health. Anthropologists who take a long-range view of human behavior point out the effects climate has had on the evolution of culture among different peoples.

In the life of one individual, whether or not he will attain his full potential growth psychologically will depend on whether his environment of people provides stimulation, encouragement, guidance, direction, and discipline as well as love, affection, and security. A child will not grow to maturity psychologically if left to his own devices, for two reasons: it has to learn to live in a world of other people; and that world has a heritage of culture acquired through the ages. The child within a few short years must acquire the knowledge of, accept as a way of life, and assume the responsibility of carrying on that heritage, and, we may hope, he will better it.

The child starts life with the basic instincts of survival. He learns by trial and error to choose the methods to attain his goal. Thus he acquires skills in the use of his body, and, if he is to become proficient, he must subscribe to discipline and training with consistency and purpose. We have little difficulty in translating this to attaining mental maturity in the acquisition of knowledge and fitting him for assuming his responsibility in the world of others. Emotional maturity is the acquisition of skills in human relations. A child has a right to gratification for his success, but success must be earned. The aim is self-discipline and assumption of responsibility.

4. The Pattern Is Adjustable.

Behavior can be changed by experience. A child learns new patterns of behavior by forces of his environment for many reasons—survival, self-protection, or gratification. These forces are not necessarily detrimental, as we are often led to believe, but may accelerate growth to a more productive level.

Behavior patterns in children and personality disturbances in adults have been attributed almost entirely to emotional trauma in early infancy and childhood. The more pessimistic school of thought sees emotional stress as an impediment to growth or the cause of mental illness: that is, failing to be appreciated leads to an inferiority complex, failure, and frustration; lack of love to hate and hostility. There is a more optimistic view, which is also more realistic: The body has great regenerative power. It also has great resistance and great reserve power. There are many familiar examples of this. Under stress of emergency a person is capable of physical feats far beyond his usual ability. He can endure physical hardship, severe and prolonged, and return to a state of physical health. The mind also has resistance, reserve, and recuperative powers. We have examples of this also. People who have been denied appreciation and recognition and have been made to feel inferior have been spurred on to such levels of success that they had to be recognized.

5. The Process of Development Is Vulnerable.

Things may happen to the individual that bring the growth process to an abrupt halt, slow it up for a time, or distort it. The trauma may be psychological, but it can also be physical. Recent investigations suggest that some behavior problems are not due to emotional trauma, such as parent rejection, but to physical injury to the brain. Such injury may be inflicted by the trauma of birth or nutritional deficiencies or certain infections of the mother during pregnancy.

It is an established fact that some childhood illnesses, especially viral infections such as measles, are sometimes complicated by encephalitis (inflammation of the brain) with disastrous effects on mentality and behavior. It is thought that such infections may also visit minimal changes in the brain that result in impeding the natural process of growth.

6. There Is a Fluidity to Psychological Maturity.

There is no direct irreversible pathway to maturity, which must be traversed in a specific time interval. At best, as adults we have acquired the ability to behave in a mature way with a fair degree of success, a fair amount of the time. But under stress of one kind or another, we may revert to behavior that is quite immature—even infantile. On the other hand, children may exhibit characteristics of maturity such as bearing responsibility, or unswerving loyalty, that an adult might well be proud to possess.

7. There Is No Age Limit to Maturity.

The most vital quality of maturity is the ability to change, and to adapt to change—to find new and appropriate solutions to new problems, to seek new knowledge. This begins in childhood, reaches a degree of proficiency in adulthood, and need not cease even in old age.

8. Maturity Requires Nurture and Use.

"Food for thought" is necessary for mental health. Few can lay claim to exercising their brain power to full capacity even a small part of the time, much less with a fair degree of regularity. It is thought that many of the emotional illnesses that cause a large percentage of absenteeism in industry are due to the monotony of oft-repeated tasks that allow no change and require no new mental effort on the part of the worker.

Many people are unhappy and poorly adjusted because they are bored. They do not experience the stimulation or the urge to learn new things. They accept whatever happens to cross their paths, without question, without wonder, without curiosity. They do not know how to like people, to be interested in people, and in turn to have people like them. This inner urge is in part a product of education, but it is not derived solely from or completely dependent on formal education. Little children are the ones most filled with wonder at the smallest things about them. They find new marvels at every turn and are the most curious about the "hows" and "why." We need to hold on to this innate ability to be curious and to wonder, to be interested in the world about us and the world of others.

MENTAL ILLNESS

"One person in four is destined to suffer mental illness." "One half of our hospital beds are filled with the mentally ill." "Americans are consuming each year tons of the new tranquilizers." "A pill for the mind can help you take it." "How to deal with your tensions." "Ninety per cent of people who go to doctors have no physical ailment—they only think they do."

These are the headlines. What are the stories behind the headlines? Too often they are not completely told.

In this day of excessive communication—daily, weekly, and monthly reporting and analysis of everything that touches our lives—it is the startling that makes the headlines, and only bad news is really good for a story. Many times there is no analysis but only elaboration of facts that are half-truths because they are incomplete or out of context. As a result, our self-evaluation seems to be suffering from an inferiority complex. This applies to our mental health as well as to our material resources.

Certainly mental illness is our number-one health problem—even our number-one problem. But this is nothing new. It always has been, and always will be for any individual or for any nation.

It is not within our purpose, or potentiality, to delve into the intricacies of psychiatry. This is the province of those who deal with the mentally ill. However, a general understanding of the facts concerning mental illness should be within our grasp as intelligent and interested individuals. Such facts will enable us to recognize society's responsibility not only for the care of the mentally ill but also for supporting research in the field of mental illness. They will remove the stigma so often attached to mental illness and will bring the realization that its victims are ill, that many will recover, and that they should be accorded the same consideration during and especially after the illness as in any other sickness. The truth will dispel unreasonable fears and contribute to our quest for equanimity.

To have the truth, we need definitive answers to certain basic questions such as: What is mental illness? What are the criteria for considering a person mentally ill? How much mental illness is there today? Is there any concrete evidence that this age of rapid change and peculiar kind of stress has increased the number who are mentally ill? As there have been attempts in some sources to attribute woman's problems to neuroticism, we might add: Is a woman neurotic because of her sex? The most important questions are: What are the causes of mental illness, so far as are known? What can be done in the way of both prevention and treatment?

What Is Mental Illness?

Mental illness has always been a fact of life in every type of human society or culture; and the treatment accorded it has varied with man's concept of its meaning. Some primitive people, believing that the unhappy victim was possessed of the devil, buried or burned him alive to destroy the devil within and release the soul of the victim. Others, witnessing his seizures, his babbling in unknown tongues, his trances with voices from the unknown and visions of the unreal, attributed to him supernatural powers, and he became the oracle of wisdom. But mostly in the past, the mentally ill have been considered unacceptable human beings, even dangerous members of the community. They have been treated as wild and dangerous animals, which should either be driven away or restrained by chains. Only within modern times have the mentally ill come to be accorded the status of human beings and had their chains removed. But many are still behind iron bars with little being done to relieve them of their illness. There is still a stigma attached, and treatment has been more for the benefit of society (by exclusion) than for the individual.

The concept that mental illness may be due to changes in the structure and function of the brain is not new in medicine. It dates back to the time of Hippocrates. ("The brain is the organ where madness is born.") It has been voiced again and again through the centuries by doctors with questioning minds, but they were unable to prove their theories and had to content themselves with treating symptoms. There were never more than a few who were even interested in the problem of the mentally ill because there was so little that could be done, and most cases were considered hopeless.

Then came Freud whose teachings aroused such interest that the results have been called the first revolution in psychiatry. Freud's theories dealt with the psychological structure of the personality—the conscious and unconscious forces that account for normal and abnormal behavior. The tool for exploration was analysis of the psyche. Here was a tool that doctors could use. Some did with great enthusiasm, enlarging on Freud's concepts, changing them but still using the one tool—psychoanalysis. The soma was forgotten and ignored, although Freud had warned: "All our provisional ideas on psychology will some day be based on organic substructure." Others were and have remained skeptical of this concept.

The analytic school of psychiatry sought the answer to mental illness in the "stratification" of the personality, psychosexual development, suppressions, regressions, and complexes. Thus it came to speak its own language, one that other doctors could not understand (and were not supposed to unless they themselves submitted to analysis). Psychoanalysis assumed the characteristics of a cult paying homage to the psyche. Its initiates were devoted to the continuous examination of the content of their own emotional life, which in some mysterious way qualified them to detect and explain flaws in the personality of others.

This concept of mental illness caught the public fancy, possibly because of its mysticism—the fact that it dealt with ideas that could be expressed in imposing terms without requiring any scientific documentation and therefore were not easily refutable. Amateurs have taken it up and exploited it. There has been a deluge of novels, plays, and biographies dealing with mental illness and psychoanalysis. These have stressed the misbehavior of a small element of society in acts of incest, adultery, nymphomania, and homosexuality, which makes the murder mystery and the western gunfighters appear good clean behavior.

The phase of the science of medicine that deals with mental illness is now entering a new and revolutionary period, with a dramatic change in fundamental concepts based on sound experimental evidence that places mental illness on an organic basis. The way was paved for this change by experiences of the Second World War. These revealed the large number of people who suffered some degree of mental incompetency or emotional inadequacy. They also helped to remove the stigma and bring society to the realization that the mentally ill person is not someone to be ashamed of but a human being in need of a medical specialist.

The change in concept of mental illness is comparable to the new eras we have spoken of as accomplished facts in the fields of metabolism, endocrinology, nutrition, and surgery. That there has been a lag in developments in regard to mental illness is both understandable and justifiable. Advances in every science must wait until appropriate and effective tools for investigation become available. Since the science of the mind deals with structure of highly specialized tissue and function of an intricate and intangible nature, investigation and the solution of the mysteries of the mind have been the most difficult. These had to await the accumulation of knowledge of structure and function of less highly specialized and more accessible organs, tissues, and cells.

Mental illness is being re-integrated into the practice of medicine, as medical doctors feel the need for psychiatric help for many patients, and psychiatrists have realized the necessity of coming to grips with the soma. Thus both have come to look on the mentally ill person as a human being living in a painful way (sometimes with his survival in jeopardy). The initiating stimulus may have been applied to either the psyche or the soma, but the whole personality reacts. This is the physiodynamic concept of mental illness.

Mental health, as already implied, is a state of well-being in which the individual is able to function in a productive capacity within the framework of his environment with a degree of acceptability and without jeopardy to his associates and to himself. Mental illness is the loss of this ability to function in one way or another and to some degree. The stumbling blocks that bar the way are many and diverse. The range of mental illness from sanity to insanity, with intermediate inadequacies, is broad and the lines of demarcation vague.

Who and How Many Are Mentally Ill?

The headlines listed previously are startling. They may be ominous if we accept them literally as a prediction that we as individuals face the possibility of becoming mentally ill. If we go behind the headlines, we will not find neatly assembled and correctly correlated statistics. We will find some facts that lessen the impact. The reason is not obscure, for mental illness is a broad term encompassing many different conditions. This is best exemplified by those who are hospitalized for mental illness. They fall into several large groups.

There is one group of mentally ill with various symptoms that have one thing in common—some organic damage has been visited on their gray matter. We can have an illness of almost any part of the body, except the brain, and carry on a useful life. An offending gall bladder can be removed, or diseased lungs and hearts can be treated. Amputees or those crippled by polio are still able to work. But illness of the brain, such as infection, injury due to hemorrhage or trauma may and often does deprive the person not only of physical health but also of the faculty to run his life—his sanity. Old age may cripple our joints, and we can continue to be well-adjusted citizens; but when it hits the arteries of our brain and deprives that vital organ of nourishment, we become senile and sometimes demented. Malnutrition may today be only a hidden cause of poor health and mental inefficiency, but it used to be the cause of one form of insanity—the psychosis of pellagra.

There is another group found in mental hospitals who were cheated from the start. These are the mentally deficient—the imbeciles, the morons, and others whose misfortune has come by heritage or injury in the early formative period of their lives.

The largest group (more than half the total) are the functional psychoses of which schizophrenia is a familiar example. In the past these individuals, in whom there was no demonstrable cause for their mental illness, have remained in mental institutions with little help available. Today the picture is brighter. Research is suggesting that these illnesses are due to chemical factors—disturbed metabolism. The symptoms have been induced in normal persons by the administration of certain chemicals. If the cause is found, there is hope that a cure will follow. Moreover, the discovery of the new drugs for mental illness, including the tranquilizers, have found their greatest usefulness among these patients.

There is a fourth and itself a heterogeneous group because of the different reasons for which they were confined and why they have remained. Mental illness has in the past been a legal and a social problem as well as a medical one. A person was "adjudged insane" and "committed" often to overcrowded institutions where medical attention was inadequate. Many stayed the rest of their lives. The degeneration of family ties and responsibilities account for some of these. They may have been committed for an acute episode from which they could have recovered if adequate care had been available. They might have been released if they had a meaningful place in society awaiting them. A few of this group should never have been committed in the first place.

The fact that half of the hospital beds of the country are required for the mentally ill might suggest that a large proportion of illness is mental, which, of course, is absurd. A person who is hospitalized for a mental illness stays for at least a matter of weeks, sometimes months, and sometimes years. Physical illness requiring hospitalization is short—a few days, a few weeks, and rarely a few months. The actual admission of the mentally ill accounts for only about 2 per cent of all hospital admissions. Hospital stays in the past few years have been reduced by the introduction of new forms of therapy, including new drugs, group therapy, meaningful occupation, and the provision for occupation and social acceptance after their discharge.

The vast majority of those classified as "mentally ill" are not to be found in hospitals. They include those who visit various kinds of clinics—such as mental health or psychiatric clinics—or are under the private care of psychiatrists. These individuals are equally heterogeneous. Some go for diagnostic purposes to rule out mental illness, and some go for help in problems of everyday living.

With these many factors contributing to the incidence and severity of mental illness, it becomes apparent that there are many causes and many different kinds of mental illnesses. But mental illness is designated in terms of symptoms—the behavior of the individual—and not in the nature of the incompetency.

There are two main divisions. In the first are those who are not acceptable to society, cannot be productive members of society, and may be dangerous to society—the psychotics. These are for the most part segregated in institutions. In the second are those who continue to live within the social framework but are at odds within themselves—the neurotics.

Neurosis

"Neurotic" has become a word that we use indiscriminately to mean behavior of an individual that is queer, mixed-up, nervous, high-strung, indecisive, unpredictable, unreasonable, complaining, despondent, or pessimistic. It is also applied to tantrums, imaginary illnesses, or just some act or trait in another person that we don't understand or don't approve of. Generally speaking neurosis refers to personality problems—that is, those that arise from a person's inability to meet the problems of everyday living in a mature way. This inability gives rise to anxiety, which may be expressed in behavior patterns that are quite different from normal.

Neurotic is thus applied to a group, which is set off on the one hand from the normal and on the other from the psychotic. The dividing line between normal and neurotic is a fine one indeed. In fact, they merge one into the other. Neurotics may be quite normal in many of the facets of their personality and may have emotional difficulties in only one. All of us who consider ourselves normal are guilty of neurotic behavior some of the time.

The difference between neurotic and psychotic is more definitive. The neurotic lives, frequently unhappily or painfully, in the world of reality but is at odds with himself and is held responsible for his acts. The psychotic lives in a world of unreality, sometimes quite happily and is not held responsible for his misbehavior. If neurosis is a caricature, psychosis is a nightmare. The same elements of behavior are present but in a world of unreality and aloneness. To be nervous or upset even to the point of being neurotic is not the pathway to insanity or psychosis. A previously well person can become psychotic but not via the process of neurosis. Psychotics do not worry about losing their minds.

Psychiatrists are far from agreed on what has happened to a person's mental and emotional make-up that makes him inadequate and makes him express his anxiety over his inadequacy by neurotic behavior. This lack of agreement as to the causative mechanism of neurosis is the natural product of the divergence of opinion on what constitutes the normal pattern of growth and development of the personality, and what the driving forces are that accomplish these changes from infancy to maturity.

Also there are various degrees of neuroticism. Some psychiatrists say that one person in eight is neurotic, others that the ratio is one to four, and still others that everyone is neurotic. The pessimist looks on neurotic behavior as compulsive, or inward forces that the person is both unconscious of and unable to control. The optimists, while granting that there are inward forces that are the bases of growth and development to maturity, also recognize that these forces can be thrown out of gear by disturbances in physical function. More important, they recognize that men and women are endowed with a will and a conscience to aid them in achieving mature behavior a good percentage of the time. Thus the attributes of neuroses such as aggressiveness, hostility, anxiety, and drive for perfection are at times also components of healthy normal behavior. There could be no true love, for example, without times of anxiety for the welfare of the loved one. Evil would prevail if rightminded citizens did not rise up in anger and hostility to those guilty of wrongdoing.

Psychological Immaturity

It has been said that the world is populated by a high percentage of "immature people"; that of the 170 million Americans, only one million are mentally healthy, that is, mature. Certainly we encounter people every day who seem always to meet life in an immature way, and we see in ourselves instances in which we approach our problems of living in an immature way.

The question comes—what is the cause of the prevalent immaturity, and what can be done about it? There is no one cause and no one answer. What would be an answer for one person would not be applicable to another. All the factors of growth are vulnerable, and injury that may be either psychological or physiological will affect the pattern of growth, either retarding it or distorting it.

We make no pretense of offering a solution to this problem, but there are certain things worth thinking about. The goals of maturity are not the products of the new age of psychology and psychiatry. They are the same standards set up by philosophers and religious leaders throughout recorded history. For the most part, man, when he has appeared to heed, has in reality only given lip-service to these standards and has not made them a guiding force of his life. The fact is we have set our goals of maturity too low. Success is measured in terms of material wealth and the achievement of dominance over others, not of finding our own aptitudes, doing our work well, caring for the welfare of others, and of the quality of our own inner happiness.

In searching for the cause of immaturity we have stressed the emotional and neglected the physical aspects. We look for evidences of emotional trauma and not for earlier physical experience in life that may have contributed to behavior problems. Because emotions are something intangible we have been fearful of directing them (for fear of injuring them) and rather give them full reign. What is psychological trauma for one is not necessarily so for another. It may have an emotional basis, but it may also be physical.

The Psychosomatic Concept

"Psychosomatic" is a word frequently used and as frequently misused and abused. Its derivation is simple—psyche means mind; soma means body. Thus psychosomatic should mean that there is a fixed, indissoluble bond between the two. Whatever force affects the one will affect the other. There is nothing new about this basic concept. The familiar slogan "a sound mind in a sound body" goes back to the days of the Romans and implies that health in one area of the personality, the mind, is dependent on the health of the body and vice versa. The recognition that disturbances in one have repercussions in the other is also not new. Everyone has experienced bodily discomfort due to uncomfortable mental experience. For example, when you are frightened you can't get your breath, shivers go up your spine, you tremble, and your feet get cold. Or, if you worry, your stomach hurts, you can't eat, you can't sleep, and your head aches.

The psychosomatic concept of illness has come to be limited to a one-way affair—mental disturbances causing physical symptoms. Starting with the premise that emotional disturbances can be the cause of physical symptoms, there has evolved one concept of psychosomatic medicine some of whose advocates go to the extreme of attributing all illnesses to a basic emotional disturbance. This, of course, is not based on scientific facts, accurately tested and undeniably corroborated, but rather on random observations and elaborate theoretical fabrication. This need not worry us, for most doctors will first look for physical causes of illness and treat them before he sends a patient to a psychiatrist.

Psychosomatic medicine should have quite a different meaning. It should seek to understand the mind-body relationship in all illnesses. It should recognize that psychic disturbances can cause physical symptoms, but it should not stop there. It should also recognize that the reverse is true—that the disturbances of physical body functions can be the cause of psychic disturbances. Thus, psychosomatic is not a one-way street that must be followed in the pursuit of the cause of man's illnesses; it is a dual highway.

Every illness has two components—the psychic and the somatic. An illness may be serious in proportion to the patient's emotional reaction

to it. For instance, an operation to one woman may be an opportunity t
have something to talk about, to another it may become a serious ris
to her life because of her fear of surgery, concern about finances, or worr
over a home situation.

When we apply the one-way psychosomatic concept to illnesses i
women, we are in danger of getting into the woods and losing our wa
It is true that the physical manifestations of being a woman, her feminin
sexuality, is an inescapable, ever-present part of her feminine personalit
and that it causes an emotional impact. It is no wonder, therefore, tha
the cause of her physical disabilities, not only in the sexual sphere bu
in all other aspects of her physical being as well, has been sought i
her emotional make-up. Her illnesses have been attributed to her failur
to accept her womanliness in a mature way or to her propensity to us
it as a means to escape reality. Woman therefore has been called neuroti
because she is female and not because she is a human being caught u
in the complex of circumstances. Her status as a human being has, o
course, colored her behavior. When she was man's property withou
social or civil rights, she used whatever means were at hand to establis
her identity and to attain her ends. Today, American woman has achieve
a status—freedom, rights, and privileges, and in turn responsibilities—
never enjoyed by woman before.

Does modern American woman still use, albeit unconsciously, her femal
sexuality to gain her own ends? Does she cash in on the time-honore
title of the weaker sex to avoid responsibility and unpleasant duties
Or, perhaps not so unconsciously, but to please the male, does she assum
these attitudes? In turn, are many of her illnesses due to the emotiona
conflict within herself and with the world about her?

Many are saying yes. Her somatic complaints such as headaches
sterility, frigidity, the physical discomforts of adolescence and menopause
menstrual abnormalities and discomfort have been attributed to psychi
causes. These things have been repeated so often that woman hersel
is asking, "Am I neurotic?" "Are my pains and discomfort psycho
somatic?" "Am I losing my mind?"

This leads us to the consideration of the other line of psychosomati
medicine, which recognizes that somatic illnesses do produce psychi
manifestations. The delirium of fever is an obvious example. A newl

emerging concept is that disturbances in endocrine function cause disturbances of woman's equanimity. We shall meet with examples of this in all the ages. It will be worthwhile to examine the somatic basis of a few conditions which superficially may appear to be psychogenic, such as "inferiority complex," "neurasthenia," "neurosis," and the physiologic basis of them.

INFERIORITY COMPLEX VS. HYPOTHYROIDISM

Ida did not ask: "Am I neurotic?" although she was far from being happy or physically normal. Rather, her personality was such that her associates might have thought she was neurotic and carelessly ascribed her condition to an "inferiority complex."

Ida had few of the attributes of feminine attractiveness. Her short height was accentuated by her broadness of beam and bulges in the wrong places. Her dull and lifeless hair was a characterless color between blond and brunette and was unresponsive to her efforts to arrange it. No amount or kind of cosmetics could conceal the puffiness of her features or the coarse muddiness of her complexion, which was further marred by pimples. Nor did her manner add anything to her personality for she appeared shy, embarrassed, and perhaps a trifle bewildered. While she lacked animation and sparkle, there was no doubt that she was anxious to be understood and to find help.

When questioned as to what was bothering her, she hesitated before each faltering and sometimes indefinite answer. Putting her thoughts into words seemed to be a difficult process for her, but eventually her problem emerged. Ida wanted help so that she could be like other girls of her own age. She derived no pleasure from her work or play because she was tired all the time. She could not say when her trouble started— perhaps a few years previously. She was now twenty years old and a clerk in the candy section of one of the large department stores. High school had been too difficult, so she dropped out when she was sixteen. She lost one small job after another because of forgetfulness, slowness, or lack of dexterity, which made simple unskilled jobs too difficult for her to hold.

Ida did not go out socially because she was just too tired. At times she felt irritable and nervous, at others depressed. She had no serious physical complaints. The fact that her menstrual periods were quite irregular, every two or three months, and were scanty did not seem to bother her. But she was concerned about gaining weight. She admitted that her meals were haphazard and that she nibbled at the candy she was supposed to sell.

If we stop here in Ida's story, we might be tempted to view her as a problem in personality adjustment and mental retardation—a neurotic and a stupid one at that. She seems to be filled with anxiety about herself and unable to find her place in life. But let us not be hasty. Let us leave her psyche for a moment and examine her soma. What physical signs could we find that would throw some light on her problem?

On physical examination, no single extraordinary abnormality was found. But there were many subtle deviations from normal, which when added up became quite significant. She was short, 62 inches, but she weighed 135 pounds. The weight was fairly evenly distributed. Her hair was sparse, coarse, stringy, and dry. Her nails were brittle and short. Her skin was coarse, lacking in vitality, color, and clearness. Along the back of her arm, it felt dry and scaly with permanent little goosepimples. Her blood pressure was low, and her pulse slow. All her responses were slow.

The summation of her physical symptoms was also revealing. She was tired all the time. She hated cold weather, couldn't seem to keep warm, but she liked the summer. She never perspired. She was troubled with constipation. Her menstrual periods were irregular and scanty. She was slowly gaining weight.

As we review these findings, there are many vague symptoms that refer to every organ and system of her body, in fact to all elements of her personality. The over-all picture is the significant clue—a lowered efficiency of all types of function that may be summarized in one word, hypometabolism, which usually means hypothyroidism. The supposition of hypometabolism could be verified by specific tests for thyroid function such as the BMR, and administration of the thyroid hormone should relieve her difficulties.

It would hardly be fair to place the whole burden of correction on the thyroid extract, however, as the hypometabolism had led to faulty habits and behavior patterns. These Ida would have to correct by conscious and serious effort. This does not negate the diagnosis of hypometabolism, as no illness is ever purely physical. Ida was placed on thyroid extract, she began to feel better and became interested in doing the things a young woman usually enjoys. The thyroid extract made her lose some of her puffiness, and with her increased energy she used up more calories, but the thyroid extract alone would not cause her to lose weight. So she was placed on a high protein, low calorie diet.

The change that emerged after a few months was for Ida a Cinderella story. She slimmed down to a smaller size and looked well in her clothes. Her hair, which previously would not hold a curl, was glistening and manageable. Her complexion was fresh and clear. Her eyes had a sparkle, and she answered questions with enthusiasm, even bubbled with the news that she was now a member of a girls' bowling team and that she had been asked out on a double date. Her "inferiority complex" had vanished.

It may seem farfetched to suggest, as we have with Ida, that hypometabolism could ever be taken for a personality disorder. But hypometabolism affects every cell in the body. Its over-all action is to lower the efficiency of every system of the body and the body as a whole. The intensity of the changes, of course, varies with the degree of thyroid deficiency. Hypometabolism may be severe enough to be incapacitating or may be just enough to produce subtle changes that are difficult to evaluate. In such cases, the woman is conscious of her lack of well being and becomes anxious about herself. Many of woman's functional problems, such as menstrual irregularities, sterility, and miscarriages, which have emotional components, are due to thyroid deficiency and are amenable to thyroid therapy.

NEURASTHENIA VS. HYPOGLYCEMIA

Doris did ask: "Am I neurotic?" And she asked it in all earnestness, because she was deeply worried. She was worried about her health, or rather the lack of it, about her marriage, and about her children. She knew that she did not feel well, and she blamed her family difficulties on her own inability to cope with their everyday problems. She was rapidly demonstrating to herself that she was a failure as a person, as a wife, and as a mother.

Doris had reason to ask this question, for in her story are seemingly all the components of a neurosis—anxiety, fear, shame, coupled with the physical complaints of headaches, tremors, fatigue, and asthenia. The question was: Did her family problems result from her emotional conflicts, and were her physical ills the expression of this inadequacy? Or, was she physically ill? Let us examine the facts of her case.

"I'm so tired all the time," she said, "and I look so terrible. I'm just a horrid scarecrow, I'm so skinny, and it is not because I don't eat. I eat all the time, but I never gain any weight. I'm so irritable and cross that I am ashamed of myself. But the thing that really frightens me are the spells that I have. I get confused and depressed. I'm light-headed and dizzy. I forget what I am doing. I drop things and then suddenly I break out in a cold sweat. And then I start trembling like a coward."

"My poor husband," she continued, "I love him, but I don't know how he puts up with me. Our love-making is wonderful when I'm not too tired, which is not very often any more. But look at me—I'm certainly no prize to come home to, and I never feel like dressing up and going out."

The thing that had really frightened Doris and made her seek help was that recently she experienced spells of "blacking out." At first they had been momentary, but the day previous to her visit she had really passed out.

"I don't remember exactly what happened. I was alone with the baby—thank heaven he was in his play pen. I sat down to have another cup of coffee and a cigarette and to read the morning paper after my husband had gone. I didn't feel well, so I dawdled. When I made myself get up and start the morning chores, my hands began to shake, my heart to pound, and I was frightened. Things began to spin around and that was the last I remember till I came to and found myself sprawled out on the kitchen floor."

Doris was age thirty-four, a college graduate, who had achieved a fair degree of success as a reporter and feature writer before her marriage. With the birth of her son, she gave up her job to devote her full energies to making a home and taking care of the family. In this she had not been so successful because she had been sick all the time and physically unable to be an efficient housewife. Was she a failure because she resented the demands on her time and energy as a housewife, which left very little for herself as a person? Was she in revolt because she found cooking and housecleaning less stimulating and rewarding than doing a profile of the new lady congresswoman or a sob story for the Sunday supplement? Perhaps, but do not jump to conclusions.

Doris's story so far might suggest that she was—as she feared—verging on a nervous breakdown or even that she had some organic disease of her nervous system. A diagnosis of an emotional or nervous disorder might seem more likely than a metabolic disorder. But before searching for signs of a brain tumor or seeking to expose the hidden facets of her subconscious conflicts there were other things to be done—a thorough physical examination, appropriate laboratory tests, and the evaluation of her symptoms in the light of these findings.

The physical examination revealed nothing significant except that Doris was nervous, tense, and appallingly underweight. She was 65 inches tall and weighed only 98 pounds. The usual laboratory tests were normal except for a moderate anemia. Going back to her history, the sequence of events leading up to her illness and the relation of the symptoms to her everyday routine might reveal a pattern of some significance.

The onset of her illness had been since the birth of her son. At first when the baby was small, she had felt well and had been happy in her new role, which allowed her time to herself and the opportunity to do what she had always wanted to do—creative writing. This was suddenly ended when the baby got sick. Occupied as she was with his care day and night, her life lost all semblance of routine. She worried, lost weight, and of course was nervous and upset. The baby had in time completely recovered, but Doris continued her haphazard routine of living.

Her day went something like this. She got up in the morning, often dizzy and headachy, always hurried, had breakfast of coffee with sugar and cream, a sweet bun, or toast with jelly. She drank six to twelve cups of coffee during the day. Lunch was only a snack, and by dinner she was too tired to eat. She had a peculiar craving for sweets. They seemed to make her feel better for a while, and she was now consuming two or three of the large pound-size milk chocolate bars a week.

The fact that eating a piece of candy made her feel better was one clue which suggested that she was having periodic attacks of hypoglycemia or low blood sugar. This could be verified either by doing a test of her blood sugar when she was having an attack or doing a sugar tolerance test at a later date.

What causes spontaneous hypoglycemia? It is a combination of two factors—nervous tension and faulty eating habits. Nervous tension has been mistaken for neurosis, and the statement is made that spontaneous hypoglycemia occurs in neurotic individuals. That is not necessarily the case. Rather, emotional stress calls on the body to be ready for instant action—the alarm is sounded, the endocrine system is alerted. It becomes supersensitive and overactive, and as a result too much sugar is used too fast for comfort.

With faulty eating habits, sugar is not available in a slow steady stream over a period of hours. This is not the result of failure to take in sufficient food but from taking in the wrong kinds of food, and paradoxical as it may seem, it is from taking too much carbohydrate rather than too little. Proteins which deliver the sugar slowly, cause a slower, less marked rise, but it is maintained longer.

In a normal person, going without food does not cause hypoglycemia, but merely hunger and weakness, because the body calls on its storage of carbohydrates in the liver and muscles for the sugar necessary for energy. If abstinence from food is prolonged, the person loses weight but does not become hypoglycemic. But a normal person can throw this mechanism out of balance by the wrong kind of diet—too much sugar. Such a person starts the day off in the morning after a long fast with a meal of pure carbohydrates, the blood sugar rises quickly, but the rise is not sustained. It falls again very rapidly. Each rise in the blood sugar from ingested food calls on the sugar metabolism mechanism to remove it from the blood stream, which it does very quickly. In times of stress, the endocrine mechanism is supersensitive and overactive, and too much sugar is used so that the blood level falls below normal. Anything that adds to nervous tension (stress), such as too much stimulation of the nervous system by coffee, tobacco, or the lack of sleep and rest will aggravate the situation.

In the light of these facts Doris's problem is understandable. The groundwork for her hypoglycemia was laid by her period of worry and anxiety over her baby's illness with loss of sleep and no regular meals. It was established by the faulty eating habits, which persisted after the crisis had passed. She adhered to no routine of eating, but ate mostly carbohydrates when she felt hungry. She had found that eating candy seemed to help. It did momentarily but in the long run made her worse.

There was no medicine for Doris to take. She had to cure herself by restoring a normal environment for her endocrine function. This required the application of the triad of good health—diet, exercise, rest and relaxation—and insight into her problem. The result was restoration of her equanimity.

Many conditions of ill health, which are in fact the result of violations of good health habits, have the appearance of neuroticism.

NEUROSIS VS. PREMENSTRUAL TENSION

"Am I losing my mind, am I going crazy?" was the question that Juliet asked. "Surely there must be something terribly wrong with me. I do such awful things. I scream at my husband, I scold my children, I slam things around. I cry if anyone even so much as looks at me. I have these spells when I seem to be someone else. After they have passed, I can't believe that it could have been I who behaved so, and I vow that I will never let it happen again. But it does. This other me unobtrusively slips in and takes over, and I am helpless to do anything about it. It's worse because I can't seem to realize at the time that it is the other me that has engulfed my mind and body or that the real me has ever existed."

As Juliet appealed for help with such urgency and desperation, she sat with her body tense and rigid, her hands clasped tightly together to hide their tremor. Her eyes were pleading for understanding as the tears welled up and overflowed.

After the storm had passed, she told her story. She was thirty years old, had been married ten years, and had two children. Her husband had a good job, and they lived in a nice house in the suburbs. This should have been a happy family, but it was not.

Since girlhood Juliet had experienced days when she was blue, depressed, nervous, and irritable, but she had managed to live with this discomfort and not pay it too much attention. In the last few years these "spells," as she called them, had gradually been getting longer and the symptoms more intense. They lasted a week or ten days during which she was moody, depressed, and cried at the slightest provocation or none at all. At times a simple incident might throw her into a temper tantrum. The spells she now realized always preceded her menstrual period. Each month she was relieved and was herself again just as soon as the flow was well established but not before harm had been done. Quarrels and misunderstandings were recurring with monotonous regularity in her family. The wounds of angry words and unreasonable actions were becoming more slow to heal and because they were reopened each month were becoming quite serious. They were threatening the very life of her family relationship. The climax of her story had occurred on the same morning that she appealed for help.

Juliet was in the kitchen trying to fix breakfast and get the children's lunch ready, but everything seemed to go wrong. She burned her hand, spilled the milk. Then the children came into the kitchen and started squabbling—nothing more than the usual children's arguments—but it was the trigger that threw her into a temper tantrum. She screamed at the children, grabbed them and shook them, all the time scolding them for their misbehavior. They managed to free themselves and ran to their father for protection. Juliet, her rage spent, ran to her bedroom and flung herself on the bed limp and shaking. Lying there exhausted and miserable she heard her husband get the children off to school and then slam the door as he hurried off to his work. In the quiet that followed, she realized that she must find help before it was too late.

Was Juliet neurotic, or as she phrased it "losing her mind?" Did her psyche need help? No, it was her body and its infinitely complicated chemical mechanism that was playing tricks on her. She was suffering, and the suffering was both real and acute, from a definite physical illness, which has come to be called "premenstrual tension."

Medical Recognition

Woman has traditionally been characterized as moody, unpredictable, and vacillating, and man has been puzzled by her seemingly unreasonable sensitivity—the flow of tears, the flush of anger released by the slightest incident or no incident at all. Woman herself may have wondered at the change that at times comes over her when the world looks different and attributed it to part of her lot of being feminine. Rarely, if ever, did she ascribe her discomforts to figments of her imagination or her actions to willful misbehavior.

The periodicity of these symptoms and their relation to the menstrual cycle has long been recognized by professionals, to whom woman was an intriguing biological enigma—either a psyche to be analyzed or a soma to be explained. It is natural that no agreement as to the cause was ever achieved. On the one hand were those who considered the symptoms purely psychic in origin—woman's unconscious rebellion against the experience of menstruation and its implications to her life. She was described as feeling degraded and inferior by the recurring necessity of submission to this period of uncleanliness, or as living in a state of anxiety over what the end of each month would bring—fear that she might be pregnant, or might not, depending on what she wanted. Others attributed the symptoms to a disturbed physiologic state such as might be caused by an unidentified toxic substance which accumulated premenstrually, or by allergy to some chemical component of the menstrual cycle. Only recently has the condition been recognized as a true medical problem, frequent in occurrence and amenable to medical treatment.

Premenstrual tension was described as a medical problem in the early years of female endocrinology. The symptoms were attributed to an imbalance of the ovarian hormones, which resulted in retention of fluids. The validity of this thesis was demonstrated by the relief obtained when ammonium chloride (a simple drug that doctors have long used to reduce excessive fluids in the body) was administered premenstrually. Unfortunately this information was not used to any great extent in the relief of woman's discomfort. Research continued in the effort to find what was the actual disturbance in chemical and nervous balance, all of which was of interest to research physiologists but of little help to women. The significance of premenstrual tension was not brought to the attention of doctors in medical literature. Women did not tell them about it because they thought there was nothing to do about it.

In the last few years, there has been considerable clinical study of premenstrual tension searching out its true symptomology, its frequency and importance, its physiologic basis, and finally methods of treatment. The study of this condition was probably brought about because woman has emerged from the home, where she could take time out when she felt indisposed, to the world of industry and business, where a record of her indisposition was kept. Perhaps more important, she realized that this condition was a handicap to her and her determination to do a good job.

The most interesting and revealing study on premenstrual tension was conducted on women inmates of a prison. Such a set-up is as near a controlled experiment as will ever be obtained with human beings. First the "test subjects" were known. Their mental ability had been tested, their social behavior observed and recorded. The routine of daily living—activity, work, play, rest, and diet—is uniform for all and is also a matter of record. Such a group can be tested for changes in efficiency, as well as clinically tested for changes in body chemistry and function. And finally different forms of therapy could be tried and compared as to their efficacy.

It was found that over 50 per cent of these women said that they had some of these symptoms. An interesting finding was the relation of premenstrual tension to their being in prison in the first place. A review of their records indicated that 62 per cent of the crimes of violence that sent them there were committed in their premenstrual week. Symptoms were relieved most frequently in the group who were given medication to restore fluid balance and maintained on a high protein diet to prevent the incidence of hypoglycemia. The benefit of such treatment was demonstrated by increased output, improvement in behavior, and fewer requests for medication.

Symptoms

There are two groups of symptoms of premenstrual tension—the physiological and psychological. Both vary in intensity in different women and may vary from month to month for any one woman. But probably every woman has at some time experienced some one of these symptoms, and most women have enough each month to be warned a day or even two weeks in advance that a menstrual period is imminent.

The psychological symptoms may be mild depression—just "the blues" —or they may be so severe as to cause complete personality change, which mimics a mental illness or psychoneurosis. The woman is filled with anxiety about things that usually do not bother her and for no reason that she can give. She becomes restless, unable to concentrate, forgets things that she should have remembered. She cannot sleep, or her sleep is restless and disturbed. She is always on the brink of tears. She doesn't sing the blues, she cries them and without provocation. She may be irritable, she takes affront at the slightest word, and a mild question sets off a tantrum. Or perhaps along with feeling a little blue, the day's work takes on mountainous proportions. She loses her manual dexterity— for household chores or office tasks. Her day as she looks back on it has been one of muddling, inefficiency, frustration, and lack of accomplishment.

Along with this loss of feeling of well-being and comfortable adjustment to her life, she does not feel well. Some women have severe headache or backache. Abdominal discomfort varies from a dull heaviness in the lower abdomen to severe cramps. Nausea and vomiting, swelling of the feet and ankles and hands, and puffiness of the face certainly do nothing to add to her pleasure or her attractiveness. Swelling and tenderness of the breasts may be mild or severe to the extent that she has to resort to a larger bra and may find it more comfortable to sleep in one. Her abdomen swells perhaps just enough that it feels hard and uncomfortable or to the point that she has to seek out her loosest fitting clothes to be comfortable. She gains weight. Unless she is watching her weight very closely she may not notice it. But if she is dieting to lose weight she may be disturbed and unhappy to find that she has gained occasionally as much as six to eight pounds.

These symptoms are gradual in their onset, starting only a day or two before the period, but in a few women they begin twelve to fourteen days in advance. The insidiousness of the onset and the variability of their intensity and character are probably the reason women fail to recognize them for what they are. Just as characteristic is the abruptness of their disappearance within a few hours after the onset of the menstrual flow. It is as if a veil has been lifted, the world again has become bright, and life is meaningful and good.

The Cause

What is the cause of this periodic change that women experience in regular recurring cycles? There has been considerable research in the past two decades, but the answer is not as yet completely defined. Investigators, however, including gynecologists, physiologists, and psychiatrists, all agree on certain fundamental facts:

1. Premenstrual tension is a clinical entity, which is somatic not psychic in origin. That is, it is due to disturbance in woman's body function, not in her mind or emotions.

2. This disturbance is a complex mechanism. It has its origin in disturbance of the ovarian cycle and the balance of the hormones, but it reaches out to involve other endocrine gland function and both the autonomic and central nervous systems. This is quite understandable when we recall the earlier discussion of the mutual dependency of the means of control of the body.

3. These disturbances of endocrine control and the repercussions on the nervous system lead to marked changes in the physio-chemical equilibrium of the body. The predominant alteration is retention of fluids.

Retention of fluids means that the body loses its ability to maintain the balance between intake of fluids and excretion. Rather it holds on to more than it should even though there is no excessive intake. There is rarely any deficiency in intake, for our food has such a high percentage of water. This excess is stored in all parts of the body and accounts for many of the symptoms. The most obvious is the gain of weight. Fluids in the abdominal organs cause heaviness, irritability of the intestinal tract, bloating, nausea, and vomiting. Fluids in the tissues surrounding the brain and in the brain itself cause the nervous symptoms of irritability, depression, and nervous tension.

The Treatment

The control of premenstrual tension is the woman's own problem. The responsibility rests on her to recognize it for what it is and to see to it that it does not interfere with her ability to maintain a normal, consistent pattern of social behavior, which is acceptable to her associates. She must recognize that periodically she may be subject to symptoms that are unpleasant and make her an unpleasant person to be around. She must further realize that there is a physiological basis for this. This knowledge she must take as a challenge to do something about it. We are not completely creatures of our emotions. Each of us has a mind and a conscience and should use them.

To help control premenstrual tension, a woman must also maintain a high degree of physical well-being by proper attention to her health. This does not mean just when her period is due but every day of the month. As the premenstruum approaches, cutting down on the fluid intake and restricting salt in her food will help lessen the retention of fluids. There are available simple medications which she may safely use. They contain a diuretic to remove the fluid, to which may be added a mild sedative for control of instability, and vitamins of the B-complex, which are important to the metabolism of the ovarian hormones.

If these measures are not enough, and she is still uncomfortable premenstrually, she should see a doctor, taking care to find one who is really interested in the problem and knows something about it. Doctors who have studied the problem thoroughly and thoughtfully do not always agree on what constitutes the best method of treatment. But they do agree that premenstrual tension is not psychic but somatic in origin and that the causative mechanism is endocrine imbalance. There is no specific hormone therapy to be administered. However, thyroid medication, if indicated, may be quite helpful by increasing the efficiency of all body function, with relief of fatigue, increased activity, and a feeling of well-being.

There are several types of medication from which may be selected the ones most appropriate for the individual case. If the fluid retention seems to predominate, there are many drugs, some quite new, which will reduce the excess fluid. If the nervous symptoms are troublesome, there is a choice of the old standbys, the mild sedatives, or the newer tranquilizers or mood elevators, or a combination of drugs may be used. The drug companies have recently recognized the significance and prevalence of premenstrual tension and have put on the markets their proprietary combinations of drugs.

Although premenstrual tension has only recently been accorded the status of a clinical entity—that is, something doctors should diagnose and treat—there is perhaps no human ill that has a greater impact on our modern culture. It may affect woman and her reactions not only to herself as a person who is ill, but in relation to the people around her, as a wage earner, and as a responsible member of society.

There are no statistics that give a definitive answer as to what percentage of women have premenstrual tension symptoms. Some investigators have suggested that as high as 75 to 80 per cent of women have a moderate degree, and most agree that at least 50 per cent of women of the Age of Maturity experience this recurring syndrome. What part it plays in the difficulties of personal relationships with family and friends, ability to get along with people, to perform her role as wife and mother, what misunderstandings and family quarrels had their beginnings in minor incidents precipitated by woman's irritability, impatience, loss of insight and perspective at the premenstrual period we do not know. It is hoped that the dissemination of knowledge not only to woman herself but to those about her will be of great benefit in helping her carry out her role in life.

THE AGE OF MARRIAGE AND MOTHERHOOD

IX

MARRIAGE

SOME YEARS AGO two young women, both of whom were about to be married, came to me for medical consultation. To Mary and Suzanne life seemed to promise a new meaning as each approached the fulfillment of her maturity in love and marriage. They presented such a striking combination of similarities and contrasts that they have remained a vivid picture in my memory.

Suzanne and Mary, although unknown to each other, had much in common. They were both in their early twenties, attractive, and well dressed. They were from families of moderate means, and their lives of school, beaux, and parties had been much alike. Now they were planning to be married and had come for premarital examinations. Here the similarity ceased, and their differences became obvious. Marriage would be a turning point, and thereafter their lives would be vastly different.

Suzanne and her attitude toward marriage should have come as no surprise. Her mother, in making the appointment, had revealed a great deal, not only about Suzanne as the bride-to-be, but also about herself as a mother.

"Doctor," she said, "Suzanne is going to be married next week. She is still so young and inexperienced in many ways that her father and I have great misgivings about this marriage. But she is so determined this is what she wants that we have had to give in to her wishes. So, I want you to talk to her very seriously, tell her all the things she needs to know, and of course give her a thorough physical examination. She is so busy with shopping and fittings, showers and parties, and all the things a bride has to do, she just hasn't had time to think of seeing a doctor—much less make an appointment. Poor child, she is just exhausted and frantic that she won't get everything done. But I told her she just had to take time to see you. Please, won't you give her a good talking-to?"

Knowing that a mother does not always have her daughter's confidence and that daughters are sometimes much more responsible and better informed than their mothers realize, I gave Suzanne the benefit of the doubt and waited for her to speak for herself. But I was in error. Suzanne was just what her mother had implied—a child playing at being grown up. To be married was her only goal in life, and she was on the verge of achieving it. Courting had been fun, the engagement exciting. She had captured her man, and she expected that he would see to it that she lived happily ever after. He was good looking, had a good job, and she was going to be his wife. As far as she was concerned that was all there was to it. She had been the spoiled darling of her family, and she expected to be the same to her husband.

Suzanne came to me because her mother told her she must, not because she felt any need for medical consultation or any other advice. In answer to questions, she told with enthusiasm of her wedding plans, but when that was finished, animation left her. She sat silent without one question, waiting for whatever unpleasant facts might be forthcoming. She did not want a physical examination, and because she was resentful, prudish, and unco-operative, an adequate examination was impossible.

In contrast to Suzanne, Mary made her own appointment, a fact indicative of her seriousness. My first impression—that she was an attractive, intelligent, well-poised young woman and one with a purpose—ripened into respect for her as a person of considerable maturity as she told her story. She and John, her fiance, expected eventually to live on a farm in Pennsylvania. His father was giving them the land with an old house on it, and they knew it would take a lot of work for a long time to make it both a home and a profitable business. They had plans for remodeling the house and establishing a dairy herd, plans they hoped to carry out gradually as they earned the money. But even the start must be postponed a year until John had completed college. Mary had graduated from college the previous June and was already working, and John had a part-time job, which would enable them to build up a little reserve fund for the beginning of their venture.

The most important of their plans was the family they hoped to have and the home life they dreamed of. This too would have to wait, but they had concluded that waiting, although difficult, would have its compensations. The year or so would give them time to learn to live together, to work together, and to love together. In short, Mary was looking forward to her marriage as a new way of life to be shared with the man she loved. She was seeking all the help available and some specific information. She had a list of questions for which she wanted answers.

Suzanne and Mary represent extremes in the concepts of marriage. Between them are all degrees of variation. Marriage has an individual meaning for every woman, and this meaning changes as the years go by. If we should question women already married, we should find their experience of marriage ranging from joy, happiness, and fulfillment to sorrow, disappointment, frustration, and disillusionment. After years of marriage, some women may view their marriage with complacency; some accept marriage with resignation and submissiveness; some continue to strive to make it a good way of life with optimism and determination; some have revolted at a bad bargain; some have reneged on their promises; some suffer in silence; and some do not have to speak, for their radiant happiness speaks for itself.

It is not our purpose to explore the problems of marriage. They are individual problems for which there are no classifications or specific answers. We shall consider here the meaning of marriage to the mature woman, her preparations and qualifications for it, and how a premarital examination and marriage counseling can be helpful to her.

THE MEANING OF MARRIAGE

Every woman considers marriage a desirable goal. Even a little girl, mothering her doll babies, speaks glibly of some day having a house and babies of her own, with a vague and unimportant father as part of the background. In youth, these childish fancies fade and she dreams of her ideal man, who will be responsive to and appreciative of her attractiveness, love her above all else, and with whom she will find happiness. But as she achieves maturity, marriage and love, children and husband take on a different meaning.

To the mature young woman marriage is a way of life that promises fulfillment of her maturity in all the facets of her personality. It is an age in which the joys will be greater and the sorrows less because they will be shared by the man she loves. She recognizes that this age has as its purpose the establishment of a home and the rearing of a family. Her role as wife and mother is a privilege and responsibility—not only to be loved but also to give love, not only to possess but also to give of herself. Moreover, she recognizes that marriage is a tried and proven state of human relationship, in which there are three basic ingredients necessary for successful achievement—social (including legal), physical (sex), and emotional (love).

Marriage first of all is a social state, and legality is its basic foundation. Without it there can be no useful structure. When legality is the entire structure, however, marriage can only be cold, barren, and devoid of human values. But the significance to woman of legality is variable. Happily, the day has passed, for American women at least, in which a woman had no choice, but might be given in wedlock, sometimes for a consideration, and was expected to perform her wifely duties for her lord and master uncomplainingly. Today woman herself decides whether she will be a wife to any man. When she does marry, legality rarely subjects her, rather it protects her. In fact, by it she holds the whip hand, and, we must admit, occasionally uses it vindictively.

Legality in marriage has been given other interpretations. In a recent voluminous dissertation on women, called by some a "modern classic," legality is depicted as the one great flaw in marriage, and if woman is to fulfill her true sexual significance, she is advised not to submit to the legal bondage, which makes her the second sex. Such a caricature of the meaning of womanhood and marriage is derived largely from mythology, fiction, poetry, case histories of neurotic females, and sick minds— male and female. It is fired by a fertile imagination, but presented as scientific fact, and is expressed by a facile pen in the jargon of a cultist. But it hasn't the slightest semblance to the true image of mature womanhood and marriage.

There are marriages in which legality is the only bond holding man and woman together. Most of these probably started with high hopes and expectations on the part of the couple but either never matured or degenerated to legal bondage and failure.

Marriage is also a physical state, but mating does not constitute the sole basis of marriage. We might think so if we accept the concept of marriage as it is presented to us by modern means of communication. Newspapers, magazines, novels, theater, radio, and television seem to be preoccupied with sex attraction and sex problems to the exclusion of other aspects of marriage. Even some marriage manuals, books that propose to be scientific guides to successful marriage, reduce the ideal of marriage to the attainment of proficiency in sex technique.

Marriage is distorted by the pseudo-sophisticates, who see no truth, no interest (in reality no sales value) in any human relationship which exemplifies achievement of ideals and morality. They stress human vices, weakness, and depravity, particularly on the physical level. Too infrequently do we find marriage depicted as a relationship based on the ideals of love, compatibility, and responsibility.

Marriage is not merely license for sexual union, and based on sexual attraction alone it is destined to failure. This is pointed up in the cases of some of the many times wedded celebrities. Such marriage vows, taken so casually and frequently with one mate after another, serve only to legalize and publicize sexual promiscuity and should not be dignified by the name of marriage.

Physical relationship outside of marriage never fulfills the needs and ideals of a mature woman in our present culture. She may accept it as second best in the attempt not to let life pass her by, but she knows that she is missing the rich and important experience embodied in being a wife. Marriage is a human relationship which, to flourish, must bear the stamp of approval of society. A woman can experience the maturity and fulfillment of her sexuality only in such a union, which proclaims she is wanted enough to be a wife, grants her the prestige of home and family, and assures to her children a respectable place in society. Such a union, marriage alone can provide, but this is not enough. A mature woman does not give herself sexually without love.

Marriage is an emotional and spiritual state and must be above all else the fulfillment of love, which encompasses, among other things, mutual regard and respect, concern for the welfare and happiness of the mate, and companionship. Sexual union becomes a means of expressing this love. Such a marriage has as its goal the building of a way of life together—a home and family. How well it will succeed depends on the emotional maturity of both of the partners—the maturity with which they meet life together with honesty, integrity, compassion, tolerance, understanding, hopefulness, perseverance, determination, and unselfishness. The ideal marriage is not a natural heritage, but a responsible career with certain qualifications, which are acquired through preparation and training.

QUALIFICATIONS FOR MARRIAGE

Society makes no demands, sets no standards of preparedness for young people wishing to embark on this career. Yet there is no career in which preparation is more important if success is to be achieved, and no career in which society has a greater stake than the institution of marriage, home, and family. In the professions, trades, or even in semiskilled jobs, there are some requirements as to intent, suitability, knowledge, and skill. But in marriage the one requirement is the expressed desire on the part of the couple, and the only qualifications are those that assure a degree of physical maturity and a modicum of good health. The laws of the states require that the woman be of some minimum age, usually eighteen but sometimes (with the consent of her parents) twelve or fourteen. The only prohibitions are positive serology (indicating syphilis), which need be only temporary, and mental deficiency of a severe degree.

Our culture is guilty of a greater fault than the lack of specific requirements for marriage, in the sorry spectacle of marriage as it is advertised in stories of divorce and marital tragedies that make headlines. Our mass media depict the preparation for marriage as sexual sparring (which frequently does not stop there), in which casual encounter and mutual physical attraction are the only essentials and the time required but a day, a week, or rarely a month.

The qualifications for marriage in any couple are to be found in the degree of maturity they have attained. Their chance of success will depend on the preparations they have acquired during the years of growing up and may be measured in terms of their motivation, training, and ideals.

Motivation

The reasons a woman wants to marry are probably never single, clear-cut, and completely ideal, but are a mixture of the mature and immature, arising from different needs in each individual, and compromises with reality. If she has achieved a degree of maturity in her thoughts and judgments, she has a fair concept of the true meaning of marriage and believes that she has found a mate who will share and strive to attain with her the ideal of love and marriage. On the other hand, if she is immature, she may marry for what she thinks marriage can give her. She may be seeking the security that a husband with a good job and satisfactory social status will provide, an escape from an intolerable or unpleasant home environment, or relief from the necessity of working at a job she does not like. She may be child-like, unrealistic, and play-acting. She may see no further than the ceremony in which she has the leading role, and any personable young man willing to play the supporting role may be acceptable. She may also, if she is immature, confuse infatuation with love. She may be blind to the faults of the man she wants to marry as well as to their dissimilarities and their incompatibilities. They may have scarcely had time to know each other and may have nothing in common but the urge to possess, which is the powerful and sometimes blinding force that leads them to marriage.

Most young people, however, probably want marriage on a mature basis —for love, home, and family—but they may be unsure of their abilities to assess their motives or oblivious to the necessity of making judgments. Although it is important that they have a mature motive and mature judgment in the choice of a mate, an equally important motive is to be a good mate and to make a full contribution to marriage. And this motivation must be strong, true, and lifelong.

Training

A young woman reaches the Age of Marriage with an accumulation of knowledge. How this may contribute to her qualifications depends on the kind as well as the amount.

There is first the general knowledge about marriage acquired through her own experience. This is informal, intangible, and unmeasurable but probably is the most important of all, for on this is built her ideal of marriage. There are many facets of this knowledge, reflecting her experience with people, with ideas, in reading and from school, but especially from her home. If her experience has been that of a child of a good, sound marriage and a responsible member of a happy home, she will accept this as what marriage should be and expect the same for herself. But if her experience has been that of a child of an unhappy marriage, a broken home, she may expect less, have a poor regard for, or be afraid of marriage. On the other hand, her early experience may strengthen her resolve and determination to make a good and lasting marriage for herself.

The second kind of knowledge is that which she has of sex. There is a tendency to blame failure in marriage, promiscuity, illegitimate pregnancies, and other problems, social and personal, on lack of knowledge of the purely physical facts of sex. As a result there are controversies over sex education in the schools—the what, when, and how of presentation of the facts of life to youngsters before they get into trouble. And for the older age group as "premarital training," there is a deluge of information on the physical aspects of the relationship between the sexes—the technique of "love," "ideal marriage," being a "vital wife," and "fulfilling woman's sexual responsibility."

Sex education is not a topic that can be taught as a specific subject, segregated and alone, for so many class periods at any one age level. Children are getting sex education every day of their lives. The important thing is to add to this not only sound factual material but also appreciation of the true meaning of sex, in which it is integrated with other aspects and ideals of life. The trouble comes from the mass of misinformation that is passed on. On the one hand, there are the fears and taboos of sex—the concerted conspiracy of the elders to ignore sex or to consider it something unspeakable or unclean. On the other hand, sex is stripped of the mysticism of love in "frank" and "realistic" discussions that reduce it to the purely physical level and interpret it as a drive that dominates our lives and that we are helpless to do anything about other than to perfect its techniques.

Both of these concepts fail to recognize the true significance of sex—that it is a powerful force within everyone for great good and happiness or great harm and sorrow. It is the responsibility of each of us to use this force with discipline and self-control and to integrate it with a purposeful life. The achievement of this is true sex education.

A third kind of training for marriage is acquired through general education. Modern woman has access to all the avenues of learning, and she is availing herself of the opportunity of acquiring an education. A large percentage of girls finish high school, and many go on to college and professional training. Formerly, it was accepted that there were only a few things a woman needed to be taught—the simplest fundamentals of formal education and the practical side of running a household and caring for a family. To this, the more affluent added the art of being a lady. Even today there still remains the feeling that somehow a woman in making the most of her intellect loses something of her femininity and that she really does not need higher education to fulfill her feminine role of wife and mother.

Many young women who choose marriage as a career see no need for higher education. Equality of education, between husband and wife, however, makes for greater stability of marriage, which increases with the amount of education they have received. Divorce rates are lowest among college graduates. While marriage as a career brings no regular salary, hours of work, vacation, advancement by title and citations, it is the most demanding in skills, training, and knowledge if success is to be attained.

Ideals

In days gone by, family ties and tradition were strong, and the social areas in which young people moved were circumscribed. These provided guidance in the suitability of a marriage. The choice of a mate was limited to young men of similar backgrounds, training, and ideals. Today with larger cities, larger schools, lessening of the hold of the family, and woman's early entrance into the working world, which takes her away from home at an early age, she comes into contact with many young men of all types of background. They have only each other to judge and appraise, not a family to please or a social status to uphold. And they have only their own ideals to guide them regarding what they want and expect of marriage, and only their own determination to realize these ideals. The realization of the importance of qualifications has led many young people to seek counseling before their marriage.

PREMARITAL MEDICAL CONSULTATION

The practice of a couple consulting a physician before marriage is becoming fairly common. This is a constructive step that gives some assurance that their marriage may be a successful one. Statistics have been presented that show that fewer marriages end in divorce among couples who seek medical advice before marriage. But it is incorrect to attribute the success of these marriages entirely to the intrinsic value of the consultation. In large part success in marriage derives from the character of the couple who seek advice. It is not only the information they receive about themselves and marriage that is significant but also the fact that they want information. The desire for guidance and information indicates that they are approaching marriage with maturity and seriousness and that they recognize that a good marriage will come only as a result of continued, consecrated effort on their part.

Not all premarital examinations are actuated by such earnestness of purpose. Suzanne, for example, was sent for "sex education" in one easy lesson. Her lack of maturity was not essentially her fault but was the result of lack of proper guidance and of sex education. No doctor can give the "facts of life" in one or a dozen consultations, even with the help of a stack of marriage manuals. Sex education is a way of life, which is learned step by step through the years. At maturity one should have achieved some understanding of and respect for one's own self and the ability to love and live with others, giving fully of one's self, receiving joyfully from others, and sharing both the good and bad.

There are those whose purpose in seeking medical advice may not seem to reflect the ideal of maturity. Some want only advice on the technique of contraception. This is a valid reason, if it is the expression of the desire to plan their marriage and the time they are ready for parenthood. If their marriage is based only on physical attraction and seeks only sexual indulgence free from the penalty, as they see it, of pregnancy and parenthood, it will eventually add one more case of failure to the statistics.

What is a premarital medical consultation? In what ways may it be helpful in starting marriage off right? It consists of three parts: a medical history; a physical examination; and a certain amount of marriage counseling. By these the doctor seeks to evaluate the couple's physical fitness to assume the responsibilities of marriage, their physical ability not only to have children but also to pass on to their children the heritage of sound minds and sound bodies. The counseling is directed toward helping them to achieve a happy adjustment to the married state. To put it another way, the doctor seeks to answer questions such as Mary had on her list.

"Am I normal?"

"Am I physically able to have a happy marriage?"

"Will I be able to have children?"

"Will my children be normal?"

"How can I plan my family?"

Let us see what is meant by each of these and how the doctor arrives at the answers.

"Am I Normal?"

Most young women approaching marriage are normal physically. They have attained their full growth to body maturity and show no evidence of a present illness or of abnormality due to a past illness. Some are not as robust as they should be, but this is at times partly due to the stress of the engagement period and preparations for marriage. It adjusts itself when the ceremony is over and the woman settles down to a normal routine again.

Physical maturity on the sexual level may be presumed if the girl has started to menstruate at the normal time and has had regular cycles for several years. Almost every doctor has had the acquaintance of a young woman who has been told previously that she had an "infantile uterus" and could not have babies—and who was therefore amazed on being told that she was pregnant. It is risky ever to tell a woman who has her normal complement of pelvic organs that she cannot conceive. The uterus may appear smaller than normal at premarital examination and still be hospitable to a pregnancy. In some rare cases a girl may have a truly infantile uterus (this is usually associated with menstrual abnormalities), and treatment should be started immediately and not delayed until she has tried two or three years to become pregnant.

Physical abnormalities such as heart disease or diabetes, when present, are not a deterrent to marriage or even to a future pregnancy. But it is important for the woman to know of these handicaps before marriage so that she may take proper care of herself, have medical advice in planning her pregnancies, and obtain adequate medical care at the very start of her pregnancy.

Nervous disorders, such as previous nervous breakdowns or illnesses, may be important from the standpoint of the woman's ability to make a successful adjustment to marriage and motherhood. If the woman does not appear to have recovered from such ailments, the marriage counselor may advise further investigation and treatment before marriage.

The doctor will always look for evidence of the venereal diseases, syphilis and gonorrhea. Both diseases are transmitted by sexual contact but are vastly different in the way they affect the body. The laws of many states require blood tests before a marriage license is granted, and persons having positive serology must have adequate medical treatment before the marriage can be consummated. The doctor may recommend a blood test for each, even though the law does not require it, if neither has previously been tested. Most young couples, however, have had blood tests before their premarital examinations, as it is part of the physical examination that the Armed Forces give to all their members, and all blood donors to the Red Cross are tested for syphilis.

If on examination gonorrhea is demonstrated in either of the couple, marriage should be postponed until it is cured, as it can be. And if either has had gonorrhea in the past, the doctor will make a thorough search, and institute treatment if he thinks it necessary, to prevent its transmission to the other partner. A quiescent case contracted years previously can be reactivated by the increased sex activity of marriage. The most serious aftermath of gonorrhea is sterility, and one of the tragedies that every gynecologist sees frequently is the sterile marriage due to closed tubes in the woman who has contracted gonorrhea from her husband, on her honeymoon, because he failed to be rechecked before marriage to see if he was completely cured of the gonorrhea contracted years before. He, too, may be sterile or of reduced fertility as the result of the disease.

In young women, an ovarian cyst is occasionally found in a premarital examination. If it is causing no trouble, the doctor will usually advise that it be watched. Removal may become necessary at some later date. In an older woman other forms of pelvic pathology, such as fibroids, may be encountered and evaluated in terms of the woman's health and her ability to have children.

"Can I Have a Happy Marriage?"

By asking if she is "physically able to have a happy marriage" a woman usually wants to know, first, if she can have sexual intercourse on her wedding night without pain and, second, how she can achieve a happy sexual adjustment in marriage. The doctor does not find the answers to these questions by a pelvic examination alone, indeed if he can give any answer at all, because so much depends on the woman—her knowledge of sex and her attitude toward it. In the cases of Mary and Suzanne we could hazard a guess, before examination of either, that to Mary the answer would be "yes" and to Suzanne "no," because we know that success in marriage depends more on emotional readiness than physical ability.

Women approach the consummation of marriage with a vast array of preconceptions of what it will be like, what physical sensations and emotional reactions it will bestow on them. Some will be full of fear and dread, because they have heard and believed the stories that others have passed on to them. Some who consider themselves modern and informed put aside these fearful concepts and naïvely expect a soul-shaking, exalting experience. They do not realize that love-making is an art, proficiency in which is attained only after much practice. One must learn it to earn its reward. Finally, there are those who have had previous sex experience and think they know it all. But if they are marrying the man they truly love, they still have something in store for them, which only marriage can give—the deep warm satisfaction that comes with belonging together before all the world.

Great importance has been attached to the premarital pelvic examination as a necessary part of preparation for marriage. But the limitations in its usefulness must be fully realized. The pelvic examination yields informa-

tion as to the degree of physical maturity, which most women hav
adequately attained, and as to the presence of physical abnormalities, whic
most young women do not have. Its greatest value is reassurance to th
woman that she is normal.

It is true that doctors who are experienced in premarital examinatio
can get a pretty good idea of how mature a woman is in her concept of se
by her reaction on the examining table. If her attitude is one of acceptanc
and co-operation, it would seem to indicate that she accepts her sexuali
in a mature way. In contrast, the immature woman makes examinatic
impossible by her anxiety, shame, and false modesty. But the examinatic
alone, while revealing to the physician, does not materially make ar
change in the woman, unless it is accompanied by desire on her part f
knowledge and understanding and effort on the part of the doctor
contribute that information.

Frequently an adequate pelvic examination cannot be made because
the presence of the hymen. What should be done about this is entirely
question for the young woman to decide. The hymen is a soft elast
membrane, which stretches easily and occasionally tears but is usually r
impediment. Only in very rare instances is it a tough occlusive membran
which must then be cut.

The more serious problem is an intact hymen associated with rigidi
of the muscles which embrace the vaginal opening. This rigidity is du
partly to nervous tension because the woman is apprehensive about th
new experience and its implications. It is also due to the fact that this
one of the most highly sensitive spots in the whole body, and just touchir
it may cause reflex spasm of the muscles, which in itself is painful.
such cases, the doctor will advise premarital dilatation of the opening of th
vagina, not merely cutting the hymen. This may serve a double purpose ;
a help to the attainment of normal sexual relations. The gentle massag
will relax and stretch the muscles as well as the hymen, and the experienc
becomes a part of the education of the woman to the acceptance of th
part of her body. For this reason, the doctor does some of the dilating an
teaches the woman herself how to assist by gentle massage with her fing
or a dilator made for the purpose. Because dilatation may be necessary i
a fair percentage of women (less often since women are using the intern
tampon for menstruation and have already accomplished the desire

results), the premarital examination should be made well in advance, about six weeks, of the date of marriage.

Only a part of the groundwork for a happy sexual adjustment in marriage is laid in the premarital examination. How well the edifice will be built depends on many factors.

In answer to the woman's question, "how can we achieve a happy sexual adjustment?" there is one bit of helpful advice that the doctor can give:

"You must find out for yourselves what constitutes a happy sexual adjustment for you as individuals. Don't try to measure it by descriptions in books or by what others tell you about their sex life. You have to establish, by earnest effort, trial and error, what is right for you, what brings to both of you the greatest happiness and satisfaction. This is true not only of the frequency of marital relations but also of your own physical and emotional reactions to it. There is no criteria to which all must conform. To reach this understanding of yourself and your mate, you must put aside prudery and false pride and be truthful and self-revealing. And remember the greatest joy is in giving—giving of yourself fully and giving pleasure to the one you love. The satisfaction that you achieve will be measured by the mutual joy of giving and sharing. If either of you is selfish, demanding, and disregards the other's needs and feelings, which also includes withholding yourself with any degree of frequency, your marital adjustment is doomed to failure.

"Your sexual union is the way you express your love to your husband. It therefore has two components, the physical and the emotional. So much has been written about woman—her ability to achieve a climax and her frigidity—that stresses only the physical aspects and ignores the emotional that you probably have an erroneous idea of what climax should be. You may think that you will have that reaction each and every time you mate. But that will not be true. Let's look at another human experience, which we can be quite matter-of-fact about, and see why this is so. Listening to music is a good example because it also involves the physical and emotional. And this is not as far-fetched as it might seem. Music is not just a part of our culture; it is a part of all nature. There is music in the woods, in the waves, in the fields, in the quietude of eventide. So also music is a part of you. You may be a person who reacts with intense emotion, lifted to the clouds of happiness, or moved to tears of sadness. Your reactions may be an acute physical reaction or a quiet inner satisfaction of a beautiful experience. Sometimes when you are in the mood, you react intensely, sometimes when you are not, it leaves you cold. And so it can be with your marital relations. The only standard is whether it is satisfying and fulfills your needs."

"Can I Have Children and Will They Be Normal?"

In the vast majority of cases, the doctor will find little to suggest that a family of normal children is impossible to the woman preparing for marriage. There are only a few physical conditions apparent to the doctor on examination that may tell him whether the woman will be unable to conceive. Infertility is common in marriage, but it is not usually apparent on premarital physical examination.

Every mother wants her baby to be perfect, and she starts wondering about this long before she becomes a mother. When she asks the doctor at her premarital examination whether she will have normal babies, she is asking him to evaluate the weak lines in her family tree and to tell her what, if anything, she has to fear. Maybe there was an aunt who was in a mental institution, a cousin who had fits or was a cripple. The doctor should discuss heredity with her more for the purpose of reassuring her that she has nothing to fear than of forewarning her. Very rarely will he advise against pregnancy. He will point out that many of the diseases that people fear are hereditary are not. A disease may be prevalent in one family even in several generations and still not be hereditary. There are in the strict sense of the word no hereditary diseases. There are only hereditary weaknesses, defects, imperfections.

Diabetes, however, is a problem that deserves consideration premaritally. It is a metabolic disease resulting from the deficiency of function, the inadequacy of essential mechanisms of the body. This trait may be transmitted, but not invariably. The occurrence of diabetes in the family of one of the couple does not mean that their children will have diabetes. Even if one of the couple is diabetic, their children may not be. But the union of two diabetics will almost always result in children with a diabetic tendency. Whether such a couple should marry and have children is a question for them to decide.

Mental disorders and insanity are the conditions couples most frequently fear may be hereditary. But this is a false idea. Insanity is a general term applied to many types of mental disorders, as we have already learned. The fact that some member of the family has been in a mental institution does not mean that "insanity runs in the family." What has been said about insanity applies generally to epilepsy.

Heredity as a premarital problem has been discussed to allay the fears that come from misinformation and not because it is a deterrent to marriage and parenthood. Marriage is not a breeding experiment, to produce superior offspring. It is doubtful if it ever could be, for we are all varied mixtures of physical fitness and defects, of potential strength and weakness.

"How Can I Plan My Family?"

The fact that women are asking this question today and the equally important fact that doctors are able to give the answer and are recognizing the importance of rendering this service mark a tremendous step forward in the emancipation of woman. It also affords a means of betterment of life for all mankind in the future. The knowledge and application of the science of contraception must be counted as one of the truly great medical advances of our lifetime.

This does not mean to imply that avoidance of motherhood is emancipation. But for woman to be able to plan her family—to space and limit the number of children she will bear—with consideration for the welfare of the whole family—this is emancipation. By it, she achieves freedom of choice to be a healthier, happier mother better able to care for her family. She achieves freedom from fears of too frequent pregnancies with their unfortunate effects on herself, her marriage, and her children. She achieves freedom from want for that family. It is emancipation that allows her to fulfill the potential trinity of her personality—person, wife, and mother.

Important as this knowledge is in the life of woman, it is also potentially important to the betterment of life for all mankind. The life of a nation depends on its ability to balance its human needs with its natural resources. The application of this knowledge can help ensure population growth that will not exceed the means for satisfying the basic needs of that population.

There is great need for this in some of the underprivileged areas of the world today. But widespread dissemination and use of this knowledge is a thing of the future.

When man's knowledge progressed to the point where he recognized the cause-and-effect relationship between sexual intercourse and pregnancy, he began to invent devices to prevent pregnancy from being the natural consequence of his sexual behavior—and the practice of contraception came into being.

The term contraception means the use of some procedure or appliance before, during, or after sexual intercourse for the purpose of preventing conception. There are, as this definition implies, many different methods used for the purpose, and they vary greatly in effectiveness. None are methods of "birth control," which is a misnomer. No one controls, in the sense of preventing birth once pregnancy has started, except by abortion.

Contraception became a science, a part of medical science when two things happened: when woman sought medical advice on the subject; and when the doctor, realizing her need and the validity of her request, sought to expand his knowledge so that he might be able to give sound advice. He soon realized that any method he could conscientiously recommend must meet the three requirements of effectiveness, acceptability, and harmlessness. It should be a method that could be expected to accomplish the desired purpose, that would be acceptable to both partners, and the prolonged use of which would not do harm to either.

Only a generation or so ago, contraception was far from being scientific. Because sex was taboo, couples did not discuss the planning of a family, and children were simply accepted as they came. The few methods then used were usually ineffectual and sometimes harmful. A woman would not have even considered asking a doctor for advice. And, if she had, she more than likely would have been rebuffed by the doctor who considered her "unwomanly" and her request an affront to his dignity.

The change in attitude to that of today did not come easily. It came as the result of courage, determination, and fortitude of pioneers battling ignorance, prejudice, and intolerance, and the battle is not yet won. In a few of our states the dissemination of the facts of contraception is still prohibited by law.

The devices used for the purpose of contraception have been until recently of two general types: the "natural method," in which intercourse is restricted either as to time or manner; and the "technical" (mechanical, artificial), in which some external device is used to prevent the entry of the male cell into the uterus. Recently a third method is being investigated —biological contraception. This seeks to find some way of temporarily reducing the fertility of one of the partners. This must be differentiated from "sterilization," whereby the individual is permanently deprived of fertility by some surgical procedure for a specific medical or social reason. None of those now used completely satisfies all the requirements, and all have some disadvantage. But the search continues for better methods. The natural methods include continence, incomplete or interrupted intercourse, and the rhythm method.

Continence, or abstinence from intercourse, is of course a sure way of preventing conception, and it is the only 100 per cent effective way, but it hardly satisfies the requirements of being either acceptable or harmless. It is one that few individuals would follow, and it certainly is not one that any physician with his knowledge of the importance of sex in marriage would recommend. Incomplete intercourse is mentioned only to be condemned. It fulfills none of the requirements, and its habitual use is harmful to both parties. It is not safe or efficient, nor is it acceptable or satisfactory.

The Rhythm

The rhythm or natural method of contraception is based on the fact that a woman can conceive only within a few hours after ovulation, and ovulation occurs only once during each menstrual cycle. The short space of time in which she might conceive is called her fertile period, and the rest of the cycle her sterile or safe period. If abstinence is practiced during the fertile period, conception is avoided. But it is not that easy. The problem is not only determining when the fertile period normally occurs, but of predicting it for each cycle. It is this necessity of predicting accurately the time limits of the fertile period that makes the method difficult to use effectively and gives rise to some of its failures. For one attribute that can never be applied to woman is predictability.

Extensive research has shown that ovulation occurs about two weeks before the onset of the menstrual cycle, not at mid-period. In other words, there is a fixed time relationship between ovulation and menstruation which follows. Since two weeks is about mid-period in a twenty-eight-day cycle, you might think this is unnecessary quibbling, but it is not, as we can easily demonstrate.

In a regular cycle of twenty-eight days, ovulation may be expected to occur fourteen days before menstruation, which is also fourteen days from the first day of the preceding menstrual flow and also mid-period. But we have seen that regular twenty-eight-day cycles are rarities rather than the rule. If the cycle is only three weeks long, ovulation may occur at the end of the first week. If the cycle is six weeks long ovulation occurs at the end of the fourth week, neither of which are mid-periods. These represent marked irregularities, but the same difficulty occurs also for most other women. We have noted before that women who considered themselves regular experience some variations, being sometimes a few days early and sometimes a few days late. Such women therefore can only predict that the next menstrual period will start anywhere from twenty-five to thirty days after the onset of her last period. Therefore, her fertile period may also vary by five days. In women who are irregular to the point of having periods every four to seven weeks, there is a corresponding irregularity in the time of ovulation, and it therefore becomes completely unpredictable.

It is not even this accurate, for the interval between ovulation and menstruation is not fixed at fourteen days, but may be thirteen or twelve or as short as ten days. So the fertile period will have to be considered as lasting not just one day, but three or four days. Actually, the woman is fertile only about twelve hours out of the four days, but the trouble is that we have no way of knowing (from calendar dates alone) when those few hours occur. The uncertainty of the duration is compounded by our uncertainty of how long the sperm (male cell) can remain fertile and lie in wait for the ovum. It is probably at least twelve hours, and may be much longer. So, to include all the possible variations, we must say that the fertile period is potentially three days before and three days after the day we think ovulation should occur.

This seems quite complex and difficult to apply to a specific case. To

do so, the woman must first know something of the variability of her
cycle, which means that she must have a calendar record accurately and
regularly marked for at least one year. Let us follow through on a case.
The dates of the first day of each cycle are listed in the first column, and
the duration of the cycle in the second:

January	10	
February	7	28
March	5	26 (shortest)
April	1	27
May	1	30
May	29	28
June	27	29
July	27	30 (longest)
August	24	28
September	21	28
October	18	27
November	13	26
December	13	30

We note that the shortest cycle is twenty-six days and the longest
cycle thirty days. The potential fertile period we may represent graphically
this way:

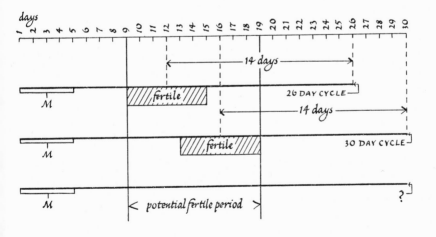

In the shortest or twenty-six-day cycle, ovulation is expected to occur fourteen days before menstruation, on the twelfth day of the cycle. Allowing for variation of three days either way, the potential fertile period for each twenty-six-day cycle is from the ninth to fifteenth day. In the longest or thirty-day cycle, ovulation occurs fourteen days before menstruation or on the sixteenth day. Allowing for the three-day variation, the potential fertile period for each thirty-day cycle is from the thirteenth to nineteenth day.

This woman will have no way of knowing or predicting how long the oncoming cycle will last, twenty-six, twenty-eight, or thirty days, so she must allow for all possible variation. In other words, she must consider that the fertile period can start on the ninth day because it may be a short cycle and can last until the nineteenth day because it may be a thirty-day cycle. This makes the potential fertile period ten days. Some women do have signs of ovulation such as pain, increased mucus discharge, or even slight bleeding, but these are rarely constant or characteristic enough to be reliable.

Other means of determining the fertile period have been devised such as observing basal temperatures, examination of vaginal smears, biological testing of the urine, and determination of changes in vaginal acidity and chemistry. These will be discussed in the chapter on infertility.

The rhythm is obviously a difficult method to use. It is difficult to work out, even with slight variations, as we have seen. It imposes a long period of continence to which young married couples will find it difficult to subscribe. With pronounced irregularities it is almost impossible of application. There is only one consoling feature, if it is consoling, and that is in cycles of marked irregularity it is probable that many of the cycles are anovulatory—physiologically sterile cycles.

Contraceptive Devices

There are many contraceptive methods commonly known and practiced, but there are only a few that are approved as satisfactory and safe by the specialist. The vaginal douche has undeservedly been used with confidence by many couples as a contraceptive device, and frequently has failed them. This in spite of the fact that all kinds of chemicals have been added to kill the sperm—chemicals widely advertised as a boon to "feminine hygiene." The reason for failure is not hard to understand if one remembers that the sperm, empowered with relatively rapid motion, are usually deposited directly on the cervix at intercourse, and some have made their way into the protective shelter of the mucus secretions of the cervix in a matter of seconds. Thus they are soon out of the reach of the devitalizing and sweeping force of the fluid wave of the douche. Thus, the vaginal douche alone cannot be considered a reliable contraceptive technique. This is so widely accepted by doctors that many interested in the problem of fertility-sterility believe that couples who have relied on the douche alone with apparent success are actually of relatively low fertility.

Barriers of one form or another that the woman placed in the vagina before intercourse were one of the earliest contraceptive devices. Sea weed and sponges soaked in vinegar were used in this manner. With advent of modern chemistry, foam powders, creams, and suppositories have been advocated for "feminine hygiene." The undesirability of some is obvious. The ineffectiveness of others is due to the difficulty and uncertainty of placing this barrier directly over the cervix. The newer creams and gels, which are dispensed with applicators, still have an incidence of failure too high to make it the technique of choice. They are recommended by marriage counselors when the diaphragm cannot be used or is unacceptable.

The condom is a mechanical barrier used by the male. This is the only technique involving a protective device used by the male, although all the natural methods are dependent on him—and his self-control. The condom is not an invention of modern times but goes back at least to the days of the Roman Empire. Today it has the most widespread use of all contraceptive devices. It is a sheath made of rubber or animal tissue worn by the male. When properly used (tested for leaks before applying and worn throughout intercourse not just before ejaculation) it is reliable— but it has some disadvantages. It is unaesthetic, it may reduce the satisfaction of normal marital relations, and most men dislike to use them. It is inconvenient, for a supply must be kept on hand because a single condom is usually used only once.

The vaginal diaphragm, pessary as it is sometimes called, is the contraceptive device recommended as most nearly fulfilling the requirements of effectiveness, acceptability, and harmlessness. When used with a spermacidal jelly or cream, it has been effective in about 98 per cent of the couples that use it. And it is likely that some of the failures in the 2 per cent are not failures of the method but rather failure on the part of the person using it, either inserting it improperly or not at all. "Taking a chance" just once may result in conception. It should not, if properly fitted, disturb the natural course of marital relationship. It has no harmful effects on either partner. It is aesthetic because the woman may insert it in privacy, and thereafter neither partner is conscious of its presence.

The vaginal diaphragm consists of a ring—usually a coiled steel spring, over which a dome-shaped sheet of rubber is attached. The ring is flexible to conform to the contour of the vaginal canal. It must be of the size to fit snugly diagonally across the depth of the vagina, that is, it covers the anterior wall of the vagina and the cervix. This means that each woman must be fitted with the proper size and taught not only how to insert it but also how to check to see if it is in place properly. A jelly or cream containing a highly efficient spermicidal agent is used on the diaphragm and is a very important part of the technique; so much so that some authorities have referred to the diaphragm as merely the agent for placing and holding the spermicidal agent in the proper location for an adequate length of time. In other words, the relative importance of the diaphragm and jelly (or cream) is a fifty-fifty proposition. Since this is a chemical-mechanical barrier, it must be left in place until it is reasonably certain that all the sperm cells are dead—six to eight hours. A douche is usually recommended at the time of removal of the diaphragm (half before and half after removal) purely for aesthetic reasons. It has no importance in the technique of contraception.

Thus, when a young woman asks her doctor, "How can I plan my family?" he will usually recommend that she be fitted with and instructed in the proper use of the vaginal diaphragm. This can be done before marriage in about 50 per cent of women without any dilation of the hymen. If the hymen is partially occlusive, and time allows, he may recommend dilatation. The doctor, after he has provided her with a diaphragm and is assured that she has mastered the technique of its use, will tell her to come back three months after marriage for a check on

Marriage 189

the size. Usually a change to a larger size is unnecessary, but if she originally required a smaller than average size before marriage, she may need a larger one.

Women often ask, "Can the diaphragm be used only at the fertile period?" The answer is "no." The diaphragm must be used at all times, and that means every time, for it takes only one time to conceive, and one can never be sure when the fertile period is. Such consistent use prevents the worry of uncertainty and becomes an accepted part of married life.

Practically all women who have not borne children can be properly fitted and can successfully use a vaginal diaphragm. The only exceptions are those with developmental defects and pelvic pathology such as tumors. Retroversion (tipped womb), contrary to the thoughts of some, does not make its use impossible. And most women can still use a diaphragm after they have had a baby—or several babies—because obstetrical care today seeks to avoid undue stretching and tearing of the birth canal, which would make it hard for the diaphragm to be retained in place. But a woman must be refitted after each child.

All the methods listed have some merit and all have some shortcomings or disadvantages. How they might be rated as to effectiveness and acceptability depends a great deal on the individual couple and their inclination as well as ability to use them correctly. Perhaps the most important single factor in the effectiveness of any kind of contraceptive is the couple's motivation—whether they really want any method enough to learn how to use it properly and to use it consistently. The report of a fairly high degree of success with some of the less effective methods and the failure with the more efficient would seem to indicate that it is not only which method is used but how carefully and consistently any method is used.

Biological Contraception

The ideal of a simple, effective, and entirely harmless method of contraception has yet to be found, but the search continues, and has turned to another entirely different approach—the biological. By this a way is sought to render one or the other of the partners temporarily infertile with some assurance that at the discontinuance of the method, fertility will return.

Recently there have been popular articles announcing the discovery of "a pill to prevent pregnancy," which is premature exploitation for its news value of this new field of basic research. The investigators had no intention of presenting their findings as a new discovery that provided the ideal method of contraception but presented them merely as a progress report.

After the chemical identity of the naturally occurring steroid hormones was ascertained, biochemists have continued their search for others of more powerful and more selective physiological activity. The synthesis of new adrenal corticosteroids has been the most fruitful and most spectacular. But there have also been many new steroids having the biological properties of the sex steroids. Among these has been one that taken by mouth has a progestational-like activity two to twenty times that of progesterone-like products, although it belongs to the testosterone group of compounds. Its most dramatic property or action is that it will prevent ovulation. (It has been used experimentally as a form of "shock therapy" in menstrual abnormalities and infertility, and was also reported in the popular press as a new drug to relieve sterility.)

This new steroid has been tested in several series of women with the results indicating a fairly high degree of effectiveness in preventing ovulation and, in turn, pregnancy. The tablet is taken by mouth daily, starting the fifth day of the cycle and continued for twenty days to the twenty-fifth day of the cycle then discontinued. Bleeding occurs two or three days later. If the medication is continued indefinitely, bleeding is also delayed. The investigators, and the drug companies who have made the product available for clinical trial, do not claim it to be the ideal contraceptive or even recommend it for that use. For one reason, the drug (and it is a drug, not a natural hormone) causes in some women such unpleasant side effects as nausea and vomiting, headache, loss of appetite, enlargement of the breasts. Another is that it is not infallible, for it must be taken every day or failure may occur. The most important drawback is the possibility of damage to the intricate hormone mechanism of menstruation with long-term use. Women who have used it for a few months have subsequently become pregnant, but no one knows what would be the effect of its use over several years. Therefore its possible application would be restricted to women in their forties who already have their families.

And even in these cases there is doubt of the physiological wisdom in interfering with normal body function.

Whereas this method has been tried in several hundreds of women, it has been tried on only a few men (mostly in jail). It has reduced spermatogenesis to the point of infertility in some of these men, but it also resulted in loss of libido (sexual urge) and potency (ability) and demonstrable degenerative changes in the cells of the testes. It is doubtful that there will be much enthusiasm on the part of investigators or the male recipients to pursue this further.

The Ideal of Contraception

The search for the ideal method of contraception and the means of making this available to the largest possible number of couples are important and legitimate facets of medical science. The significance of contraception should not be evaluated from the negative and narrow aspect, which sees as its goal merely the prevention of pregnancy, but by its higher ideal—the achievement by more couples of a happy, healthy family.

One danger of contraception to the average couple is that it will be used too long. For many reasons the time for a couple to have their babies is in the early years of marriage when they are young, because physiologically fertility is highest in the early twenties and gradually declines as the years go by. If the couple postpones the starting of a family until certain other things are accomplished, such as paying for a new car, buying a home, or getting ahead in business, there may be no end to their wants, and the day will never come when everything is propitious. Or, delaying too long, they may be faced with the dismaying fact that they are no longer able to reproduce.

Another danger in the prolonged use of contraception is the threat to the stability of their marriage. While they pursue the material gains, they are missing out on the richer human experiences. These may bring more problems but also bring greater fulfillment of their marriage—an appreciation and understanding of each other in parenthood, home, and children. The tangible proof of this is in the fact that divorce rates are lower among couples with children than among childless couples.

ACHIEVEMENT

How is the achievement of the ideals of marriage to be measured? In days gone by, when marriage was "for keeps" and divorces rare, marriage was considered successful if the couple established a home, acquired a respectable place in the community, and had the usual quota of children. Family ties were stronger then, and couples accepted their responsibility as parents in the guidance and discipline of their children and the maintenance of the home, but perhaps not always with consideration of whether or not they were also achieving their ideals of happiness in marriage. Today marriage is not always "for keeps," and we see instances of marriages that had all the outward appearance of success suddenly breaking up after one year or twenty-five years. One marriage in three today ends in divorce. The grounds are no longer the harsh realities of adultery, physical cruelty, or desertion, but by mutual consent on the vague reason of incompatibility. This may seem to be a pessimistic view of marriage, but there is a more optimistic interpretation: two out of three do not end in divorce. The important thing is not to measure achievement in terms of the number of failures but rather in analysis of the cause of failure.

These failures do not represent the couple's disillusionment with the institution of marriage. Most of them marry again or would be willing to do so if a promising opportunity presented itself. Rather, failure is based on the fact that they wanted more than they were getting from their marriage. We Americans are extremists and to a certain extent perfectionists—we want the most and the best that is to be had, and this holds for marriage as well as for jobs, automobiles, and acclaim as a nation. We want to be happy and comfortable. Some see the necessity to work for everything that is worthwhile, but some expect it as a constitutional right to enjoy without effort. The trouble comes in our concept of what is the best in marriage, what brings true happiness. In marriage, as in other areas of living, failures are the result of lack of proper qualifications—in motivation, education, or ideals.

There are reasons to question whether many young people have a strong and lasting motivation and also the necessary acceptance of responsibility. There is a strong trend, within the past few years, to earlier marriages.

This is demonstrated by the fact that over half of the women who enter marriage for the first time are between the ages of eighteen and twenty-one, and half of the men are between twenty and twenty-four. These ages were adequate for the preparation for marriage a few generations ago, when life was comparatively simple (and shorter). People lived on farms or in small towns, and individual enterprise or business was the rule rather than the exception. Then the woman was expected to stay within the home, and the husband's need for extended training or formal education to earn a living was limited. In our complex world of today, these ages are reached before either of the couple has acquired the necessary education and training to make or assure a future for themselves.

This might seem to indicate that the younger generation are expressing their independence and determination to fulfill themselves at the normal time (physiologically) for having a mate and children. A few have achieved this mature concept. However, it would seem more likely that the trend toward younger marriages is more an expression of conformity in behavior to the immature standards of the "gang"—the "thing to do because everyone else our age is doing it, and so should we." Youngsters have taken into their own hands the early recognition of the attraction between the sexes, and parents either have been unable to stop them or have abetted them. This is exemplified in early dating, mixed social activities, and even in the pre-teen-age institution of "going steady." Without guidance and direction in the use of their time along other lines, what is left for them by the ages of eighteen to twenty (ruling out sexual promiscuity, which is not acceptable to them) but marriage? In fact, there is evidence of more promiscuity in the increase in teen-age pregnancies.

The concern over what may be the effects of the trend of marriage at early ages is intensified by the fact that divorce rates are highest among the younger age groups and among those with less education.

Young people marry early not only because it is the thing to do but because it is easy to do. The responsibilities are light, and if they do not like it, they can get a divorce and try again. It is particularly true that the responsibilities have been lightened for the man, more so than for the woman. It used to be that the male accepted the responsibility in marriage of earning the living, providing a home and support for his wife and children, and he expected to stay married to the same wife. Marriage was a fateful step, a long-term commitment and acknowledgment of social and economic responsibilities. It was postponed until the couple, particularly the man, was able to undertake these responsibilities.

The man has been relieved of responsibility by many changes: Marriage is not irrevocable because of the ease and acceptability of divorce. Children are not the natural consequence of marriage because of the availability of contraceptives. He has been relieved of financial obligations by many factors so that he not only does not have to assume full responsibility of support for his family but can continue his education with assistance given by G. I. grants, scholarships, and the willingness of parents to continue the support of their married children, and of the wives to work. (And "children" is used advisedly, for most of them are playing at being grown up.) The most alarming aspect of this situation is that the girls are assuming a share of, if not the total, financial responsibility. Both husband and wife may be working, but often she stops school to work and help him through school. She gives up willingly the chance for an education, which is not only available but which she should have. This is not to blame the man or to point out his shortcomings but to lament the fact that both boy and girl are being cheated of something fine and important—the achievement of maturity to some degree to guide them in the choice of a mate and to equip them to assume the responsibilities and appreciate the significance of the meaning of marriage.

The young man is denied his age-old prerogative of being the head of his household—the provider and protector of his home and family—and every woman needs to feel the warmth and security that the respect for his assumption of this responsibility brings. This carries no implication of male dominance, which woman does not want and in most instances will not tolerate, but neither does any woman find happiness in assuming dominance herself. Moreover, in assuming the role of provider, for a time at least or in part for always, she is denied her own female prerogative —that of the care of home, husband, and children and the making of a strong family group.

But this is not the only threat to the happiness of the very young couple. When the girl stops her education at an early age, she is prepared to work only in the lower level jobs, and there she will stay. She does not have the training to use fully her capabilities, which is a great loss to herself and to society. If she is to continue to work throughout her marriage, and a large percentage will have to do so, she should have the right to work at a job which is interesting to her. It should be a challenge to her capabilities and should bring her the satisfaction of having done something worthwhile, not just routine work the only reward of which is a pay check at regular intervals.

There is still another facet in this need for a girl to continue her education, even though she never goes into the business world. She needs education to fulfill most fully the role of wife and mother. She must have some foundation for growth to continue to be a companion and helpmate to her husband as he progresses in position and experience in the world. As a mother she guides and directs her children with intelligence and knowledge as well as by mother love and instinct. Furthermore, the period in which all her time and effort will be required for running the home and caring for the children is relatively short in terms of years. She begins to have free time as the children go to school, and the job practically ends as they finish high school. She should be prepared to use this time fruitfully.

There are those who contend that failure of satisfactory sexual adjustment is the most frequent and the most fundamental cause of marriage failure. They have examined only the superficial aspects of sex and have placed undue emphasis on the importance of technique in the physical enjoyment of sex. Sex failure is the cause of marriage failure when it is an expression of immaturity. Those who marry only because of sexual attraction or infatuation are destined to disillusionment. As the novelty of conquest wears off, as desire is assuaged, there is nothing left unless there is some seed of maturity, which they have the patience to nurture. Youngsters who go into marriage for romantic love can translate this to mature married love (which encompasses a great deal more than sex) if they have the determination, try to understand their difficulties, and seek guidance which is available to them. Sex is a natural part of our being, but only a part; it can be and must be integrated into the whole. It becomes a trouble-maker by the emphasis and distortion of its meaning that our culture visits upon it.

There is another aspect to be considered, that of sexual maladjustment as a cause of failure in marriage. In a good marriage, sex is the most profound expression of giving—because both want to give of themselves to commune with each other—it is the tool of love. On the other hand, when misunderstandings occur for any reason, this mode of communication may be cut off, and they become cold to each other. Then sex becomes the tool of hostility, used to hurt.

In factual analyses of causes of divorce, difficulties have been found in many areas of disagreement that make life together no longer desirable. These include problems of finances, housing (living with one or the other's family), in-law interference, religious differences—none of which have proved to be insurmountable in mature individuals if they try to solve their problems.

The rising tide of divorce, juvenile delinquency, crime, broken homes and marriages, unhappiness in home life, and mental illness has brought into focus the need for strengthening the ties and improving the qualities in the experience of marriage. This has led to the establishment of marriage counseling agencies sponsored by churches, civic organizations, local courts, and schools. Advice and admonitions, which are available on every hand from amateurs, often do more harm than good. Advice must come from persons whose experience, training, and human sympathy equip them to see clearly and help the couple understand. No one person could possibly have all the answers. Marriage counseling agencies include doctors, lawyers, religious leaders, social workers. They counsel with the husband and wife, separately and together. They go into the home and seek to find all the areas of conflict and misunderstanding with the purpose of saving the marriage. But their aim is much more. They also seek to help couples recognize danger signals and so avoid the storms that might destroy the marriage. Ideally, they aim to prevent rather than cure. This is attained through education of young people for the career of marriage before they get too involved emotionally. Such education, as has already been stressed, is the primary responsibility of parents and should start in the home. This provides the strong foundation of ideals to which schools and marriage counseling can add factual material on the social, economic, and physiologic aspects of marriage. But there is also another responsibility of the parents: protection and restraint until the young people are able to handle the sexual aspects of their personality with responsibility, self-discipline, and understanding—that is, in a mature way.

Marriage counseling should not be restricted to dispensing facts about sex—the art of love. Those who see failure of marriage as a failure of sex adjustment would seek to correct this by giving more sex information—counseling on the technique of marital relationship. The peculiar thing is that this is offered as the "modern" approach to marriage and its problems. If we take a casual glance into the past, as recorded in the literature of other times, we find there is far more explicit data on the "art of love," meaning the technique of sexual satisfaction, and a tremendous variation in the meaning of love as related to the attraction between the sexes. There have been times when sex was ignored, as in the age of chivalry, or concealed, as in the victorian age of prudery, or flaunted, as in our jazz age a few decades ago, or considered a sin, as by our puritanical ancestors. There have been times when woman was merely man's instrument of pleasure, and her very life depended on her ability to please. There have been times of lusty sexuality when restraint was unthought of, and times of licentiousness. It would seem therefore that the technique of love is not something new that moderns must learn.

Today, we are dealing with a situation different from any previous one because there is more equality between the sexes, and the younger people see love as a partnership based on companionship and compatibility as well as physical attraction. To be a vital wife does not mean that she is an accomplished sexual sparring opponent, but a mature woman who is able to communicate with her husband—a mature man—on all the levels of their maturity.

X

PREGNANCY

WHEN DOES PREGNANCY BEGIN? At what moment is a new individual conceived? No one can ever know the exact instant that marks the beginning of the creation of a new life. The fateful event occurs at a time that is unrecognized, unproclaimed, and unrecordable. Because this is so, age is dated from birth, not from the beginning of a new life. It is true that, measured by time alone, there is a difference of only a few months. But in that short time a chain reaction is set off that transforms a single cell—a tiny dot of living matter—into a squirming, crying infant. The trigger of that chain reaction is sprung not by the physical union of the mother and father but by the union of their cells, the ovum and the sperm. This unheralded, undated beginning of a new life is called "conception" or "fertilization."

THE DRAMA OF CONCEPTION

The ovum that is to play the leading feminine role in fertilization is one of many similar cells provided by the ovary. Each is housed in a cluster of protecting and nourishing cells that constitute the follicle. Each is immature and quiescent, awaiting its turn to start on the fateful journey to seek its mate that can end only in either death of the ovum or the creation of a new life. Although each month a few of these follicles grow, and are ready to answer, only one ovum with its follicle, is singled out each month to grow to full maturity. The others achieve some degree of maturity—understudies who stand in wait and serve a useful purpose in doing so. How this selection is made we do not know. When sufficiently mature, the follicle breaks and the mature ovum is thrown out from the ovary (ovulation). It is then "on its own." This is a precarious moment for the ovum, because it has lost its connection with the ovary, which has provided it with food and shelter. It must now quickly find its mate or it will die. A perilous journey to the place of rendezvous (the Fallopian tube), which must be accomplished within about twelve hours (twenty-four at the most), lies before it, and, to make the situation more critical, the ovum has no means of locomotion. It has to depend on forces outside itself to get there. What are these forces that propel it?

The ovary is not connected directly to the Fallopian tube. There is a space between them. The crossing of this chasm is the first hazard that the questing ovum must overcome. When the follicle ruptures, there is an escape of fluid, and the ovum is carried along in the current. If it happens that the direction of the current is toward the tube, the ovum has a chance of successfully making the jump. Then the tube will help out. The end of the tube is like a hand with fingers (fimbriae) outstretched to catch it. The motion of these fingers draws the current toward it. If all goes well, the ovum is safely in the tube a few minutes after expulsion from the follicle. Undoubtedly, many times the ovum fails to make the jump. In that case, it perishes and is absorbed. In rare instances, the ovum may travel across the pelvis and enter the tube of the opposite side.

Once the ovum reaches the Fallopian tube, transportation facilities are more dependable. In the first place, the passage-way of the tube (lumen) is about the size of a bristle, so the route is laid out. Moreover, the tube is lined with secretory cells to provide some fluid and other cells that have cilia (hair-like processes) extending into the lumen. These move back and forth like paddles in water and set up a current that moves toward the uterus. The force of this current is increased by rhythmic contraction of the walls of the tubes. The ovum is borne on this current toward the uterus.

But all is not clear sailing. The tube is not like a straight water pipe with a smooth inner lining. It is more like a rubber hose, which lies in curves, and whose inner lining is cracked and furrowed. The passage way is tortuous, and its walls are thrown into many folds or wrinkles with numerous dangerous crevasses in which the ovum might become lodged. Here there is another great hazard to be met. The current may carry the ovum over the falls into the cavity of the uterus before it has been fertilized by the sperm. The ovum must be stopped here by the sperm, or it will die. The sperm therefore must reach the ovum deep in the recess of the mother's body and at just the right time.

In many ways, the sperm's journey is more difficult than that of the ovum. To assure such a meeting, nature has made two provisions: first, she has equipped the sperm cells with the power of locomotion (they swim like tadpoles); and second, whereas she sends out only one female cell at a time, she sends out many millions of male cells. At intercourse, the male contributes about one teaspoonful of fluid (semen), which normally contains about 300,000,000 sperm cells. While the ovum is the largest cell in the body—almost large enough to be seen by the naked eye—the sperm cell is the smallest. Each sperm consists of a head, which carries the life-giving elements that it will contribute to the ovum, and a long whip-like tail by which it moves, with an intermediate connecting zone. The head is small comprising only $\frac{1}{10}$ of the total length. Placed head to tail, it would take four sperm cells to reach across the ovum. It has been estimated that 2 billion sperms could be contained in a grain of wheat and 2 billion ova would be required ·to fill a thimble. From such tiny structures a new life begins!

Sperm cells are started on their race to find a mate by being deposited high up in the vagina close to the cervix, some on the cervix and perhaps a few directly into the opening of the cervix. The fluids of the vagina are slightly acid, and this acidity seems to activate the male cells—that is, to make them move faster and more purposefully—but it also imposes a penalty. If they do not get out of the acid vagina into the friendly alkaline reaction of the cervix in less than six hours, they will die—as many of them do. But millions do reach the comparative safety the uterus provides.

From the cervix the sperm must ascend through the body of the uterus and into the tube. They have to buck, with all the strength they possess, the same current on which the ovum placidly rides. This is a distance of about six inches, which does not seem far until we consider the minuteness of the cell making the journey. It is made more difficult by the folds of the lining of the uterus. It becomes a journey of up hill and down vale.

But by their rapid vibratory motion, the successful ones reach the tubes—some to the right and some to the left—in about an hour and a half. Here, if the ovum has not yet arrived, they must lie in wait for it. Time is limited for them, just as it is for the ovum. No one knows how long sperm cells can live once they pass into the uterus, but all indications are that it is twenty-four to forty-eight hours at the most. Of the millions that start only a fraction of this number reach the goal. Perhaps the hazards of the journey are nature's way of ensuring that only the strongest, most vigorous will survive to meet the ovum.

When the ovum comes into view, the swarming mass of sperms race toward it—as bees to a flower. The ovum does not necessarily accept the first sperm to reach it. By what means it makes its selection we do not know. Those that are rejected and fated to die have served a necessary purpose, for it seems that the male cell to be successful must have escorts to sanction the union. The one sperm cell, of all the millions that started the quest, becomes attached to the ovum. The head burrows through the cell wall of the ovum, losing its tail in the process, and its nuclear material blends with that of the ovum. Its portal of entry is quickly closed and the whole outer covering (cell wall) of the ovum becomes thickened so that no other sperm may enter. Fertilization has been accomplished—a new life begins.

Fertilization is the fulfillment of the biologic purpose of sex in all living creatures—the blending of the contributions of a male and a female to produce a new life. This is true whether the creature be a simple one-celled animal or the complex human being. It might help us to understand the nature and meaning of sex to consider for a moment the forces necessary to the successful union of the single male germ cell and the single female germ cell.

These two different kinds of cells do not just happen to come together. There is a powerful attraction one to the other, and there is a deep-lying mutual need that compels them to seek each other. The placid journey of the ovum might suggest that the female role is passive, while the hazardous journey of the single victorious sperm completed in competition with millions of others, might entitle it to be called the active role—its journey even a conquest. But there is nothing that suggests that either cell is superior or inferior to the other, or even that they are equal. Rather this union is an expression of mutual dependence, co-operation, blending, and contribution.

The moment of fertilization is of tremendous significance in the lives of the offspring, the father, and the mother. At that instant the fertilized ovum becomes a new life, distinct from that of either parent. From then on it follows its own predestined course of growth and development. At that moment, the father has made his sole contribution to the new life— a single sperm, one cell from millions. His part in procreation is over. Thereafter, his role is only that of an onlooker; interested, perhaps deeply concerned, but still only an observer. But the mother's role is only beginning. To her is given the duty and the privilege of nourishing and protecting the life of the developing embryo. Within her body the single cell will divide and redivide millions of times and step by step without a slip, organs will develop, the body will take form until there emerges a child—differing from all others in its potentialities, but racially resembling its parents.

This prelude to the drama of pregnancy—the expulsion and migration of the ovum, the quest of the sperm and their fortuitous union, which is conception—as it actually happens in a human has never been witnessed. How then do we know that this is the way it occurs? The outline has been drawn from facts that have been observed in the human, and the missing features filled in from the many actual observations in various laboratory animals. The changes that lead to ovulation in the human are well understood, for a wealth of material for study has been provided in ovaries removed from women by surgical operation. The appearance of the mature human ovum during its sojourn in the tube has also been established by examination of ova obtained during surgery by washing out the tubes. One such ovum was obtained on the fourteenth day of a patient's menstrual cycle and probably had been expelled from the ovary only a few hours previously. The information pertaining to the mechanism of ovulation and migration is drawn from laboratory animals. For instance, movies have been taken that magnify and reveal most vividly what happens during ovulation in a live rabbit. Here the follicle could be seen growing to maturity, breaking, the ovum floating out, and the tubes reaching out to receive it. This much of the process is probably much the same as that in the human.

The changes that occur in the ovum as it passes into the cavity of the uterus, settles down, and burrows into the wall are known facts observed in human material. Such material for the most part has been obtained quite recently by deliberate and diligent search either at the time of surgery by injecting fluid into the tubes and washing the contents (if any) toward the vagina, where it is collected for study, or by careful preparation and examination of these organs removed for other reasons (such as tumors or infections). By these methods, ova only recently fertilized and still free have been obtained as well as ova in different stages of implantation. This is a most remarkable accomplishment for two reasons. First, the chance that a woman coming to surgery has conceived in the day or week preceding is remote, and therefore many examinations and searches were destined to be failures. Second, the minuteness of the structures being searched for make the finding as difficult as looking for the proverbial needle in the haystack. The ovum in the tube and even after it reaches the uterus is hardly visible to the unaided eye and must be greatly magnified to be positively identified. The youngest implanted ovum so far obtained was less than eight days old (obtained the twenty-second day of the woman's cycle). It gave no indication of its presence other than a small indenture in the lining of the uterus hardly larger than a pinprick—and that in a velvety surface. Prior to these studies the only human material consisted of a few early ova found by chance in surgical specimens or products of early abortion.

These few early ova have yielded sufficient information to reconstruct what actually happens in the human being. The ground work for these interpretations had been laid by the vast amount of information concerning embryologic development obtained from laboratory animals including the chick, which is so accessible for study, and the monkey, which has a reproductive cycle most closely related to that of the human.

Implantation of the Ovum

Fertilization marks the beginning of a new individual, still only a single cell, which must now find a suitable place to grow, where it will be protected and nourishment will be readily obtained. As we have seen, such a haven has been prepared for it in the lining of the uterus. By the third week of the cycle, the endometrium, thick, soft, and rich in nourishing material, is ready to receive the fertilized ovum. The ovum floating through the tubes reaches the cavity of the uterus about three days after fertilization and then spends three leisurely days in settling down. Six days after conception (on the twenty-first to twenty-third day of the cycle) it attaches itself usually on the back wall of the uterus close to the top. But by this time, it is no longer a single cell.

A new kind of activity—intense and purposeful—is started within the ovum by the entrance of the sperm and the blending of the life-giving elements of each. The new cell (still called the ovum) divides and redivides, and these new cells cling together to form a ball—called a "morula" because it is said to look like a mulberry. By the time the ovum reaches the uterus, it consists of six-to-twelve cells encased in a mucilaginous covering, which makes for easy transportation. But it is not much larger than the single original cell since with each division there is reduction in size of the cells. These few small cells of the morula look alike, but they have far different destinies. Thereafter as the cells increase in number and the ovum in size, some powerful force will set each cell on its own course of specialization. Only a few cells, a small cluster within the ball, are destined to become the embryo. All the others must develop into structures fitted to nourish and protect it.

The first apparent change is the accumulation of fluid within the ball, which increases until the morula is transformed into a hollow sphere filled with fluid. This occurs at about the time the ovum is attaching itself to the wall of the uterus (the sixth day). Its walls consist of a layer of cells called the "trophoblast." Underneath this layer of cells at the pole of attachment (the point of contact) with the endometrium is a cluster of cells called the "inner cell mass." This first sac of fluid is the "yolk sac." But soon fluid appears between the inner cell mass and the trophoblast to form another cavity—the "amnionic sac."

The trophoblast is entrusted with the business of anchorage and food getting. The ovum, which is embarking on a course of prodigious growth, must have food and have it quickly and abundantly. So the trophoblast sets about its task in a ruthless way. The first thing it does is to send out little finger-like projections (villi) all over its surface. These seek out the crevices between the endometrial cells. At the same time, the cells of the villi secrete chemicals that dissolve and digest the endometrial cells. This serves to open the way for further entrance, and the tissue juices provide food that the villi absorb. By this time the fertilized ovum has burrowed deep into the succulent endometrial tissue.

The trophoblast becomes the "chorion" by the acquisition of another layer of cells and blood vessels. Each chorionic villus has a distinct structure, a solid layer of cells covering a looser core of cells. In the early villi, small blood vessels lined with only a single layer of cells, and a lumen large enough for a single blood cell to pass, are formed. The first embryonic red blood cells are formed in "blood islands" or clusters of cells within the villi, which continue this blood-forming function until the embryo has developed to the point that it can produce its own blood elements.

The chorionic villi have now dissolved endometrial gland cells and opened small venules so that each villus extends into little lakes of fluid consisting of blood elements and tissue juices. Shortly thereafter the maternal arterioles are also opened, thus adding fresh blood (containing more food and oxygen) to this pool. Meanwhile, arrangements are being made in the villi for circulation of its newly formed blood elements toward the embryo. On the seventeenth day the small blood vessels in the villi make contact with each other and begin to form continuous channels which collect the villus blood and transport it toward the embryo. Thus embryonic circulation is established. This is the basic and only contact between maternal and fetal circulation—a villus bathed in a pool of maternal blood. There is no direct connection between maternal and fetal blood. The only substances that can pass from mother to fetus are those that can go through the cells covering the villi, just as food is absorbed in the digestive tract and oxygen in the lungs. The cells of the villi seem to have a selective power, allowing some large molecules to pass through and holding back others. The transference of waste products from the fetus to the mother is also reduced to this chemical level. (Recently investigation has shown that, late in pregnancy, there may occasionally be areas in which a few fetal cells pass into the maternal blood stream and vice versa.) The connection between the mother and fetus is thus primarily anchorage, which also provides a mechanism for chemical exchange. There is never any kind of nerve connection.

By the time the ovum has burrowed deep into the endometrium and the chorionic villi are functioning, changes have occurred within the ball of cells. The inner cell mass has become a distinct plate (the embryonic plate), consisting of several layers of cells between the two cavities—the amnionic cavity above and the yolk sac below. It now has reached the stage of development or differentiation whereby all the forerunners of each of the elements of pregnancy are present.

The ovum thus so amply nourished and protected grows rapidly, and the direction of expansion is toward the cavity of the uterus. It appears first as a blister on the surface of the endometrium, then as a sac extending into the cavity, and by the third month it is the size of a goose egg that completely fills the uterine cavity. The first mechanism of supply is no longer adequate, and changes have taken place in the chorion and endometrium to meet these needs. Each has developed into two distinct structures having similar functions; the fetal membranes and decidua provide the housing, and the placenta becomes a specialized organ for fetal-maternal exchange.

Physical Components of Pregnancy

The changes that take place after implantation are directed toward one ultimate goal—the formation of the structures that are present at birth. These physical components of pregnancy are the baby (the fetus), with its bag of water (the fetal membranes and amnionic fluid), the afterbirth (placenta), to which the baby is attached by the cord (umbilical cord). How do these structures evolve from the simple little sphere implanted in the wall of the uterus?

The inner cell mass will grow and develop into the embryo by the third week; after the fifth week it will be called the "fetus." As it grows, it floats out into the amnionic fluid, but retains its attachment with the outer wall by a structure, the body stalk, which will become the umbilical cord. The molding of cells into tissues and tissues into organs while the whole takes on human form is the fascinating story of the Age of the Unborn.

The amnionic fluid, which soon completely surrounds the fetus, provides a perfect environment—a constant degree of moisture, temperature, and pressures. It allows the fetus freedom to grow and to move about as it learns to use its muscles. Later it is useful in other ways. After the fourth month the fetus drinks the fluid and takes some into the bronchial tree, thus assisting in the functional development of both the digestive and respiratory systems. This fluid world in which the fetus is submerged is not like a dead sea but rather a fresh spring, for it contains many chemical elements (protein, sugar, calcium, vitamins, and digestive enzymes), which may be useful to the fetus, and it is constantly changing. It has been demonstrated that in the latter part of pregnancy (which is probably also true from the beginning), half of the fluid is replaced each hour and a half. Where it comes from and where it goes, no one knows for sure.

The yolk sac is quite prominent in very early embryonic life, when it appears as a distinct sac attached to the under surface of the embryo. It has a very short, but probably useful, life as a source of nourishment and then disappears within the first few weeks.

The endometrium at the time the ovum is settling down is at the height of its cyclic secretory activity. It does not break down, as in the menstrual cycle, but undergoes further changes to become the "decidua." It increases in thickness and becomes more succulent with more complex glands and a richer blood supply. These decidual changes involve the whole lining for a while, but there is soon a difference between that which is under the implanted ovum and that which lines the rest of the uterus. The basal decidua becomes part of the placenta. The true decidua, which lines the uterine cavity, continues to increase in thickness until the third month, when it is about a half-inch thick. As the fetus and its membranes fill the uterine cavity, and the uterus becomes distended, the true decidua becomes compressed and thinned so that at the end of pregnancy, it is a very thin sheet.

The placenta is the exchange post between the maternal and fetal circulatory systems and therefore must consist of elements of each. The fetal portion of the placenta is derived from that area of the chorion that is directed toward the wall of the uterus. Here the villi—each with its small arteries and veins, branch and rebranch—and these blood vessels unite to form the artery and veins of the cord. The endometrium increases in thickness in the placental area to supply better attachment and provide by more and larger blood vessels a more profuse blood supply.

At birth the placenta is a thick rounded structure about the size of a layer of a cake. When it is dislodged at birth, some of the maternal tissue is torn off with it. The placenta is a most versatile organ; it serves as a means of attachment and of chemical exchange; its cells have a selective action and some digestive and elaboratory function; it has another entirely different purpose—it becomes the important endocrine gland that maintains pregnancy.

The fetal membranes are derived from that part of the chorion that covers the embryo as it bulges into the uterine cavity and the amnion, which lines this sac. As the fetus grows, this part of the chorion becomes thinned out, the villi disappear, and it loses its food-getting capacity and devotes itself to containing the fetus. When the sac fills the uterine cavity, this adheres to the decidua.

We have considered pregnancy so far only from the standpoint of the child-to-be. We have seen how a single cell, becomes a ball of cells that burrows into the lining of the uterus. Soon these cells begin to become specialized, some to be the forerunner of the baby's body—and others to be the appendages (placenta and membranes) that will provide attachment to the mother, from whence comes nourishment and protection. The force that directs the transformation of this single cell to a living, crying baby at birth comes from within the cell itself. The nature of this force, the ability to grow and develop, is a mystery we cannot fathom; we have no knowledge of it except the name by which we call it—life.

While we do not know what this life force is, we do know a great deal about the processes by which it accomplishes its purpose (which will be told in "The Age of the Unborn") and about the factors of the environment necessary to promote growth and development. The provision of this suitable environment is the mother's contribution to a successful pregnancy. What changes take place within her body to provide these needs? What is the force that directs and guides these changes?

In seeking to understand the changes that occur in the mother's body during pregnancy, a host of questions immediately come to mind. How does the uterus go about providing nourishment and protection? What prevents it from continuing its cyclic function of menstruation, which would sweep pregnancy away? How will it accommodate its structure o the expanding size of the fetus? By what mechanism does it placidly house the baby-to-be for ten lunar months and then suddenly and purposefully exert the strength necessary to expel it? How does it use its strength forcefully enough to expel and yet gently enough to do so without injury to mother or baby? What preparations are made for a birth canal, a passage that previously was in some places no larger than the lead of a pencil, and is at birth as large as a baby's head? How can all these things be done in such a way that after the birth of the baby, a return to the conditions that existed before pregnancy may be accomplished?

The changes that these questions foretell are those that occur in the reproductive system. But pregnancy affects the whole body in its demands for physical adjustment to the growing baby within. Likewise, it affects the whole personality, constituting as it does a transition period to that phase of human relationship, which, with all of its responsibilities, joys, and sorrows, is summed up in the one word "motherhood." The study of pregnancy, in all these ramifications would fill many books. However, we can get a satisfactory concept of pregnancy if we confine our discussion to three aspects: (1) pregnancy as nature directs it—physiological changes, what they are and how they are accomplished; (2) pregnancy as the woman experiences it; (3) pregnancy as the doctor supervises it.

PREGNANCY AS NATURE ORDERS IT

There are many demands the mother's body must meet to ensure a successful pregnancy. It must provide the baby with shelter, warmth, and protection from physical forces that might be harmful. All the materials necessary for life and growth must be supplied in adequate amounts, sometimes at the expense of the mother's body. A bountiful supply of oxygen must be available continuously from implantation to birth. Waste products must be eliminated. Because the fetus rapidly increases in size, there must be changes in the mother's body to give it the necessary room to grow and adjustments in her body mechanism to take care of the increasing weight that is localized in one spot. While her body is accommodating itself to the needs of the growing fetus, it must also be undergoing other changes that will allow this new individual to make its entrance into the world. When the time comes for the grand entrance of the baby, her body must supply the necessary forces to expel it through the small birth canal gently, firmly, and without harm.

Nature—the wisdom of the body—in meeting these needs by change in structure must also provide new and different levels of stability not only of the reproductive function but of every other function of the woman's body as well. Moreover, these levels of stability must be healthful to the woman during pregnancy and the changes involved temporary so that she may revert to the previous level of stability or normalcy when pregnancy is ended. The physiologic needs of pregnancy that nature must meet in this way are threefold: physical housing of the pregnancy and the building up of a physical mechanism for effective delivery when pregnancy has reached maturity; provision for the metabolic requirements of the mother's body in its new role as well as those of the developing child; and finally, an over-all control mechanism that maintains the pregnancy for the time necessary—ten lunar months.

The Housing Is Built

The housing of a pregnancy is, of course, the function of the uterus but provisions must also be made for the moving-out process at the appointed time. To serve this dual role, the uterus consists of two parts, the expanded upper two-thirds—the body; and the lower one-third—the neck or cervix.

The body with its endometrium, prepares each month for a pregnancy. When pregnancy occurs, the body must make the necessary accommodations to maintain it. At the beginning of pregnancy, the body is a small, hard, almost solid muscular organ. At the end of pregnancy, it is a large thin-walled (but still muscular) sac. It has increased its capacity five-hundred times, for within it must be room for a seven-pound baby, a one-pound placenta, and a pint of fluid. The weight of the uterus increases from one ounce to two pounds. The change in size and proportions of the uterus is not due just to stretching. There is an increase both in the size of each individual muscle cell and in the number of such cells. A similar growth occurs in the size and number of blood vessels and supporting and connective tissue. With this growth, the body of the uterus retains its function as a muscular organ, holding this activity in abeyance during pregnancy until time to bring it to full force at birth.

The cervix, on the other hand, appears to take little part as the body is growing and expanding. Even at the end of pregnancy, it has increased only slightly in size and looks like a useless appendage. But it has not been idle or uncooperative. It, too, has been undergoing changes to make it better fitted for its role. Because it has no part in either the housing or the expulsion of the baby, it has no need to increase in size. Its part is to constitute the exit from the uterus to the birth canal. In other words, during pregnancy it must serve as an almost completely closed support to the uterus and its contents, and at birth, it must open wide—it must dilate. To serve this double purpose, it becomes quite soft and spongy, and the lining thick and honey-combed. At birth the lining is swept away, and the soft swollen muscular wall is slowly stretched until the whole tube becomes just a ring around the opening of the uterus.

The vagina must serve as the passageway during birth. Its walls become thickened, swollen with fluid, and more loosely constructed so that it, too, can be easily and widely stretched. The vaginal fluid is increased in amount and is highly acid, thus providing an effective barrier to infection. The tissues surrounding the outlet (skin, muscles, and connective tissue) also become softer and distensible to allow for the stretching incident to birth.

These are the physical changes in the reproductive organs. We shall see more of their nature and purpose when we follow the process of birth.

Necessities of Life Provided

Metabolism, as we have seen previously, is the sum total of all the chemical processes of the body participated in by all the tissues and organs. Moreover, in normal metabolism, nature maintains a stability that is optimum for the welfare of the body as a whole and of each of its parts. In pregnancy, nature maintains stability at different levels to meet the needs of the mother's body with the physical changes incident to pregnancy and the needs of the growing and developing child.

The metabolic processes of the growing and developing infant are sustained by an adequate supply of oxygen and the essential nutrients and by the efficient elimination of waste products—all mediated through the mother's blood stream. As pregnancy advances, there is an ever-increasing vascularity—an increase in the size and number of blood vessels in the uterus. Stability of circulatory function is maintained by a corresponding increase in the blood itself. To keep these blood vessels, as well as those of the mother's general circulatory system, filled there must be an increase in the total volume of the blood. Furthermore, to maintain the stability of blood function, there is an increase in both the fluid or plasma and the formed elements, especially the red blood cells.

The increase in blood volume is an important change in maternal physiology. The increase on the average amounts to about one-third more blood (three pounds or six cups) in the mother's circulatory system, but this may be considerably more or less in individual cases. The importance of this is the burden placed on the heart. To keep this larger amount of blood circulating, the heart has to work harder. The heart, as all other organs of the body, has considerable reserve power, and, when normal, it is able to perform the additional work adequately and without undue strain. The stress on the heart is greatest in meeting the needs of pregnancy rather than in labor, as has been commonly believed.

An increase in blood volume alone would not be sufficient to meet the needs of pregnancy. There must also be an increase in the number of red blood cells by which oxygen—the breath of life—is carried to the placenta. The mother's blood-forming tissues are thus called upon to produce a much larger quota of blood cells (a continuous process since the life of the red blood cell is limited) in order to maintain a normal blood count.

The function of the kidneys is to filter the blood and by a selective process remove the waste products and hold back and return to the blood stream the useful chemical elements. Their work is increased by the greater volume of blood to be filtered as well as by the presence of more waste products incident to pregnancy. The kidneys therefore have to do about 50 per cent more work than usual during pregnancy.

The materials necessary for normal metabolism in pregnancy are provided by the elements of nutrition. There is no great increase in the amount of food the mother needs as measured in calories, but there is considerable change in the kinds of foods necessary. She needs more protein for the growth of the uterus and the increased blood production as well as for the growth of the child. She needs more iron for more blood, her own and the child's, and more calcium, for the baby's bones, and more vitamins. She needs these in the right amount at the right time.

The most interesting thing about the metabolism of pregnancy is the way nature assures that these needs will be met. She does not depend on a day-to-day supply as pregnancy progresses but starts early to build large reservoirs from which she may obtain the proper amount at the time it is needed. We have seen this same system as she used it in normal nutrition. Here it is extended for the nutrient requirements of two. And nature is a little partial—if there is not enough for both, the child's needs come first.

The most important fact about diet, and one that women are apt to overlook, is that the reservoirs should be filled to normal capacity before pregnancy starts. This obviates the necessity of making up a deficit at the same time the increased needs of pregnancy are being met. It also assures adequate supplies in the early weeks of pregnancy when the form and structure of the baby's body are emerging and before the woman is sure that she is pregnant.

The control of metabolism is the function of the endocrine glands. It is not surprising, therefore, to find a change in these glands during pregnancy. The thyroid enlarges to the point that swelling in the neck is obvious in most women, and the BMR is increased. The parathyroids, which control the metabolism of calcium, become enlarged to fulfill their increased function. Similarly, the adrenals become enlarged, and the anterior pituitary increases to twice its normal size. The changes in structure and function of the endocrine glands are directed toward maintaining normal metabolism at a different level to supply the needs of the mother and baby. But the actual maintenance of pregnancy resides in another endocrine gland, which evolves during pregnancy, and whose life span is the duration of this one pregnancy—the placenta and its precursors the trophoblast and chorionic villi. It is in these that we shall find the explanation for the endocrine mechanism of pregnancy.

Controls Are Established

The stage is set for pregnancy at the end of the third week of each menstrual cycle. At that time the corpus luteum is working at top speed, pouring out estrogen and progesterone, which in turn have transformed the endometrium into a succulent bed. But this is not just another menstrual cycle, for one week previously the ovum has received its mate, joined forces with it and started to grow. Now the fertilized ovum has just reached the interior of the uterus and is ready to settle down in the place prepared for it. The direction must be given that this is not just another rehearsal. The curtain is about to rise on the greatest of all dramas, the evolution of a new life. But where will the call for "action" come from?

In this crucial moment nature again shows her versatility and practicality. She calls on the ovum itself! It must supply the force that will sustain the corpus luteum. The trophoblast becomes a miniature endocrine gland that produces the necessary gonadotropins. These gonadotropins prolong the life of the corpus luteum, and the corpus luteum in turn maintains the endometrium and prevents menstruation, which would sweep the pregnancy away.

This mutual dependence of the growing embryo and the corpus luteum lasts through the first two months of pregnancy. (If the corpus luteum is removed surgically early in pregnancy, abortion almost invariably follows.) But by the second or third month the corpus luteum is no longer needed because the pregnancy's own endocrine gland, the placenta, is by then producing estrogen and progesterone in sufficient quantities to maintain pregnancy.

Ascheimm and Zondek in 1928 discovered one of the first clues to how the endocrines control pregnancy and, in doing so, gave us a reliable test for pregnancy. They found a certain substance in the urine of pregnant women, which, when injected into immature mice would stimulate their ovaries. It was therefore a gonadotropin. The questions were: Where did it come from? What was its use?

At first, investigators thought that it was the same as a gonadotropin of the menstrual cycle, which is secreted by the pituitary gland. But soon, they found that this urinary gonadotropin of pregnancy was different from the pituitary gonadotropin. They traced its origin to the placenta, and to the cells of the trophoblast, which are actively secreting long before the placenta is formed. In a pregnant woman, this gonadotropin appears in the urine very early, sometimes even before she misses a period and almost always by the time the period is two weeks overdue. It is therefore an accurate test for pregnancy, which will be positive long before the prospective mother or her doctor can be sure that a pregnancy exists. This is the basis of the Ascheimm-Zondek test and others such as the rabbit or frog tests for pregnancy.

The finding of a new gonadotropin peculiar to pregnancy did more than give the doctors a test for pregnancy. It established the fact that the placenta was an endocrine organ, that it produced hormones that were necessary for pregnancy and were thrown into the blood of both the mother and child. Further study revealed that the placenta produced not only gonadotropin, but also estrogen and progesterone in quantities much greater than are present during a menstrual cycle. By determining how the amount of each hormone varied as pregnancy progressed, and interpreting this in terms of the known physiologic properties of each, some indication of their function in pregnancy was obtained.

The appearance of gonadotropin in the mother's urine within a few days after the ovum becomes implanted indicates an early and urgent need for it. Apparently this need lasts only through the second month, because at that time the gonadotropin decreases in amount so that by the third month the level is low and remains so throughout pregnancy.

Estrogen is evidently needed in an ever-increasing amount. There is a rapid increase in early pregnancy and then a slow steady increase as pregnancy advances. Production reaches its peak just before birth and almost disappears immediately after the birth of the baby.

Progesterone is not found in the urine, but another substance (pregnandiol) derived from it is excreted in the urine and may be measured. Such tests indicate that progesterone is also produced in gradually increasing amounts throughout pregnancy and disappears after delivery.

There is thus an optimum ratio between these hormones as pregnancy advances, but it is a changing one. Since we know what kind of action each hormone is capable of, this changing ratio helps to explain the hormone mechanism of pregnancy.

The dominant role of endocrine function in pregnancy is played by estrogen and progesterone. Their interaction for the maintenance of pregnancy and their integration with other hormones for maintenance of metabolism constitute a complex mechanism. Without going into detail, we may summarize their continued and combined action as follows:

They maintain the functional life of the endometrium to meet the needs of the ovum and later the growing fetus, at the same time restraining the musculature of the uterus so the fetus will not be expelled until term. Other ovarian cycles are also suppressed, which otherwise might interfere with the course of pregnancy. They induce growth in all the reproductive organs but especially in the uterus to accommodate the expanding fetus and render the tissues of the birth canal soft and elastic so that it can be adequately dilated at delivery. They prepare the breasts for lactation and probably play some part in the onset of labor. Many theories have been advanced as to what causes the onset of labor, but the truth is we do not know why labor begins at the appointed time.

PREGNANCY AS WOMAN EXPERIENCES IT

Modern woman has emerged as an independent person who can choose whether she wants a baby and, if so when, and the important fact is that, rather proudly, she still chooses marriage and motherhood in preference to all other roles. There is a wealth of knowledge of the functions of mind and body now available to help her attain success in this role.

As an experience, pregnancy differs for each woman. Its character will be determined by her past experiences and present life situation, her attitude toward being pregnant, how much she learns, and how much misinformation she has accepted as truth. Even the physical changes that she sees and feels, while following a general pattern, are made different by individual variations.

Pregnancy is a transition period in the life of a woman to another level of maturity, that of motherhood, and as such it involves every aspect of her personality. The richness of it as a human experience, as an adventure in living, depends on the degree of maturity she brings to it. Just as she must achieve maturity as a woman on the physical, psychological, and sexual levels, so also must she achieve the true maturity and real meaning of motherhood. Nature sees to it, as a rule, that she does not undertake this adventure until she is physically ready and has assurance of a fair degree of success, but this is not necessarily the case for the psychological and sexual aspects.

The Signs Are Revealed

Nature does not announce the initiation of her most profound and meaningful endeavor with great fanfare. Rather she allows the information to come gradually by signs and symptoms. Occasionally, she is quite evasive, even deceptive. Perhaps this is her way of helping woman in her transition to motherhood—assuring her that it will be gentle and allowing her time to become accustomed to the idea. It also gives nature a chance to be sure she has made a successful start, thus saving the woman disappointment; for undoubtedly many pregnancies start, are lost, and their presence never known or even suspected.

How does the existence of pregnancy become known to woman? It depends to some extent on the woman's concern about being pregnant. She may begin to wonder days or even weeks before she has the first sign—failure to menstruate—sometimes with hope, sometimes with fear. She may skip one or even two periods without giving it a thought, or she may reject the possibility for reasons of her own. This first sign of pregnancy, the absence of menstruation, is only suggestive, not proof positive, that pregnancy is on its way. When she fails to menstruate a second time, she has good reason to believe that a pregnancy has started. There will be other signs to help confirm this.

The breasts give the second sign of pregnancy. They become swollen, heavy, and tender. There may be throbbing or pain in the whole breast and tingling or prickly pain in the nipples. Such changes are experienced by many women each month premenstrually and therefore are only suggestive. But as the weeks go by, this fullness persists, and other changes become apparent that are characteristic of pregnancy. The nipples become larger and darker. The areolar (brown area around the nipple) becomes broader and darker, and scattered through it, little white lumps about the size of a small bead appear. These changes in the appearance of the breasts persist after pregnancy is over and are therefore significant signs only in the first pregnancy. The changes within the breasts—turgescence, growth, and increased secretory capacity—are under endocrine control in preparation for lactation. The actual secretion of milk, which is withheld until the baby arrives, is preceded by a sticky clear fluid (colostrum), which appears in the early months and may increase as pregnancy advances.

Frequency of urination may afford another clue to the existence of pregnancy. It may be increased to the point that the woman is concerned that she may have a bladder or kidney disturbance. In this instance, however, it is without pain or discomfort. Increased frequency is due to the pull the growing uterus exerts on the bladder, which subsists after the third month.

These physical signs and others that appear later are but reflections of the changes and adjustments nature is arranging for the perfection of her goal—the hospitable environment for the growth of the new life. There are other symptoms that occur in early pregnancy, which are vague, variable, and unpredictable. In the past, they have been attributed to the woman's emotional reaction to pregnancy. But in the light of present-day conceptions of the interrelationship of body chemistry and physiology to the mind and emotions, they more likely represent the normal adjustment—of the soma and the psyche—to the changes and needs of pregnancy. They therefore are normal, not neurotic, symptoms. The most commonly experienced ones are morning sickness, cravings for food, lassitude, and the "blues."

Morning sickness is the symptom most women associate with pregnancy and is expressed in the frequently heard remark—"but I can't be pregnant because I feel fine." This is, of course, false information and reasoning. A woman does not have to feel sick to be pregnant, nor are nausea and vomiting necessary accompaniments of pregnancy. Many women never have these symptoms, and many feel better during their pregnancy than ever before. Morning sickness, when it does occur, may be only waves of nausea in the morning, or it may be bothersome with vomiting, and occasionally the woman is unable to retain any food. This symptom may appear as early as the second week and usually does not last more than a month or so.

The craving for foods, usually for one particular kind of food, is one of the accepted hallmarks of pregnancy. In some instances it is the reflection of the body needs, sometimes it is a whim arising from an emotional need that the woman seeks to satisfy by some unusual or exotic food. Occasionally, it is a bid for attention. Whatever its cause, there is no harm in assuaging the peculiar appetite as long as she does not allow it to interfere with her normal nutrition—which means that she does not slight the essential foods and does not eat excessively and gain weight.

Lassitude is a rather indefinable symptom that is often present in early pregnancy. The woman finds that she tires more easily with her ordinary activity. She is drowsy at times and may drop off to sleep during the day, although she has had more sleep than usual during the night. She may find it difficult to concentrate and find herself daydreaming. Within a few weeks, these symptoms disappear, and the woman is her busy, energetic self again (if that is her usual characteristic and she is meeting the physical needs of pregnancy).

"Having the blues" is the way a woman describes the moods that sometimes engulf her, suddenly and for no apparent reason. Then her feelings are easily hurt, and she may burst into tears for no apparent reason. There are moments of morbid thoughts, unaccountable depression, and foreboding. These moods are a common experience of pregnancy although most women make every effort to control and conceal them.

During the first three months the signs of pregnancy that the woman recognizes by the changes in the way she feels and functions are presumptive. After that she begins to have more positive evidence. The growth of the uterus is concealed until the third month of pregnancy, but after that she can feel it, and see it as it grows. At first it is just a little pear-shaped knob above the pubic bone. It expands to a rounded melon and then becomes oval. By the fifth month, it has reached the umbilicus, and her pregnancy becomes obvious to others. In the ninth lunar month, it seems to fill the whole abdomen, reaching up to her breast bone. A few weeks before birth, it may drop down as the baby's head descends into the pelvis preparatory to birth.

Quickening or "feeling life," is the first time the mother feels the movement of her baby, and it occurs with variation at four and a half months. At first it is only a feeble, indistinct fluttering, but eventually it is quite vigorous kicking. Of course, motion of the baby kicking its legs and moving its arms does not suddenly start at four and a half months but has been present from almost the beginning, as we shall see in "The Age of the Unborn." In the early months, because it is small, cushioned in an abundance of fluid, and its motions weak, they are not perceptible. But by the fourth month, the baby has increased so in size that its living quarters are cramped, and its motions, now vigorous, no longer escape notice.

The time that the mother "feels life" is fairly constant, but the degree of activity that she feels thereafter is variable. Some babies are very active, others quite placid, and both are normal. It has been said that the degree of activity may give some indication of the sex of the baby—that boys kick harder than girls. As this is not characteristic after birth, why should it be so before? The thumps probably are not visible to others, but they are apparent to her doctor as he examines her, and they give him some indication of the position of the baby—whether it is "lying" in the best position for a normal birth.

Pressure changes occur, as pregnancy advances, due to the weight of the pregnancy. The woman is a little less steady on her feet, walks with a different gait, and is more apt to fall. The weight of the distended uterus and its contents pressing on the pelvic brim may compress the veins of the legs and impair circulation, resulting in swelling of the feet and ankles and causing excessive varicosity of the veins, as well as pressure on the rectum and constipation—and hemorrhoids, which are also varicosities. Most of these unpleasant symptoms and resultant permanent damage can be avoided or kept at a minimum by proper prenatal care.

Weight gain is a normal aspect of pregnancy, but it does not have to be excessive or distort a woman's figure. Rather it should be only so much as will ensure that the woman's weight will return to normal after the loss incident to delivery and recovery from the changes of pregnancy. If, at the beginning of pregnancy, she is underweight, she may profit by acquiring a few extra pounds. If she is overweight, she will do well to gain less, and even lose if her doctor so advises. When she starts pregnancy at a relatively normal weight, she should not gain more than the requirements of pregnancy, about 14 to 20 pounds. The extra pounds may be accounted for in a quite definite ratio between the products of conception and the changes in the mother's body. In the first group, the baby's weight accounts for 6 to 7½ pounds, the placenta one pound, and the amniotic fluid 1½ pounds. In the second, the growth of the uterus amounts to 2½ pounds and of the breasts, 3 pounds. This still leaves approximately 7 pounds that are due to: increase of her body fluids, 4 pounds, and her stored proteins, 3 pounds.

One of the interesting signs of pregnancy that women quite naturally dislike are striae and pigmentation. Striae are the lines that appear on the abdomen, breasts, and thighs. They are at first red, later become white, but remain after pregnancy. They give the impression that the skin has been stretched beyond its endurance and has given way along these lines. The interesting thing about them is that some women have them, and some do not, irrespective of the size of the baby or the mother's weight gain, and that there is nothing much that can be done about them. Keeping the weight within normal range, proper support of the abdomen and breasts, and massaging with a cream or oil may help a little but will not prevent them.

These are the same markings that appear in girls during adolescence, particularly of the breasts and thighs. They are also typical of adrenal over-activity in Cushing's disease and adrenal hyperplasia. It would seem, therefore, that striae have their origin in the glandular mechanism of pregnancy, rather than mechanical stretching.

A dark brown discoloration due to excessive deposit of pigment, usually containing iron, appears in certain areas. The nipples and areolar of the breast become larger and more deeply pigmented, and a dark line extends downward on the abdomen from the umbilicus to the pubis. Splotchy brown areas appear on the face and neck. This increased pigmentation, associated with adrenal hyperplasia, usually disappears after pregnancy.

Bright red spots, which are not due to pigment but are dilated blood vessels, may also disconcertingly appear on the face, neck, and upper parts of the body. These are thought to be due to increased estrogen levels. They too disappear.

Prelude to Adventure

Pregnancy announces itself to woman's family and friends by subtle changes that are apparent long before her silhouette takes on the characteristics of pregnancy. There is a certain fullness about her face, her complexion has an inward glow, a heightened color, and her eyes have a dreamy look, with a new spark of happiness, a new depth of contemplativeness, perhaps even a sadness or far-away look. Her actions and moods are exaggerations of her usual self. The reason for these changes is not hard to fathom. Pregnancy is an adventure in living, participated in not just by reproductive organs, but by the whole body and not only by the physical self but the total personality. This adventure is directed and co-ordinated by the systems of control—the endocrine system and the nervous systems.

These subtle changes might be summarized by saying that she becomes "ultra-feminine." They occur because from early pregnancy her body is literally flooded with the female sex hormones, and it cannot help but respond to their beneficent and feminizing influences. And emotionally she could never have more reason to be conscious of her femininity. These are changes over which she has no control. But the effect these changes will have on her total personality depends entirely on her and her emotional reaction to her pregnancy, which is the prelude to woman's greatest adventure—becoming a mother. As with any other human adventure, whether it is planned or a turn of fate, she may anticipate it with joyful exuberance, quiet determination, serious dedication, reluctance, or open rebellion, according to her particular personality as well as to what the outcome of the adventure will mean to her life. With the realization that there is no turning back, come the emotional reactions that humans almost always experience as they face the unknown—doubt and fear.

Fear is a normal component in any situation in which the outcome is as yet undetermined. It is nature's way of ensuring that we recognize that danger lurks in some form or another. The soldier experiences it before battle, the patient before surgery, the actress before opening night of her play, and the student before examination. The fear experienced is in proportion to the threat the unknown holds, whether it refers to bodily harm to one's self or another or failure in an enterprise. The important thing is not fear, but how it is met. It should be met with knowledge, confidence, and courage.

What and how much does a woman fear in pregnancy? Not any one thing and not to any certain degree. She may have fear for her own life and health, that her baby will be abnormal, that she may lose her pregnancy, that she is inadequate to care for her baby. These are old and common fears that women may have had according to the superstitions and misinformation of their times. Modern woman may have these and new ones added by the current misinformation she has acquired as to danger to her unborn from such things as the Rh factor, heredity, measles and other infectious diseases or irradiation. She may question her own ability to perform as a woman should in "natural childbirth," fear that she will not be adequate to the psychological demands of the "child-parent" relationship, or that the coming of the baby will offer too great a complication to her life situation as a modern woman.

Most of these causes for fear will be absent in a normal woman who is happy in her marriage, wants her baby, and has enough knowledge of pregnancy to discount myths, superstitions, and misinformation, and, equally important, who places herself under the guidance and care of a doctor in whom she has confidence. Doubt comes in every adventure of significance. Sometimes we have worked and planned for something we have wanted very much, but when its attainment is in sight, we have doubts and misgivings. Similarly, there are times in this prelude to adventure that a woman doubts that she wants this particular adventure—this having a baby. Psychologists call it rejection and tell us that it happens so frequently it may be considered a normal part of the emotional reaction to pregnancy. It is a passing reaction, which a woman should recognize for what it is. It is not a reason for feeling guilty or ashamed.

"Lady-in-Waiting" or "Mother-To-Be?"

Certainly woman has sufficient reason to be conscious of her femininity —her femaleness—as the months of her pregnancy pass by. It is expressed in different ways as she passes through the various stages. There is the first period of waiting to be sure that she is pregnant, then her baby-to-be becomes a reality, her unborn sheltered by her own body as she feels life. In the last phase, she awaits the arrival of her baby. What do these mean to her? Do they make her a "lady-in-waiting" or a "mother-to-be?"

She is a lady-in-waiting if she devotes herself to the material and physical aspects of her pregnancy. Too often pregnancy is depicted as a wonderful experience only because of the attractive clothes that are designed especially for her or the showers of gifts for herself and the baby. The success of her role is too frequently measured in terms of the attention she pays to the physical aspects—her diet, her rest, her exercise, what she must do and must not do, knowledge of the physical changes in her body, acquaintance with hospital procedure and delivery rooms. Like all other ladies-in-waiting, if she accepts this as her role in pregnancy, she will be only the attendant, who goes through the motions of the ceremony, but never receives the crown—the true meaning of motherhood.

She is a "mother-to-be" if pregnancy truly serves as a transition to another phase of mature womanhood—that of being a parent. The mere physical experience will not magically change her, nor the "maternal instinct" endow her with the qualities necessary for successful motherhood. These she will attain by understanding the meaning and assuming the responsibilities of being a mother.

In the pageantry or adventure that is to follow, she will not play the single star role, although in the prelude she holds the spotlight. She is co-starred with and happily, graciously accepts equal billing with the father and the child. There will be two themes to this story, intertwined and mutually dependent, of the making of a happy family: one how husband and wife become parents, and the other how the child achieves its independent personality with knowledge of itself and the world about it. In this prelude, we see her as a mature woman, married for love, to whom the coming of a child, desired by both husband and wife, is the expression of that love and fulfills the true man-woman relationship—the creation of a family. This is only another way of saying that she is advancing to another stage of her sexual maturity.

It is important to hold on to this concept of sexual maturity. It is a mistake to try to reduce any human experience to the purely physical. To stress this importance, we shall recall the meaning of emotional and sexual maturity and apply this to pregnancy. Sexual maturity, as we have said, requires the acceptance of being a woman, as well as the experience of physical function. Here, she accepts pregnancy as her part of a partnership with her husband, and does not reduce it to its purely physical components. She does not make pregnancy a mysterious business in which he has no part, but neither does she expect or try to make pregnancy mean the same to him that it does for her. She does not blame him for her condition, nor use it as a reason for making excessive demands. She shares with him her plans for a successful pregnancy—her hopes, her dreams, and together they begin to learn the meaning of parenthood and to prepare to assume their responsibilities as parents.

The physical fact of bearing a child does not assure the sexual maturity of motherhood, which is loving and giving of herself as she meets the responsibilities to her family as a mature woman. She will not look on the child as a gift or possession to satisfy her needs, but as a person with its own rights whom she will care for during its age of helplessness, and guide, teach, and allow to learn by experience. She will neither reject it nor be overwhelmed by the responsibility, nor yield her own rights as an individual. She will not seek to dominate the child, but neither will she allow it to dominate her.

To play the role of mother-to-be successfully in terms of the welfare of the child, herself, and her family relationships, there are certain attributes woman must have, certain responsibilities she must meet. She must be realistic, she must be informed, and she must obtain adequate prenatal care.

First, a woman should be realistic about her pregnancy. A young woman having her first baby may be thrilled with the experience and may believe that it somehow sets her apart as deserving of special consideration. She is encouraged in this belief by the popular articles, books, and frequent discussions among women on the joy that is supposed to be hers in pregnancy and delivery if the "natural method" is followed. She may envision a doting husband, a doctor at her beck and call to soothe and encourage, and a circle of family and friends who stand in awe at the miracle of motherhood. But she should remember that pregnancy and birth, miraculous as it is as a performance of nature and as wonderful as it is to her as a person, are the common experience of more than four million other women each year in the United States.

It is the duty of doctors and medical personnel to see that woman has a healthy pregnancy and help her have a happy one. They are wholeheartedly sympathetic to her needs and devoted to her welfare, but ecstasy is not their business. Husbands, family, and friends have to carry on their daily lives in an ever-increasingly complex world. The mother-to-be must be realistic, therefore, and considerate, although also expecting consideration, especially from the two who will be most closely associated with her in the adventure of pregnancy, her husband and her doctor.

There is much being said about child-parent relationship. As applied to the father, it is recommended that he participate in his wife's pregnancy, labor, and delivery. This is not necessary, or an advance in human relationships or even something new. There is a custom among primitive people called "couvade" in which the husband must behave as if he were having the baby and should conduct himself in the prescribed manner to ensure a successful delivery. Injury to him is expected to cause abortion.

We have recognized that women are individuals, that no two are alike, and no two will look on pregnancy with the same feelings. Husbands are individuals too—male individuals—and the same may be said for fathers-to-be. Not much is ever said about what constitutes a mature man. No books on the First Sex, the Found Sex, The Way of All Men, have been written as companion volumes to those on women. The Seven Ages of Man is only a short poem, or part of a play, written a long time ago, and not very enlightening or complimentary. Aggression, domination, and strength are the characteristics that are extolled. The attributes that we have described for a mature woman are not specifically feminine, and the world would undoubtedly be better if man too were urged to subscribe to them. But it is folly to expect a man, especially the young husband and father-to-be, to have the same kind and degree of interest in female physiology, even of pregnancy, that a woman does. A husband may be interested, deeply concerned, and proud of his wife in her pregnancy and his prospect of being a father, but rarely is the impact of parenthood felt until he sees his offspring and becomes a father in reality.

This concept of having the male participate in the physical aspects of pregnancy is one of the ways of trying too hard to level out the sexual differences, which goes along with the effort to make women more aggressive—"sexually responsible"—and have men assume feminine responsibilities. And with this there is an attempt to measure the depth of emotion —the mystery of love—in terms of physical intimacy and knowledge. This is wrong—each has a part to play, and each should respect and appreciate the other's performance while giving force and character to his or her own role. But it is woman's function to have the baby.

Woman Needs To Be Informed

There are those who say that pregnancy and childbirth are natural processes and that there is no need for woman to have scientific information as to the mechanisms. Certainly there is no doubt that woman has borne babies long before she (or those attending her) knew very much of what was happening to her. Perhaps she fared well in the dim past when life and culture was at its simplest level and she began to exercise her reproductive function as soon as she reached physical maturity. But time has changed this. Her culture became more complicated and her life no longer a particularly "natural" one as her physical health and vigor were reduced by inadequate diet and lack of exercise, and her attitude confused by the lore of misinformation. Then childbirth, under the care of equally misinformed attendants, became the valley of death into which she descended and from which many did not return. Now doctors know how to make pregnancy and childbirth safe and what contributes to making it happy. Woman needs to share in this information so that she may do her part.

There is no doubt that most women want to know. The question is how much? The answer must be given in terms of time. Ideally, a woman should learn the facts of her own body structure and function as she is growing up and as these facts have significance to her. She should have learned how to maintain a high degree of health. In this way she is ready physically and emotionally for pregnancy. Even with this background she will appreciate further information when these facts have more personal meaning as she experiences the changes incident to her own pregnancy.

Unfortunately, few women have such schooling in physiology, nutrition, and hygiene and enter pregnancy quite innocent of any knowledge of the mechanisms of the experience that is about to be theirs. Realizing this, most obstetricians for some time have supplied the patient with a synopsis of the epic of pregnancy, which includes signs and symptoms, do's and don'ts, and a list of the danger signs. She gets other information in bits and pieces that frequently overemphasize the spectacular. This is like offering her a book review (which may be biased) and denying her the pleasure of leisurely reading the whole book, assimilating the message, and savoring to the fullest the skill and artistry of its execution.

Recently there has been a move to give women more information about pregnancy and childbirth by group activity—lectures, demonstrations, movies, and discussions, which most doctors consider are helpful, and which most women welcome. There are, however, certain dangers that must be recognized. The woman gets a distorted idea of the importance of pregnancy as a training period, making too great a production of it at the expense of her responsibilities of everyday living. She thus becomes so preoccupied with being pregnant that she slights the lifetime business of being a person. Or she may see pregnancy as a training period such as an athlete undergoes for the expert performance of some physical feat. Since she is not an athlete, she may interpret childbirth not as a normal physiological activity that she is capable of attaining by her own limited physical endowments but a contest only for one of championship caliber. Or having acquired a certain number of facts as to the usual course of pregnancy, she is led to believe that she knows all the answers and may be disturbed by her own variations within the normal, which do not conform to the average. When such training is presented as an elaborate ritual to overcome fear, she is led to believe that pregnancy and childbirth, which she had previously accepted as a normal experience, really must be something to be afraid of.

There is a minimum of information that every woman should have. She should understand and practice the rules of good hygiene, physical and mental, and proper nutrition. She should understand what are the normal changes to be expected in the way she feels and functions, partly to allay apprehension, but primarily to differentiate them from the abnormal. Above all, she must know that she should have medical care not just for delivery but from the beginning of pregnancy.

PREGNANCY AS THE DOCTOR SUPERVISES IT

It is safer now to have a baby than it has ever been at any time in history. Woman no longer need face pregnancy as an ordeal through which she must descend into the "valley of the shadow of death" to create life. Suffering and pain, as well as peril to her life, have been made the exception rather than the rule for pregnancy. This is because the doctors have made it so. It is the result of modern doctors' concept of the "Art and Science of Obstetrics" and the rigidly high standards they require of those who would practice it.

The Art and Science of Obstetrics

The art of obstetrics has been given meaning in the doctors' recognition of and accordance to childbearing the dignity that it deserves. It has as its purpose not only a healthy pregnancy for mother and baby but also a happy mother. The obstetrician in practicing his art recognizes that each mother-to-be is an individual, a personality of mind and body, both of which are important. He gains her confidence by his sympathetic interest and understanding of her problems and by making her feel that he regards her as a person as well as a physical body in the process of reproduction. He removes her fears, partly by instruction, but more by impressing on her that he has the ability and the determination to see her safely through her pregnancy. Some of this art is as old as we know human institutions to be. The midwife through the ages was able to give woman some help with her herbs and brews. She undoubtedly contributed a great deal in the comfort she gave by her soothing presence, sympathy, and desire to help.

For a while, in modern times, with the advent of the science of obstetrics, the art was in danger of extinction. As doctors learned how to relieve suffering with anesthetics and analgesics, to recognize and avoid the dangers of pregnancy, and to expedite delivery by manipulations and surgical procedures, they almost forgot, in their scientific zeal, that they were seeing a human being through what should be a richly rewarding experience, but which could be a prolonged nightmare of anguish, dread, and fear. Woman was tested, measured, dieted, and exercised through her pregnancy. Delivery was accomplished almost as a surgical procedure would be—under deep analgesia. Nature's part was ignored to the point that the doctor might decide when birth should occur and induce labor to suit his convenience.

Then suddenly some doctors became impressed by the fact that woman has a mind and emotions as well as a body. The pendulum was in danger of reaching the opposite extreme. Natural childbirth (childbirth without fear and pain), rooming-in (to foster mother love), early ambulation, child-parent relationship became the vogue. In their zeal of new discovery, they forgot that these practices of psychosomatic obstetrics had been all that women had until just recently, and that they had not been good enough.

But with the swings from one extreme to the other, the majority of obstetricians, whose work was dedicated not to a method or a theory but to the welfare of a human being in a human experience, quietly maintained a middle course. In their creed pregnancy and labor are a physiologic process in which nature needs the doctor's supervision and help. Every patient is an individual whose needs, physically and emotionally, are different. A woman's pregnancy and delivery must be planned and guided according to her needs. What is good for one is not necessarily good for another. Each of his patients merits not only his medical skill but his human understanding.

Obstetrics as a science is one of the youngest of the medical specialties. It is only in the past thirty or so years that the medical profession has conceded that woman needed medical supervision during her pregnancy, that doctors should have special training and experience to see her safely through her pregnancy and delivery, and that a hospital is the safest place to have her baby.

At the turn of the century the general practice was for the woman sometime during her pregnancy to notify the family doctor that she was pregnant, and he duly recorded her "time" in his little book so that he would be available. When labor started, a midwife might be called in or another woman, and the doctor arrived in time for delivery. Sometimes reliance was placed solely on the midwife, and the doctor, if one could be found, was called only in case of emergency. The only analgesia was a whiff of chloroform, often administered by the husband in the final stages of labor. What a contrast with modern prenatal care and the modern maternity sections of hospitals with their labor rooms, delivery rooms, recovery rooms, nurseries, and the care afforded by doctors, anesthetists, nurses, and many other trained personnel. How has this vast change been accomplished? Why? And by whom?

We take our modern world for granted—the scientific and technological advances that have removed much of the suffering and drudgery of life and opened vistas undreamed of a generation or so ago. We expect and demand more and better, which is right since it makes for progress. But we should be sure that the more is better. We should also pause once in awhile to be thankful for what we have and be grateful to those who made it possible. Nowhere in our modern world is this illustrated better than in medicine and the specialty of obstetrics.

Suppose we go back a century. To say a hundred years ago does not mean much unless we can visualize what people were like then, how they looked, how they lived, and loved, and died. This we can do, for we have abundant information supplied by the avalanche of novels and biographies, movies, TV, and radio stories of the antebellum days. General Lee's wife, President Lincoln's wife, and Scarlett O'Hara have become real people to us and their lives quite romantic. Ideologically they do not seem very different from women today, for they too had the right to life, liberty, and the pursuit of happiness. But medically speaking, they lived in the dark ages, which reduced their chances for the exercise and enjoyment of these prerogatives.

In those days a doctor's training was one year in a medical school or a year or so "reading medicine" with another doctor, and even that provided little scientific knowledge they could use to alleviate suffering and prolong life. Often the treatment was more harmful, such as purging and blood-letting, than helpful. The cause and nature of infection were unknown. Doctors spoke of "laudable pus" because they considered it a necessary part of the healing process. Hospitals were few, and in many instances the care they provided was of dubious benefit to the patient. Childbed fever, usually fatal, was rampant because doctors did not know that it was caused by infection they themselves were transmitting from one patient to another. Anesthesia was unknown. Operative deliveries,

Caesarean section, and abdominal surgery were performed with the woman conscious of every pain, slightly dulled perhaps by repeated swigs of brandy, until the torture exceeded her ability to endure, and she fainted away. It was not easy or romantic—a woman's life in those days.

The high standards of medical care we enjoy today have come to us not through writs legislated by Congress or by the people's declaration of their rights. It has come through the dedication of their lives, by comparatively few doctors and other scientists, to the pursuit of knowledge and its application to human suffering—often in spite of ridicule and opposition of their colleagues and adverse public opinion. Lister (1864), who gave us antiseptics, and Semmelweis (1858), who attributed childbed fever to "something" foreign to pregnancy that could be avoided if doctors would only wash their hands in a solution of chloride of lime, are well-known examples. So the truths of medical science, gradually at first but with breathtaking rapidity of later years, have been discovered.

The rigid enforcement of these standards originated and still rests within the hands of doctors. It was they (1910) who set the standards that our medical schools and hospitals must meet to be accredited. It was they who were instrumental in having laws passed to require a doctor to present his credentials of training and to pass an examination to secure a license to practice medicine. Before that anyone could call himself a doctor and prescribe and treat patients.

Obstetrics came into its own as a respectable and necessary specialty as a result of the dedicated endeavor of a few men, some of whom are still living. By their efforts, the teaching of obstetrics in medical schools and hospitals was broadened and improved, the necessary qualifications by graduate and hospital training for obstetrics as a specialty, and standards of obstetrical care and supervision thereof in hospitals were specified. We now have the American Board of Obstetrics and Gynecology, the American College of Obstetricians and Gynecologists, numerous local maternal and child welfare boards and obstetrical boards, all of which are devoted to one aim—the welfare of woman in relation to her childbearing function.

According to these concepts of good obstetrics, the doctor likes to start his care of the patient early in her pregnancy. This allows him to take stock of her assets and liabilities of physical health, to plan her pregnancy with her. As the months go by, he checks her progress, guiding her as problems arise, and is ever ready to meet any emergencies. By such prenatal care the groundwork is laid for her safe delivery of a healthy baby.

The Doctor Takes Stock

A young woman who considers herself quite healthy might think she has nothing of significance in the way of a medical history and certainly nothing that would be important to her pregnancy. She might even think it is unnecessary nosiness on the part of the doctor to ask her questions she considers entirely personal. Medical history, however, is one of the most important means a doctor has of evaluating her ability to have a good pregnancy and a healthy baby. From it he is able to make a tentative list of her assets and liabilities, which he will verify by a physical examination and laboratory tests.

What has her family history to do with her pregnancy? The woman would probably answer little or nothing, but the doctor finds it very important. There are only a few, rarely occurring, abnormalities that are truly hereditary, that is, passed from one generation to another, such as hemophilia. But there are some medical problems, fairly common, that have a familial incidence. If she has none of these, that fact goes on her list of assets. If, on the other hand, some are noticed in her family history, they may be potential liabilities.

Past illnesses, like other unpleasant things, might best be forgotten except in a medical history. Some illnesses can have an important bearing on her ability to have a normal pregnancy. Any disease which might have affected the heart, as rheumatic fever, or the kidneys, as in scarlet fever, are especially important because the two organs will have an extra load to bear during pregnancy and delivery.

A woman might think her age is her own business and that it is her privilege to fib about it if she can get away with it. But she probably could not fool her doctor anyhow, and age is important in pregnancy. It is not as important as it was once believed to be and as many women still fear it to be. It is true that the twenties are the best age to start having babies, but it is no more dangerous to have a baby after thirty-five than before. The course of pregnancy and the mode of delivery may be different, but it is not necessarily more dangerous.

Habits of every day living take on a new importance during pregnancy. They too become either assets or liabilities. If the patient already has good eating habits, that is to her credit, but if she has been careless about her diet she must now establish new habits of eating. If she smokes and drinks too much, it will be necessary for her to learn moderation. If she is an avid sportswoman, she will have to be satisfied with the more leisurely sports. If her most strenuous exercise is an occasional stroll to the corner grocery, she must make an effort to get out of doors more and really take brisk walks. If she has been careless about her rest and has driven herself beyond normal endurance, she will have to slow down and have adequate and regular rest.

The menstrual history is important to the doctor in evaluating the woman's glandular status. If her periods started at the normal time and were regular in occurrence and amount of flow, the doctor would feel that in all probability her endocrine glandular mechanism was normal, stable, and capable of meeting the demands of pregnancy. If, on the other hand, she had been late in starting, her periods were irregular and either scanty or profuse, and her pregnancy took months to achieve, the doctor would be alerted for other evidence of glandular instability especially of the thyroid, because he knows that glandular deficiencies often are the cause of miscarriages. The date and character of the last menstrual period affords the means of dating the onset of pregnancy and estimating the date of confinement.

This taking of the medical history has served a double purpose. It has given the doctor valuable information of the patient's physical potentialities for a normal pregnancy, and it has established a personal contact between the doctor and the patient. The doctor will know what kind of patient he has to care for, whether she is intelligent and can be expected to follow directions, flippant and careless, or a chronic complainer who expects to "enjoy ill health" in pregnancy and will try to make everyone else suffer for it. He will know her attitude toward pregnancy. If it is good, he can help her keep it so. If she is fearful, resentful, or rebellious, he has months to help her accept her pregnancy with confidence and happiness. The patient is also helped by this first consultation if it gives her confidence in the doctor whereby she is assured that he is someone who is interested in her as a person, and who is both willing and capable of taking care of her.

This getting to know each other makes the physical examination easier and more meaningful to both the woman and her doctor. She will be more relaxed and co-operative, and he will be alerted to follow up any of the suggestive findings in her history.

The purpose of the physical examination of the obstetrical patient is different from any other pnysical examination, for the doctor seeks not only to determine whether the woman is in good health but also whether her body is sturdy enough in both structure and function to meet the added stress and strains that pregnancy will impose on it. He must also take measurements of her pelvis to see if it is large enough for a normal birth. He must make a very careful and thorough search for any abnormalities, that might be detrimental to either the woman's health or to the success of her pregnancy.

There are two simple facts of her physical health that he will note because they will serve him as indicators of the normal progress of pregnancy. These are her weight and her blood pressure.

It is very important that a woman be of normal weight to start with and that she maintain it within normal limits through her pregnancy. Excessive weight is always a burden to the body and becomes a greater one with pregnancy. In fact obesity becomes a hazard in both pregnancy and delivery. If the woman's weight is normal for her height, she will be told how much she will be allowed to gain during her pregnancy. If she is overweight the allowable weight gain will be less, and the doctor may have her lose weight during her pregnancy. Underweight must be accounted for and corrected, as it is usually an indication of malnutrition. Weight will also be an important guide to the patient's well-being throughout pregnancy. Loss of weight is usually due to faulty habits of eating and rest. It may be from a more serious cause. Rapid gain in weight may be from overindulgence, but it may be a danger signal of impending toxemia.

The blood pressure is of especial importance because it not only reflects the condition of her heart and blood vessels but the efficiency in kidney function as well. A sudden rise in blood pressure may also be a danger signal of poor kidney function and toxemia.

The evaluation of the ability of the heart to withstand the stresses and strain of pregnancy is of utmost importance. In 98 per cent of pregnancies there is no heart complication. With close supervision and adequate therapy and with the co-operation of the patient, most women with heart trouble can be carried safely through their pregnancies.

The pelvic examination has a threefold purpose. The first purpose is to establish the diagnosis of pregnancy and to estimate the probable duration of it. The second purpose is to detect abnormalities, if present, such as ovarian cysts, fibroid tumors, and infections that might give trouble. The third purpose is to measure the bony pelvis. This is a solid ring of bones that must be large enough to allow the baby to pass through. If it is found to be of abnormal shape or inadequate measurements, the doctor will make his plans for the handling of delivery that will ensure greatest safety to both mother and child.

When the obstetrician assembles the information he has obtained by the medical history and the physical examination, he should have a pretty good idea of the woman's chances for a normal pregnancy. There are still, however, a few more things he must know. This information he can obtain by laboratory procedures.

Urinalysis is a simple procedure as far as the woman is concerned, and one which will become almost second nature to her as pregnancy progresses, for each time she goes to see the doctor, she must carry her little bottle. To the doctor it is an invaluable guide, for by it he is kept informed of the efficiency of her kidney function. He is warned of impending toxemia by the appearance of albumin in the urine. Diabetes shows up as sugar in the urine. Pyelitis (infection of the kidney), one of the complications of pregnancy, causes pus in the urine.

The blood is examined for several things. A count is made to see if anemia is present, a blood test (Wasserman) is made for syphilis, and the blood may be typed for two reasons: Transfusions are frequently used at the time of delivery as a precautionary measure, occasionally as a life-saving measure, so it is important to know her blood type. The second typing is for the presence of the Rh factor.

Rh Factor

The discovery of the Rh factor and the understanding of its significance in pregnancy has added another means of making pregnancy safer for the mother and saving the lives of babies that otherwise would have been lost. Had this knowledge remained merely another tool in the hands of physicians, used to increase the percentage of successful pregnancies—healthy and happy mother and baby—it would have been all to the good. Unfortunately, the Rh factor and erythroblastosis caught the fancy of popular medical writers seeking the spectacular, and the condition has been publicized widely. Women have acquired a distorted and exaggerated concept of its frequency and significance. It has become, therefore, a basis of fear of pregnancy or fear of having an abnormal child, a fear completely unwarranted.

Many doctors do not have Rh determinations made routinely since there is only one chance in six hundred pregnancies that there will be complications arising from the Rh factor. There is nothing abnormal about the Rh factor itself. It is a normal part of the blood in 85 per cent of people. When a woman's blood is found to be Rh positive (contains the Rh factor), there is no possibility of trouble. It is only when she is Rh negative that a potential danger exists, but even then only if her husband is Rh positive.

How is it that a substance that in itself is a normal part of the body can cause disease? It can do so because it sets in motion the body defense mechanism called the antigen-antibody reaction. This reaction is also the same means by which we become immunized to disease. For example, a person has one of the infectious diseases, as scarlet fever, and thereafter will not contract it a second time. The germ of scarlet fever is a foreign substance (antigen) against which the body must set up defenses. This it does by manufacturing specific antibodies that will neutralize or destroy the particular antigen. It takes time for the body to build up an adequate supply of antibodies, but once they are produced, they remain a fixed part of the body (of the red blood cells). So the next time the body is exposed to this antigen (in this case a germ) the antibodies are ready and prevent the germ from causing disease.

But what can this have to do with pregnancy? Rh is not a germ, so how does it come to play a part in the antigen-antibody reaction? To answer these questions, let us see what happens in a blood transfusion (a condition in which a large quantity of antigen may be introduced into the blood stream at one time). If a woman whose blood is Rh negative is transfused with Rh positive blood, the Rh factor is an antigen, and she will build up antibodies to it. This is a slow process so that with the first transfusion there is little or no bad effect. If she is transfused a second time at a later date, even years later, she then has a good quantity of antibodies. The antibodies attack the transfused red blood cells which causes a reaction as chills and fever or even more severe symptoms. Now to translate this to pregnancy.

The Rh factor is a hereditary characteristic. If the father is Rh positive, this may be transmitted to the baby, and the baby's blood will be Rh positive. If by any chance some of the baby's red blood cells pass over into the mother's blood, which is Rh negative, the reaction is the same as what happened in the transfusion—her blood builds up antibodies to the baby's blood cells. And again if these antibodies get back into the baby's blood, they will destroy the baby's red blood cells. There are a lot of "ifs" here, and they are important because they represent things that may not happen—and thus reduce the possibility of trouble. There are still other elements that further reduce that probability. Normally there is no mixing of mother's blood and baby's blood in the placenta. But occasionally, toward the end of pregnancy, the walls of the villi and of their tiny blood vessels, which separate the blood of mother and baby, may become weak and allow some of the baby's cells to get into the mother's blood. If this happens, the mother's blood may build up antibodies. But here again it is done slowly so that not enough are built up in the first pregnancy to cause any trouble. It takes more than one pregnancy to build up antibodies in sufficient quantities to be harmful to the baby. It probably never happens in most cases, for some women never build up antibodies, and so have two, three, four, or five normal babies. The probability is further reduced by the fact that because a father is Rh positive, it does not mean that the baby has to be Rh positive also. The chances are that one out of four of his children would be Rh negative.

Erythroblastosis is the name applied to the condition or disease in the baby that results from Rh factor incompatibility. It gets its name from a peculiar type of red blood cells in the baby's body (erythroblasts). In this pregnancy the mother has been sensitized by previous pregnancy or transfusion and has built up antibodies. Antibodies are much smaller than blood cells and can pass through the villi walls into the baby's blood stream. They destroy the baby's red blood cells, and the baby becomes anemic. The liver and spleen in trying to remove this debris, which consists largely of pigment from destroyed red blood cells, work overtime and become enlarged. But even so the liver cannot do a complete job, and the pigment shows up in the baby as jaundice. To compensate for the anemia, many immature red blood cells (erythroblasts) are thrown into the blood stream. If the reaction has been severe, the baby dies before birth. In less severe cases the baby is quite anemic and jaundiced.

The treatment of this disease is primarily by transfusion of the newborn, using Rh negative blood, which the mother's antibodies will not destroy. This is accomplished by exchange transfusion whereby small quantities of the baby's blood are alternately withdrawn and replaced by a comparable amount of Rh negative blood. Research is being directed toward finding a substance that will neutralize the mother's antibodies before birth. Laboratory scientists are able to measure the amount of antibodies the mother is producing during pregnancy, and when they increase rapidly in the latter part of pregnancy, the doctor may decide to induce labor prematurely in an effort to save the life of the baby.

What are the chances of a couple in which the woman is Rh negative and the man Rh positive to have normal children? The chances are extremely good. In 90 to 95 per cent of such cases the baby will not be affected. However, once a mother has a baby with erythroblastosis, it is to be expected that any subsequent babies will also be erythroblastotic, but it is not always so. A woman can have a normal baby even after she has lost a number with erythroblastosis. Many erythroblastotic babies are saved by medical care after birth, so the chances for a normal family are excellent, and the case is never hopeless.

Design for a Good Pregnancy

With the information derived from her medical history, physical examination and laboratory tests, the doctor is ready to work out with his patient plans for a happy and healthy pregnancy. There is no rigid regime for pregnancy. The days are gone when a woman secluded herself, some assuming a life of semi-invalidism for the nine months. A normal pregnancy, with proper guidance, need not disturb her usual way of life very much.

There are facts a woman should know, to take proper care of herself and ensure the welfare of the baby, as to diet, exercise, clothing, and care of the body. She should know what changes she may expect in the way she looks and feels, which symptoms are normal, which are just bothersome, and which are danger signals. These things her doctor will tell her. There are many good books on the physiology and hygiene of pregnancy. Her doctor will recommend one, pointing out what is especially important for her to know and be ready to discuss with her any questions that arise or any special problem of her own.

The doctor will also tell her of any defects or abnormalities he has found. Some, such as overweight, flabby muscles, or poor posture, she must correct by her own efforts. For some, such as anemia and malnutrition, he will prescribe means of correction. Some, fortunately rare occurrences such as a heart condition, he will watch and treat as pregnancy progresses.

The design for a good pregnancy is thus laid out. The woman knows what to expect and what is expected of her. As the design takes form, the doctor as the supervisor records the progress and stands ready to lend a helping hand at any time. Usually he likes to see his patient every three or four weeks during the first six months of the pregnancy, then every two weeks until the last month when he sees her every week. He has ways of checking to see if the pregnancy is proceeding according to plan for the mother and baby.

His units of measure for health of the mother are weight, blood pressure, urinalysis, and the way she looks and feels. The growth of the baby he estimates by the change in size of the uterus. After the fifth month he can hear its heart beat. The rate and position of the heart beat becomes important as term approaches.

In the last month of pregnancy, the doctor is concerned about the position of the baby. Normally he will be able to feel the baby's head in the lower part of the woman's abdomen with the back along one side, usually the left. If it is otherwise, he may be able to correct it.

There are other problems the doctor and patient must work out as pregnancy progresses, such as decisions regarding hospital or home delivery, nursing the baby, or work during and after pregnancy. They require individual consideration and planning to meet the woman's specific needs.

XI

THE MIRACLE OF BIRTH

THE MIRACLE OF BIRTH has always been submerged in its commonplaceness. A birth is happening every minute of the day and night, somewhere in the world. Babies are being born at the rate of 100,000 every twenty-four hours. How could anything that happens so often be a miracle? We rarely, if ever, think of it as such. We do not even consider a birth noteworthy unless it happens in an unusual place or in difficult circumstances. Anyone with the slightest experience with birth becomes an authority—the taxi driver in whose cab a baby was born, or a woman who has had a baby. They have witnessed the external manifestations of birth. Their reaction is one of excitement and self-importance because the inevitableness of birth requires that they do something in a hurry. It is not of wonder, for they do not know of the hidden forces and events taking place that are miraculous in their purposefulness, co-ordination, and delicate effectiveness.

Among some primitive people, birth was a fearful and dangerous event. However, it was not for the welfare of the woman or her child that they were concerned, but for their own safety. A woman in the process of giving birth was a menace. If a menstruating woman was unclean, the source of danger to plants, animals, and man, a woman in childbirth was infinitely more so. Therefore she was isolated to fare as best she could alone or perhaps with another woman until a safe time had elapsed after birth to ensure her purification.

When birth ceased to be a social peril, as civilization progressed, it became woman's personal ordeal. It was considered right and proper that woman should suffer to atone for the sins of Eve. But Queen Victoria thought differently, and because she was a queen, she could do something about it. Chloroform as an anesthetic had just been administered by Dr. Simpson, and she called on him to allow her to have it for the birth of Prince Leopold. He complied and was knighted by the Queen and excommunicated by the church!

Birth was long considered woman's business, and the necessary ministrations were in the hands of the midwife. Doctors considered the care of a woman in childbirth beneath their dignity, which was probably a blessing for the woman. The midwife respected the ability of nature, and while she did not know very much about how to help, at least she did not usually interfere. The doctor, almost equally ignorant, did not hesitate to meddle and often did more harm than good.

Today, we consider birth the business of the three participants who have been preparing for it throughout pregnancy. We may therefore observe with wonder at nature's performance; with respect for woman's right to dignity, safety, and comfort as she experiences it; and with appreciation for the doctor's skill and devotion to the welfare of mother and baby as he supervises and assists in this miraculous, mysterious event.

BIRTH AS NATURE PERFORMS IT

Nature starts her preparation for birth early, with the onset of pregnancy, and in her mysterious and knowing way brings about the changes that make birth possible. There is nothing haphazard in her plans. She is orderly, purposeful, and quite consistent so that the timing and actual occurrence of birth may be accomplished in the most efficient way, that is, quickest and best for both mother and baby.

As the tenth lunar month passes, her preparations are complete. The stage is set. She is ready to call for action, to set in motion the forces she has developed but restrained from action all these months. By her careful timing and varying strength of application of these forces, she will bring about the formation of a birth canal, guide and propel the baby through this passageway, and finally sever the baby's connection to the mother by expulsion of the placenta. Birth completed, she immediately busies herself in making the changes that will return the mother's body to its pregravid (before pregnancy) state.

The Stage Is Set

Birth means that the baby will be moved out of the uterus, which has placidly housed it for nine months. This will require two changes: the application of a proper force to move the baby, and the formation of a passageway large enough for the baby to pass through. These changes happen simultaneously and are mutually dependent. To make the intricacy of birth more easily understandable, we may consider them separately.

The force is derived from the contraction of the muscle cells of the uterus, which for some mysterious reason begins at the proper and appointed time. (The time of completion of pregnancy and the preparations for birth is called "term.") The uterus at term has been converted from the hard pear-shaped organ of prepregnancy to a tremendously distended, thin-walled muscular sac. This change might appear to be just stretching of the walls—the uterus increasing its capacity at the expense of the thickness of its walls. But the preparatory changes consist of a great deal more than mere distention. During all the months of pregnancy, while the uterus is expanding to accommodate the growing baby, effective contractions of the musculature are held in check. The uterus thus affords the baby a hospitable shelter. At the same time the muscle cells are undergoing change so that they will be ready to assume the prime function of all muscles, contraction and the performance of work—and, more important, work that will produce the desired result.

Nature has been precise and purposeful in the transformation of the uterus so that its contractions will be effective in the birth of the baby. In this transformation, there has been a great increase in the total number of the muscle cells and a marked increase in the size of each muscle cell. Furthermore, this increase in muscle tissue is concentrated in the upper part of the uterus. There are fewer muscle cells in the area near the cervix, and the cervix itself has lost rather than gained in muscle strength. Nature has a reason for these changes. If the muscle tissue were evenly distributed, when the uterus commenced to contract the pressure would all be directed inward. The result would be compression of the baby, not the motion of birth. What is needed to accomplish expulsion of the baby is pressure exerted in only one direction, toward the outlet to the birth canal.

This difference may be better understood by recalling two familiar objects—a rubber ball and a rubber bulb. If one should completely enclose the ball within the hands and squeeze it, no matter what its contents, the only result would be compression of the contents (provided you did not squeeze too hard)! But if you squeeze the upper end of the bulb, however lightly, its contents will be forced out the opening at the lower end. Nature duplicates the principle of the bulb in that only the upper portion of the uterus exerts forceful contractions while the lower portion remains not only passive but distensible. Another remarkable provision is that there are just enough muscle fibers in the upper part of the uterus to produce the right amount of force. If there were too many, excessive force might cause damage; and if too few, the force would be ineffective.

The second set of changes that have been accomplished during pregnancy are those that will facilitate the formation of a passageway. They prepare for the "dilatation of the cervix," which will provide an opening from the uterus to the vagina large enough to allow the baby to pass through without harm to the baby or damage to the passageway.

To simplify the meaning of these changes, we may go back to the example of the rubber bulb. If its contents are fluid or air, they would be easily expelled without any change in the size of the outlet. But if the content is a solid mass, the outlet must be stretched enough to allow passage. Whether this will be possible without injury to the neck of the bulb depends on two things: the distensibility of the neck; and the size, shape, and position of the object. A small, firm, evenly rounded object would be best as a wedge to stretch the opening without tearing it. An elongated oval, lying lengthwise in the bulb, would be like a ramrod or piston and would provide the best means of transmission of pressure from the upper part of the bulb. An elongated object lying crosswise would be impossible to dislodge. Effective transmission of the force could not occur, and the opening could not be made large enough even though stretched and torn.

Nature exhibits the same principles in her preparations to facilitate the dilatation of the cervix. She has provided increased distensibility of the outlet, the most propitious position for the object to be moved, and an efficient wedge.

During the dilatation of the cervix the size of its opening has been increased to fit the baby's head, and the cervix has been converted from a short thick-walled tube to a very thin ring, which marks the outlet of the uterus. This marked change is possible because the walls of the cervix have been transformed into a soft, spongy tissue that is easily stretched. The opening is made larger by the fact that the honey-combed lining of the cervix is detached and swept away in the early phase of dilatation.

The position of the baby is vital to the normal birth process. The only way a baby can be born is with its body lying vertical, that is with the head down toward the mother's pelvis or up toward her chest. If it lies crossways (transverse), which it rarely does, natural birth would be impossible. Doctors speak of the baby's position as "head presentation" when the head is directed downward and will be the first part of the baby to emerge at birth, "breech presentation" when the baby's buttocks are the presenting part.

The position of the baby in also important as a factor in the dilatation of the cervix. The upper part of the uterus, by contracting, exerts pressure on the baby, and in turn some part of the baby must serve as a wedge that will dilate the cervix. Obviously, the baby's head is the hardest part of its body and would therefore make the best wedge. Moreover, the process will be easier if the baby's head is in the position that requires the smallest opening to pass through. That is attained when the baby's head is flexed (bent down toward the chest). In about 95 per cent of births the baby is in that position. Other presentations occur, may slow the process of birth, and occasionally make it more difficult.

The efficiency of the presenting part as a wedge is increased by the membranes and fluid that encompass it. When contraction begins, the membranes are intact and the baby is still in the "bag of water," so that the irregularities of the baby are converted into a smooth ovoid and the presenting part forms a better wedge.

The stage is set. The baby is matured and ready to begin its independent existence, large enough but not too large. It is in the best possible position to make its entrance. The pelvic organs are ready to participate each in its own way, and nature says it is time for action. Labor, which is nature's way of bringing this new life into the world, begins. It will be accomplished in three stages. In the first, the entrance to the birth canal is opened up; in the second, the baby passes through the birth canal and is born; and in the third, the placenta and fetal membranes are expelled.

The Passageway Is Opened

The first act of this drama of birth begins when the musculature of the uterus begins to contract. It starts slowly and gently, and with gradually increasing tempo and intensity exerts its force. The purpose of contraction of the muscles is to perform work—to "labor." Thus the first stage of labor commences with the first uterine contractions and ends when the cervix is completely dilated and the head starts to pass through its opening.

During pregnancy the uterus does contract at times. These contractions are weak, have no pattern and no obvious purpose, and they are not usually painful. But with the onset of labor contractions become stronger, rhythmic, and painful. Uterine contractions, like those of other involuntary muscles—such as those of the intestines or the heart—are directed by the autonomic nervous system and therefore cannot be initiated, increased, or decreased by the will.

Rhythmicity is a characteristic of these uterine contractions. At the onset of labor, they occur at 15-to-30-minute intervals. Gradually they become more frequent until, as the end approaches, they are occurring every 2-to-3 minutes, and each contraction lasts about one minute.

The dilatation of the cervix is accomplished solely by the force of these contractions of the uterus. Each contraction pushes the baby's head against the cervix and stretches it a little bit. With this stretching, the lining of the cervix is dislodged (called mucous plug), and little tears in the cervix occur producing a little bleeding (called bloody show).

At the onset of labor the membranes are usually intact. But as the contractions get stronger and the cervix more dilated, the membranes are pinched between head and cervical ring and are ruptured. This usually occurs when they have served their purpose, and the cervix is dilated. With rupture, the fluid pours out ("bag of water breaks"), either as a gush of fluid, or a little oozing with each contraction. Sometimes the membranes rupture before labor is well under way, causing a "dry labor." If labor has not started, it usually does so within 24 hours but occasionally is delayed.

This first stage of labor nature usually starts at her own good time, and carries through at her own pace. Sometimes that is rapid, sometimes slow, but she cannot be hurried.

The Entrance

The second stage of labor is the actual passage of the baby from the uterus to the outside world. The passageway is through the vagina, which offers little resistance because it has been transformed into spongy tissue, which is easily stretched. The most important part of the birth canal is the solid circle of bone, the pelvic girdle. Its size and shape determines whether birth is possible, whether it will be easy or difficult, and, in fact, the mechanism by which birth is accomplished.

The pelvic girdle is not a circle of bones of equal depth all around and with straight sides, through which passage would be easy. Rather it is a curved cylinder, shallow in front (the pubic bone) and with a long deep curve (sacrum) in the back. It is made more difficult as a passageway because the entrance above (inlet) is not round but somewhat heart-shaped and the exit below (outlet) is oval.

It is through this curved passage that the baby must pass. Since the baby's head usually comes first, once the head is through, the rest will be easy. The problem is difficult because the baby's head is oval in shape and its measurements are almost as great as those of the bony canal. In some positions, it could not go through at all. Obviously, there must be means by which the size and shape of the baby's head can be fitted or adjusted to the size and shape of the different levels (from inlet to outlet) of the birth canal. This means nature provides by changing, as birth progresses, the position of the baby's head in relation to the birth canal—and by "molding" it to fit.

We speak of "normal delivery." What do we mean by "normal"? It means the way it usually happens—with the least difficulty, the greatest ease, and no mishaps. We do not stop to consider the wonder of normalcy —the perfection of the mechanism that has made it possible. In almost all births, the baby's head is placed in the proper position at the onset of labor with its back directed forward and a little to one side of the mother's abdomen. That is the best way for the egg-shaped oval head to fit into the heart-shape of the inlet. It is the position in which flexion (which is the direction the baby's head can be bent most) will be most helpful. Then, as the head descends, it turns so that it is facing directly backward. When it reaches the outlet, the head extends, and the baby is born.

"Molding" is another aspect of "normalcy"—a provision of nature to make birth possible. An adult's head is a solid sphere of hard bone. A newborn baby's head is made of individual plates of bones, which are joined together (at the sutures) by soft tissue. A baby has soft spots in its head, and this soft tissue allows for growth, but it is also important for the process of birth because it allows the head to be compressed and changed in shape as it passes through tight spots in the birth canal. The first sight of a newborn baby may be startling because it seems to have such a little face below the elongated dome-shape of its head. This is the result of molding, which nature corrects quite speedily after birth.

So far we have considered only the mechanics of birth; that is, how an object of one particular shape can be turned and adjusted to pass through a canal of varying direction and shape. We must next discover what is the force that causes the movement. It is again "labor pains," but now they have a new meaning.

In the first stage of labor, we saw that contractions of the uterus were the only necessary force. At the completion of the first stage, there is a short lull, and then the contractions occur with increasing intensity, force, and frequency, but they will not be sufficient to move the baby through the birth canal. Here nature calls on the woman herself to help by using her abdominal muscles. At first she consciously does this, but later it becomes involuntary, and she cannot resist "bearing down." In a "bearing-down pain," the woman, as she feels the uterine contraction coming on, braces her body, takes a deep breath, and holds it. At the same time, she contracts her abdominal muscles and thus makes a straining movement that exerts intense downward pressure on the abdominal contents. Now the abdominal muscles, which were useless in the first stage of labor, become very important in the expulsion of the child. Thus the "bearing-down pain" consists of contractions of the uterine and abdominal muscles simultaneously. The pain associated with these is due partly to uterine contractions and partly to pressure on the soft tissue of the birth canal.

"Pains" consist of a period of steadily increasing contraction until maximum is reached and held briefly. This is followed by a period of relaxation. It is only while contraction is taking place that a moving force is delivered.

Here is another instance of "normalcy." Nature calls on the woman to exert physical effort and to bear pain for a short period, which is followed by a longer period of relaxation in which she may rest free from pain. A double purpose is served; the woman's strength is conserved, and birth is a slower, more gentle process, which will cause less damage to the mother and be less dangerous to the baby.

After about an hour (it may vary from a half to two hours), the baby's head has traversed the pelvic cavity and is almost ready to emerge. The pelvic floor now begins to bulge with each pain. The opening of the vulva is slitlike, through which the scalp may be seen. With each pain there is more and more bulging, the vulva becomes more widely dilated, and the opening changes from slit to oval and then to circular in shape. When the pain subsides, the head recedes some and the opening becomes smaller. Finally, the vulva becomes stretched to paper thinness, and the head actually passes into the ring and stays. With the next pain, the baby's head is forced through. With the emergence of the head the most difficult part is over. Another contraction or so and the baby's soft body is born, followed by a gush of fluid and a little blood.

The second stage ends with the birth of the baby, but all is not accomplished yet. The cord extends from the baby through the birth canal to the placenta, and the placenta is still attached to the wall of the uterus. This is the baby's lifeline, because it continues (as it has through all the months of pregnancy) to provide the baby's needs. During the birth process, it becomes crucial from one standpoint, that of adequate oxygen supply. The baby could do without food for the few hours of the birth process and could manage with most of its waste products. But the placenta must serve as the baby's respiratory organ until the baby can take its first deep breath of air—utter that first cry of life. Therefore, it is vital to the baby that the placenta remain attached to serve this purpose. It is vital to the mother also as we shall see.

Removal of the "Props"

Uterine contractions cease for a few minutes after the birth of the baby. The abdomen is soft, and through its soft wall the uterus may be felt as a solid mass now so reduced in size that its upper margin is below the umbilicus. Then the uterus begins the last phase of its labor. It contracts, and the placenta and membranes are peeled off from its surface and expelled. Hence the name "after birth." This is followed by bleeding, which is usually not excessive, about a cupful at most. The uterus continues to contract to close off blood vessels and stop this flow. It does this efficiently and safely for the mother in the vast majority of cases.

It would almost seem that nature has great confidence in her ability to achieve birth without harm to mother or child, she goes about it so slowly and methodically. She has efficient barriers against the two great dangers of childbirth, hemorrhage and infection. There is practically no bleeding during the process of birth of the baby. The one potential source of bleeding is a severe tear of the cervix. This nature guards against by first having the head as a wedge and then slowly, gently exerting pressure, which dilates the cervix completely.

The bleeding at the end of the third stage is usually moderate in amount and not dangerous when the sequence of events is according to nature's plans. Excessive, dangerous bleeding occurs when the placenta is "prematurely separated," that is before the birth of the baby is complete. The uterus incompletely emptied cannot contract sufficiently to close off the blood vessels at the site where the placenta was attached. In the normal sequence, head presentation, this period when the uterus is only partially filled is momentary. Nature has made another provision for this normal sequence by having the attachment of the placenta high up in the uterus. Only rarely is it close to the cervix where it would be peeled off when the cervix is dilated.

Birth is completed. This is the way nature performs it. But what is this mysterious thing, this all-knowing power that we have called nature? Generally speaking it is life and the life processes. Life is a mystery we have never fathomed. Birth is perhaps the ultimate of intricacy and perfection among all the life processes. Some parts of its mechanism we understand, some are still a mystery.

The cause of the onset of labor is a question scientists have long pursued. What tells the muscular organ, the uterus, which has held its purposeful contractibility in check, at the appointed time to assume its inherent function? It must contract and expel the baby, which it has quietly housed and protected. There have been many theories, such as:

> Pregnancy corresponds to ten menstrual cycles, during which time periodicity is held in check, but eventually, corresponding to the 10th menstrual period, it no longer can be restrained and menstrual periodicity reasserts itself.
>
> Pregnancy and labor are habits of body functions that are inherited.
>
> The distention of the uterus reaches a crucial point that initiates meaningful contractions.
>
> The baby contributes some chemicals that initiate uterine contractions.
>
> The level of hormones that has fostered pregnancy is changed.

These and many more are only theories as to the cause of the onset of labor, for none gives the complete answer. Their wide diversity emphasizes the fact that we do not know what causes the onset of labor.

The endocrines set the stage for labor. Estrogen and progesterone are produced in increasing amounts throughout pregnancy. Just before the onset of labor, there is a marked decrease in both estrogen and progesterone. The posterior lobe of the pituitary, which we have not discussed, produces hormones, which you may have heard of as "pituitrin," that stimulate involuntary muscles such as those of the uterus. During pregnancy, the uterus is insensitive to this hormone. As term is approached, the posterior pituitary produces more and more of this hormone, and the uterus becomes more responsive to its action. Somewhere in the cause and effect of the shifting balance of these hormones will be found the answer to "what causes the onset of labor."

How is it that nature starts labor with the baby in the best possible position? We are told that the reasons are mechanical, that the baby, a solid object floating in water, naturally assumes that position because the head is the heaviest part of the body or that it fits the shape of the uterus better and is more comfortable in that position. The passage of the baby through the birth canal is explained also on a mechanical basis. Uterine contractions exert a definite physical force on the object (the baby), which turns as it moves to adjust to the varying shape of the channel through which it must pass. The control of the force of labor, muscular contraction, is by the nervous system. In the first stage, labor pains are due to contractions of the uterus, which is controlled by the autonomic nervous system. In the second and third stages, contractions of the abdominal muscles become necessary, and these are initiated by the central nervous system.

So "nature" as she presides over birth uses methods that are mechanical, hormonal, neuromuscular. How she selects and balances these effectively and efficiently adds up to the mystery and miracle that is the truly "natural childbirth."

When nature is doing her best, unhindered by faulty material, undisturbed by mishaps or accidents, she is successful. She goes about her task with or without the woman's help and co-operation, and whether or not a doctor is supervising her efforts. But even in the best of circumstances she can do a better job if the woman understands what is happening and how she can be helpful, and with the guidance and assistance of the doctor.

WOMAN'S EXPERIENCE

"How much pain will I have when my baby is born?"

"How long does it take for a baby to come?"

"How will I know that labor has started?"

"What am I supposed to do—and will I have all the help and care I need?"

These, and other questions, come to the mind of a woman as she watches the calendar and counts off the days until that special day when she expects the birth of her baby. She may ask these questions partly out of sheer curiosity; but her curiosity is colored by her emotional reaction to the inescapable fact that it is she herself who is going to give birth to a baby. With a mixture of apprehension and anticipation, she is anxious to be alert and ready to do her part, hopeful that she will acquit herself well and not have too hard a time. She will desire above all to have a normal, live baby. However much she has heard about birth—good things and bad—or however much she has read and studied, there is uncertainty as she tries to relate the facts to herself. The question still remains: "How will I feel when I have a baby?"

Birth is a tremendous event, and nature does not allow it to occur without first giving fair warning. To the woman having her first child, she is especially considerate and lets her know two or three weeks in advance that the time is approaching. This first signal is called "lightening" because the baby seems to drop down.

The woman notices that her abdomen, which had been rounded outward from her ribs down to her pubic bone, now becomes flattened out under the ribs and fuller in the lower part. Lightening is due to the fact that the uterus, which had been completely in the abdominal cavity, partially sinks into the pelvic cavity, and the head of the baby, which had previously been movable above the bony pelvis, now sinks into the pelvis and becomes fixed. This gives relief from pressure in the abdomen but increases the pressure in the pelvis, making walking more difficult and perhaps giving some pain in the legs. Pressure on the bladder leads to increased frequency of urination.

In women who have had children, this usually does not happen until labor is about ready to start or has already started. The actual onset of labor nature announces in one of three ways: by labor pains, the appearance of a bloody show, or the breaking of the bag of water.

When the first pains come, a woman naturally wonders how long it will be before she has her baby, whether she has time to do all the things she has left to the last minute. As a rule she will have plenty of time. Nature is usually, though not always, slow and deliberate. There is no way to foretell how long it will be for her. Each individual is different. Since there is no such thing as an "average woman," there is no meaning in "average duration of labor." But there are limits of time from shortest to longest for the duration of labor and each of its stages to which most women will conform.

How long labor will last depends on two things: the force produced by labor pains and the resistance offered by the soft tissues of the birth canal. A woman who starts off with good strong pains that get progressively stronger and closer together, can expect to be delivered sooner than one whose pains are weak and slow in developing. Also a woman who has a roomy pelvis with elastic soft tissues will have a shorter labor than one whose pelvis is smaller or whose tissues are rigid and hard to stretch. There are many things that affect one or the other of these factors and either shorten or increase the duration of labor. Perhaps the most common is whether or not a woman has had a previous delivery. Normally, it takes longer to have the first baby.

Doctors have a way of classifying women as to the number of children they have borne (their parity). Thus a woman who is having her first child is called a primipara (first parity), and a woman who has already had one or more children is called a multipara. One who has never had a child is a nullipara. It is an easy way to say a lot about the woman in just one word.

In a primipara then, labor lasts longer. Her cervix is more resistant to dilatation, making the first stage longer, and the soft tissues of her birth canal are more resistant and it takes longer for the baby to pass through it. Doctors expect a primipara to deliver within sixteen hours, with a fifty–fifty chance that she will deliver in less than ten hours. A few will go more than twenty-four hours, and once in a while one will deliver in three to four hours. The greater part of this time is occupied in dilating the cervix. The first stage then lasts up to twelve or fourteen hours with a good chance of it being less than eight hours. The second stage is much shorter, lasting about an hour and a half. But doctors can and frequently do take measures to shorten this stage—as we shall see later. The first stage can rarely be hurried. The last stage, delivery of afterbirth, occurs with little difficulty within a few minutes to a half hour after the birth of the baby.

In a multipara the duration of labor is shorter because her tissues, once stretched, never again offer as great resistance with subsequent deliveries. Doctors expect her to deliver in ten to twelve hours, with a fifty–fifty chance of it being less than six to seven hours. Occasionally, even a multipara can have a long labor when nothing is wrong except that her pains are slower and weaker. "Precipitate labor," that is of very short duration, occurs sometimes. We read of babies born in taxicabs on the way to the hospital. They are usually multiparas with small babies.

There are other things that may prolong the duration of labor. Certain positions of the baby and exceedingly large babies may make labor longer and occasionally more hazardous. Abnormalities of the pelvis, which complicate labor, are strictly the doctor's problem; and his method of handling them will vary with each woman's condition and need.

THE DOCTOR'S SUPERVISION

Safe and happy childbirth—maternal welfare—has become a "cause" sponsored by many different groups such as doctors, government agencies, and civic organizations. They have all come to realize, and are making every effort to impress on women, that preparations for delivery should be started, not when the woman goes into labor, but when she first learns that she is pregnant. Such preparation, or "prenatal care" as it is called, has as its aim a woman who is physically and emotionally ready for childbirth. When the time comes, a medical record of her pregnancy is available that evaluates her assets and liabilities. It was compiled by her doctor who knows her as a person as well as her physical potentialities for childbirth.

During labor the doctor observes, checks the progress, offers assistance to expedite the natural process and assistance to the woman in making her efforts more effective and less painful, and is on the alert for any signs of impending emergency.

Early in the first stage of labor, abdominal examination will tell him something of the position of the baby and the frequency and strength of the labor pains. As labor progresses, he will make repeated internal examinations to determine the true position of the baby's head and how labor is progressing, that is, whether the cervix is dilating properly. When the cervix is completely dilated and the head becomes engaged, the doctor knows that the woman is entering the second stage, which will be relatively short, and preparations must be made for her delivery.

As birth is near, the doctor stands ready to guide and support the baby's head in order to prevent damage to the mother's tissues—the perineum. In women who have had babies, the perineum is relaxed and offers no great resistance and the baby's head emerges easily and is quickly followed by the birth of the body. But in primiparas, these tissues are more tense and rigid, and labor is longer. If there seems to be danger of injury to the mother's tissues either by too great stretching or by tearing, the doctor may prevent this by making a short incision (episiotomy) to one side in the perineum. Sometimes he may use forceps to lift the baby's head through the lower part of the birth canal if the mother has become weakened or exhausted, and her expulsion efforts are not adequate.

The baby is born, uterine contraction pauses for a while, and the woman rests. The doctor uses this time to take the few stitches necessary to close the incision he has made and to take care of the baby. Usually as the baby is lifted up by its feet and given a pat, it will take a deep breath and start to cry. There is no great rush to tie the cord; it is to the baby's advantage to wait a few moments before bringing to an end for all time its connection with the mother and putting it entirely on its own, for there is with uterine contraction a surge of blood out of the placenta to the baby, which gives it a better start. The doctor, when ready, puts two clamps on the cord a few inches from the umbilicus, cuts between them, puts some antiseptic on the end of the cord, ties the end, removes the clamps, and applies a dressing. He may use a special kind of clamp next to the baby, which is left on instead of a tie.

The baby's air passages are cleared by suction and if breathing is not started it may be given some oxygen or other methods may be used to start respiration. Drops are put in its eyes to prevent infection. It is wrapped in a blanket and placed in a crib. It will have its foot prints taken and its identification bracelet put on before it leaves for the nursery.

During the period of rest, the uterus is massaged at frequent intervals to assure its maintaining a state of contraction to prevent excessive bleeding. After a few minutes, the uterus begins expulsive contraction and the placenta is peeled off and expelled.

Birth is complete, but vigilance and care for the mother's welfare is not over. She is sent to the recovery room and watched constantly to see that the uterus stays contracted and that excessive bleeding does not occur. If the uterus seems to be a bit lazy in doing its job, the doctor may order a drug to make it contract.

It would seem, from this description, that the doctor's part in birth is purely on the physical basis: to time and evaluate the pain, to check on the dilatation of the cervix and progress of labor, and to receive the baby as it is born. But this is only a small part of his job. He stands ready to assist.

Before labor begins, the doctor may be able to turn the baby, if it is not in the best position, or he may be able to do so after labor begins. Sometimes nature is slow in starting labor. If the doctor thinks it advisable for the welfare of the mother or the baby—and only for those reasons— he may induce labor. If nature is slow in advancing the first stage, the doctor may speed labor—again only for the welfare of the mother and baby—by medication or rupture of the membranes. If the second stage is prolonged, he may cut it short by episiotomy and low forceps. The doctor's assistance to the woman is directed toward making birth as easy and painless an experience as possible.

Since the first discovery of anesthesia, and with each new kind of drug and each new method of administering it, doctors have been eager and active in applying this knowledge to relief of pain in childbirth. But this has never been a simple problem. The basic requirements for a good obstetrical anesthetic are quite different from those of a surgical anesthetic. The surgeon has only one patient, and he needs only an anesthetic that will put the patient to sleep or deaden the sensation in the area where he is to work. The obstetrician has two patients—whatever drug or anesthetic he gives the mother will also reach the baby. Some anesthetics, which are safe and effective for an adult, may be harmful to the baby. The anesthetic must not retard the natural processes necessary for birth. He is therefore confronted with the problem of choosing a drug and a method of administering it that will relieve pain, be safe for the mother and child, and will not retard labor. His use of anesthesia is also limited by the fact that labor extends over many hours, and the pain is of varying intensity at the different stages. Some drugs, which could be used with safety for a short period, would be dangerous to both mother and baby if given over a prolonged period. Since the pains are intense for a comparatively short time, a mild drug will be sufficient most of the time, with a complete anesthetic for only a short period. The doctor must choose what is best for each patient. Often it is a combination of drugs. Analgesics properly used are safe, and woman can be confident that she can have her baby without excessive suffering and without injury to the baby.

Thus the doctor assists both nature and the woman to make childbirth natural, safe, and as painless as possible. At times nature falters and is unable to carry through her part, and then the doctor has to take over to accomplish birth safely for mother and baby. The two most important methods available to him are the use of forceps, by which the natural birth process is facilitated, and Caesarean section, which replaces it.

It has been said that forceps are the instruments that have saved more lives than any others. Whether this is true or not, they certainly serve the needed purpose of a means of assisting difficult births and cutting short what might be a dangerously prolonged second stage. It is the use of forceps that is referred to when you hear that a doctor had to "take the baby." They have, however, limitations. They can be used only at certain stages and under certain conditions. They require a doctor trained not only in how to use them, but when to use them.

Forceps have a very interesting history. They were first devised by a Dr. Chamberlen about 1600 and were kept as a family secret for a hundred years. It was a well-kept secret, because only doctors of the Chamberlen family were allowed to know even the nature of this mysterious instrument and how to use it. The Chamberlens were doctors in London who specialized in midwifery and claimed that they could safely deliver cases so difficult that other doctors were incapable of handling them and in which therefore either the mother or child or both would perish. And they frequently and mysteriously made good their claim. When one was called to assist in a difficult birth, he came with his black bag and worked in secrecy, concealing under the covering of the patient both his method and instrument. Other attendants including doctors had no idea what he was doing; the only clues were motions of his hands under the sheet and the clanging of metal.

The Drs. Chamberlen became quite proficient, attending royalty and nobility as well as ordinary women with good results. One of the later generations of the Drs. Chamberlen also dabbled in politics and as a result had to flee the country. He went to Holland and there sold the family secret to a doctor of the Medico-Pharmaceutical College of Amsterdam. The university had the power to grant licenses to practice medicine and midwifery, which grants were sold to practitioners for a price, and for a greater sum they sold also the secret of the forceps, provided a pledge of secrecy was taken by the purchasing physician. Eventually, the secret was made public, but only one blade was exhibited, which of course was useless. Whether Dr. Chamberlen or the university perpetrated the hoax no one knows. However, in the early 1700's the true secret of the double-blade forceps became known and soon came into widespread use. Many types have been devised by enterprising doctors in the years that have elapsed since then.

NATURAL CHILDBIRTH

"The new theory of painless childbirth" or "natural childbirth" has been the topic of widespread discussion and controversy. Doctors have argued it pro and con among themselves. Women have wondered what it could mean to them personally and have been eager to avail themselves of its beneficence. Furthermore, there have been many articles in the magazines and newspapers that have given the impression that here is something new and startling, a method never before known or used by doctors.

Some articles ardently advocate the "natural way" as an experience that every woman should strive to achieve. Failure on her part to elect to have her baby according to this "new" method is indicative, they imply or baldly state, that the woman lacks courage, or that she is indifferent to the spiritual significance of becoming a mother. In either case, the woman who submits to the use of pain-relievers in labor will miss "the soul-lifting experience" of the consciousness of birth, which is the foundation of mother love.

There have also been articles that just as vehemently deny the virtues of "natural childbirth" but rather insist that it is a return to the dark ages of obstetrics. Why should modern women, they ask, be subjected to this when modern science provides the means whereby she can go to sleep, experience no pain, and awaken with her baby in her arms?

"Natural childbirth" is a philosophy rather than a method of obstetrics, whereby childbirth is revered not as a physical function but as a spiritual experience. Its father philosopher was Dr. Grantby Dick Reed of England. Dr. Reed, as a young doctor attending a woman in labor in the slums of London, was impressed by her peacefulness and her apparent freedom from pain and was puzzled that she refused even a whiff of chloroform. He questioned her about her pain and she answered: "It wasn't meant to hurt—was it?" As this scene came back to him time and time again, he pondered the truth and through the years evolved his philosophy of "natural childbirth."

Pain of childbirth, according to the "natural" theory, is the product of a chain reaction of fear-tension-pain. Relief of this pain should be accomplished not by the suppression of one of these factors by drugs, but by the elimination of fear and tension. The ritual of preparation for "natural childbirth" is based on the concept that "faith relieves fear" and "faith is attained through knowledge." This epitome of faith is something that not only the woman must acquire through instruction and training, but also all of those who will in some way share the experience with her. These include the doctors, nurses, and her husband.

The Reed method advocates that the woman be taught, by lectures, demonstrations, and recommended reading, the normal physiology of pregnancy and labor so that she will know and understand what is happening at each and every moment of the experience. Such knowledge, it affirms, will eliminate fear and tension and furthermore will enable her not only to accept the workings of nature—to be passive, relaxed, and nonresistant—but also to participate joyously and actively assist nature. In addition, the woman needs to train herself physically. She must learn how to relax and how to command her muscles effectively. For this purpose she is taught special exercises, which she must practice every day beginning early in pregnancy.

The husband, according to this plan, is made an active partner during pregnancy and labor. He too must be taught the physiology and participate as far as possible in the physical training by helping his wife with her exercises, learning how to give her the massage that will facilitate relaxation. The purpose of his training is to ensure that he will not be just a distracted male pacing the corridors of the hospital during the long hours of his wife's labor, but that he will be with her in the labor room giving her companionship and encouragement and in the delivery room to share with her the moment of exultation at the birth of their baby.

The hospital set-up for "natural childbirth" requires modification of both facilities and services. There must be more room to allow the husband to be with his wife in privacy during labor. There must be more nurses so that one will be with each woman at all times. They must be trained in the faith to exhort her to unremitting effort, constantly encouraging her and never suggesting that she is suffering by referring to nature's expulsive forces as "labor pains." And, of course, the doctor must always be at her side so that he may, with patience for and confidence in the naturalness of the process, lead the woman from her elation to exultation.

This theory of "natural childbirth" may seem on cursory examination to be reasonable enough, idealistic perhaps, but basically sound. Why then should there be any controversy about it? Why are there so few doctors who are wholeheartedly apostles for it, so many lukewarm in their attitude toward it, and some actively hostile?

The objections and criticisms are based on the difficulties encountered in the practical application, and more important the difficulties and dangers that arise from human frailties. In addition to the modification of hospital facilities and services required for the natural method, it complicates matters to have the husband in the delivery room, just as it would in any operating room, in maintaining surgical asepsis, and it might happen that the hospital would have two patients on its hands instead of one. But these things are not major obstacles. Some hospitals allow the method to be practiced in their obstetrical services. All would undoubtedly strive to make the necessary expansion in facilities and trained personnel if they were convinced this was a method in the best interests of all or even the majority of women in labor. Few hospitals have been so persuaded.

The real objection to the theory comes from the human side of the picture—the frailties of the two most involved, the husband and wife. Not every husband, however much he loves his wife, has been conditioned by his earlier training to want to know the intricacies of her female physiology or will be able to use that knowledge constructively. He may find it difficult to stand by and give reassurance while his wife is in labor. He may prove to be more of a hindrance than a help. But even a completely disinterested husband or one inadequate to help would not be sufficient reason to deny women the privilege of "natural childbirth."

Not all women are physically endowed with the qualities for the successful attainment of natural childbirth. This includes the few who have some physical abnormality and also the great many in whom the short months of physical training during pregnancy could not overcome the result of years of inactivity. The best time to have babies as far as ease and safety of delivery are concerned is in the early twenties. Many women nowadays do not get around to having their first baby until much later. With good obstetrical care they go through their pregnancy and labor quite normally, but most of them would not do so well with the natural method. Moreover, many doctors who have observed cases of natural childbirth do not find that the physical training has contributed to any great extent to the woman's ability to participate successfully.

Most doctors are agreed that woman should know more about how her body is made and how it functions, and many have found it helpful in the management of obstetrical cases to give women some specific instruction by informal lectures and group discussion periods as well as recommended reading. Thereby she will know and appreciate the wonder of nature and not be haunted by the fears that arise from ignorance and false information. But a little knowledge is a dangerous thing. A woman may get the idea that she knows just when and how each event of labor should occur. When her experience doesn't conform, she may become apprehensive and unduly disturbed. No two labors are ever exactly alike. They merely follow a general pattern. It takes doctors years of experience to learn all of nature's variations of "normal" and at the same time to be alert to the perception of the first signs of nature's faltering. It is asking a great deal of woman to interpret these variations properly and philosophically in her first or second or even sixth or tenth experience with birth, especially since she is not the interested onlooker but the active participant.

It is quite far-fetched to expect a woman in our culture (or probably any other) to enter the physical activity of labor with complete emotional abandon. She has learned to control the expression of her emotions, and it would be difficult to completely unlearn this habit. She has also learned that the best way to get help is not usually by proclaiming her own self-sufficiency. She has also learned, if she has attained any degree of maturity, that joy and pleasure come from sources other than physical activity, and that there are hurts, pains of the mind and heart, which are far more intense than that of physical suffering or injury. It will be hard for her to perform in childbirth with her emotions completely unfettered.

Tension, the stumbling block to natural childbirth, can come from many sources other than fear of pain, lonesomeness, or ignorance of what is happening. Many a woman enters labor so emotionally involved by the uncertainty of what pregnancy, labor, and the new baby will mean in terms of her total life situation, either present or future, that the physical experience of birth does not seem so very important to her, and she finds it hard to concentrate on her part. There are many examples of such situations. It would be hard to imagine a woman who does not have some concern at the time of her labor other than the fear of pain.

All these tensions would mitigate only against the woman doing her part as envisioned by the natural childbirth method. She might not achieve painless childbirth, exultation of delivery, or peace of parturition, but she would give birth just the same. Nature would procede whether the woman helped or not.

Success of the method is not to be measured in terms of pain. Most women, even the most ardent advocates of natural childbirth, will admit that they experienced pain. They can only say: "It was pain with a difference." It is true that a large percentage of women who have had one baby by the natural method will enthusiastically say that they would follow it again with the next baby. On the other hand, women who are happy and well with their babies delivered with some form of analgesia will be just as enthusiastic and convinced that they have had the best method of having a baby. It would seem that the enthusiasm and satisfaction stems not so much from how they had their babies but from the fact of accomplishment—they do have their babies.

If the woman is mature, accepts and respects herself and her role and is comfortably adjusted to her life, she can take things in her stride. If she chooses natural childbirth and things do not go well, she can say "it was a good try anyhow" and go on about her business of living. To a mature woman, her joy and success in motherhood come from the broad rich experiences, which include sharing love and life with her husband. Birth is the inevitable climax that reveals the important fact that she has a live, healthy, and normal baby, not the fact that she was conscious of the mechanism of its entrance into the world and saw it the moment of its birth. Life and procreation are wonderful and mysterious, and it may be well for us not to try so hard to interpret them completely in terms of physical experience.

There are emotionally maladjusted women who may choose the natural method to fulfill their own neurotic needs. They face the possibility of disasterous results. They fail because they bring to labor fears and tensions far more devastating than fear of pain, which no amount of sympathetic environment can allay. They cannot take failure in their stride.

One wonders if perhaps some women who have apparently got through natural childbirth successfully have not in reality failed, in that they come out with an inflated sense of their own importance and accomplishment. This egotism translated into smugness and complacency of her own superiority and importance may be hard for others to live with—and especially hard on the child. For she may consider it a possession that she has earned, not a gift to be cherished or a responsibility to be fulfilled.

After all is said and done, a woman will reap in spiritual rewards in proportion to what she herself has contributed whether it be to marriage, motherhood, or any other human experience.

THE PUERPERIUM

When pregnancy terminates by the birth of the baby, there follows a transition period in which the woman recovers from the experience of birth and assumes her new role of being a mother. Nature must remove the props that were necessary for the success of the pregnancy. This is called the "puerperium" ("puer" meaning "child," and "parere" meaning "to bring forth").

The puerperium begins when the third stage of labor is completed and lasts for a matter of weeks, usually six. During this time two important processes occur: (1) the restoration of the reproductive organs to the normal nonpregnant state and the readjustment of the body to the pregravid state of physiologic function, both general metabolic and glandular; and (2) the bringing into full function of the breasts in lactation.

Involution

Immediately after birth the uterus, now emptied of its contents, is a large muscular sac which extends half way to the umbilicus. As the result of the various factors which have contributed to its necessary increase in size, it weighs about 1000 grams. This we have seen was the result of the stimulating effects of the pregnancy itself—specifically the hormones produced by the placenta. With this removed from the scene, the uterus very rapidly decreases in size and reverts to normal structure, a process called "involution." At the end of the first week it weighs only 500 grams and can no longer be felt above the pelvic bone. In the sixth week it weighs only forty to sixty grams or a reduction to one-twentieth of the pregnant and postpartum state.

This rapid change in size is accomplished by the reversal of the processes of change in pregnancy. There is a decrease in the size of the individual muscle cells and perhaps the disappearance of some. A small amount is accounted for in the change in the lining of the uterus.

The cervix, which had lost its muscular structure and function during pregnancy, gradually resumes its thick tubular structure partly by shrinkage and partly by growth of new muscle cells. The opening of the cervix (the external os) is never quite the same and varies considerably in appearance in different women. It is larger and may be rounded or a broad slit and is often made irregular by tears that occurred during birth.

The vagina is at first a collapsed bag. It too shrinks in size but never quite back to the pregravid state. If an incision has been made at its outlet (episiotomy), this has usually healed in a matter of a few weeks.

With the contraction of the walls of the uterus after birth, the capacity of the uterus is reduced about one half. The lining is piled and appears thickened and as in menstruation is sloughed off, leaving the basal area from which the endometrial tissue will be regenerated. This is accomplished fairly quickly—in just a week or so. But at the site where the placenta was attached the process is somewhat different. We have seen that here the changes were great, with the formation of large blood vessels and an increase in supporting tissue. The separation of the placenta leaves this a raw surface. The uterus contracts, and the blood vessels are closed off by clotting of blood within and the pressure of the contracted uterus. This at first is an elevated area. Eventually it atrophies and sinks into the wall of the uterus, and the surface area is covered by the ingrowth of surrounding endometrium. In this manner there is no scar left as would be the case in any other part of the body where comparable cleavage had taken place.

As the lining of the uterus is returning to normal structure, there is a discharge through the vagina called "lochia." With the separation of the placenta, there is normally only a small amount of bleeding, but the discharge remains blood-tinged for four or five days and then changes to a more watery type, which continues for a week, and finally there is a white discharge. The first menstruation may occur within a month but is usually within the second month.

Lactation

Among the first signs of pregnancy are the changes that become apparent in the breasts—the fullness, tenderness, and coloration, etc. These indicate that the breasts are alerted early to make the necessary changes so that they will be ready to fulfill their function when pregnancy terminates. As a matter of fact the breasts experience cyclic changes each month with the menstrual cycle as do the uterus and other structures of the reproductive organs, for they are attuned to the cyclic rise and fall of the various hormones that control the cycle.

With pregnancy, the functional elements of the breasts are stimulated to grow and get ready to function (begin the production and delivery of milk) by the hormones estrogen and progesterone. Some secretion begins early in pregnancy with the production of a watery-like fluid called "colostrum." After the birth of the baby this secretion is continued and increased for the first day or so, and while it differs from milk, it has important properties that render it beneficial.

When on the second or third day the milk comes in, it means that the cells not only begin the manufacture of milk but also pour it into the duct system. This is not the result of endocrine function alone but of a nerve reflex. It is instigated by the mechanical stimulation of the nipple by the suckling of the infant (or mechanical means as massage or milking or the use of a breast pump). The stimulation of the nipple and the withdrawal of milk is essential in maintaining the continuous flow. When the mother does not nurse the baby, the breasts may be full and painful for a few days. They will soon dry up and the breasts return to the inactive state. The drying up can be facilitated by binding the breasts, restriction of fluids, and the administration of hormones. But if suckling is continued the breasts will continue to secrete for a year or more.

Because the mechanism of lactation is dependent on a nerve reflex, it can be disturbed by nervous factors. A severe emotional shock can instantly stop the flow of milk, which may or may not be induced to return.

The nursing of the baby has some effect on the return to the normal status of reproductive function. It has a direct stimulating action on the uterus, which hastens involution with a quicker return to normal size. For a time it will inhibit ovarian function with a delay of the return of menstruation and fertility. But this is not absolute as menstruation may reappear in three to four months. There is a mistaken idea that lactation is a period of infertility—that as long as a woman nurses her baby she will not conceive. This is not a fact. There is another misconception that if a woman starts to menstruate, she should stop nursing the baby because the milk may be harmful to the baby. A better reason—if there is such a necessity—is that concurrent menstruation and lactation is excessive strain on the mother and probably results in poorer quality of the milk.

Lying-in, Rooming-in, and Child-Parent Relations

The puerperium used to be called the period of "lying-in," and hospitals devoted to women were, and a few still are, called "Lying-in Hospitals." The term now usually used is "maternity ward," which accords with the concept that the puerperium is a normal period, and safe delivery is followed by a period of normal convalescence with rapid recovery to a normal state of well-being. Accordingly, the period of hospitalization and bed rest has been cut short.

The puerperium marks the initiation of the mother (and father) into parenthood. At the beginning of the present era, when the belief became current that it is safer and better for babies to be born in hospitals, the intimate association of mother and baby was delayed for days or weeks.

The mother was kept in her room or ward and the babies housed in the nursery with all the other babies and brought to the mother only for the purpose of nursing. In recent years this restriction has been lessened and provisions made for the baby to be near the mother in a cubicle in or adjoining her room—an arrangement known as "rooming-in."

There has been a great deal said, pro and con, as to the necessity or value of this device. The advocates point out the value to the new mother in getting used to her new responsibility and acquiring skill in learning to care for the baby while still under guidance and supervision. They also stress the psychological value to mother and baby of this earlier and more intimate association.

Those who are lukewarm or opposed point out that woman is entitled to a few days of rest and quiet to recover from the stress of delivery and that there is time enough for her to assume the responsibilities of infant care, which she will more confidently accept when she again feels strong. They further point out that "rooming-in" is nothing new but was the only way prior to the era of hospitalization for delivery. The device is merely one of humanizing what unfortunately has become in some instances a cold impersonal atmosphere. The situation can be corrected by the kind of care the woman receives as well as or better than by the structure of the hospital.

More important than any physical device which keeps the parents and child in bodily proximity for a period of time is the love and understanding of the parents for each other and for the new child. Mature individuals will breach the few days of separation without difficulty, and the immature will not suddenly bloom into maturity in the few short days of more intimate contact. As for the baby's role, we can understand it after we have seen what its experiences are in the Age of the Unborn.

XII

UNSUCCESSFUL PREGNANCIES

MILLIONS OF BABIES are born each year. A commonplace fact it may seem, a simple matter of vital statistics, but when it is translated into terms of human experience, it takes on an entirely new meaning. Each individual of these millions represents a chain of events, from the mating of the two germ cells to the birth of the baby, which has been completed with perfect timing and accuracy because a delicate, complex, and ever-changing balance of protective and vitalizing forces has been maintained. It is amazing that this is accomplished in so nearly perfect a manner millions of times each year. Certainly there is no reason to be surprised that sometimes failure and mishaps occur somewhere along the way.

Success and failure are relative terms and must be defined. Ideally, a successful pregnancy is one that terminates with the mother unharmed by her experience and that yields a live, well-developed baby. It also implies that both mother and baby continue to thrive through the perinatal period, when both are recovering from the strains of birth. Some pregnancies fall short in terms of health of either the mother or the baby, and failures vary in kind and degree. These represent a broad array of medical problems associated with pregnancy, birth, and the perinatal period, which are beyond the scope of this book. We shall consider only the unsuccessful pregnancies that do not yield a live baby capable of survival.

These unsuccessful pregnancies, in which the baby is lost, fall into three large groups according to the degree of development of the baby and its chance of survival. The failure can occur anywhere between the moment of conception and the period of recovery from the hazardous journey of birth. The failure will have different causes according to the time at which it occurs during the changing phases of pregnancy.

The first large group are those pregnancies that are terminated before the fetus is "viable" (has a chance to live). Roughly, that corresponds to pregnancies up to five or six months. These are called by doctors abortions. In the second group, the fetus has developed into a baby, but has not attained the maturity necessary for independent existence. They are the premature babies. In the third group, pregnancy goes to term, but for some reason the baby is born dead (stillbirth) or dies in a short time (perinatal death).

The two groups involving a potentially viable baby can best be understood after we have followed the normal processes of growth and development from fetus to the mature infant. Therefore, it will be better to reserve the consideration of these to "The Age of the Unborn." So we have now the problem of the unsuccessful pregnancy that ends in abortion.

ABORTIONS

Don't be startled by the word "abortion." It probably brings to your mind such unsavory thoughts as "doing something to get rid of an unwanted pregnancy" or the recollection of sensational newspaper stories of a salesman or some other equally improbable person who had set himself up as an "abortionist" and was arrested when one of his unfortunate clients died as the result of his "services." Or, perhaps you have read of the police rounding-up an "abortion ring" consisting of doctors, nurses, go-betweens involved in clandestine meetings, intrigue, and money transactions. But this is not the true meaning of abortion.

Abortion, as doctors use the term, means the termination of any pregnancy by any cause before the fetus is large enough (1000 grams or about 2½ pounds) to have the slightest chance of living. In a way, it corresponds to the word that is familiar and acceptable to most people, "miscarriage." Abortion is a scientific term that covers the wider field of unsuccessful pregnancies. Miscarriage refers to only one kind, that which doctors call "spontaneous abortion," meaning that something went wrong within the pregnancy itself that led to failure and miscarriage. This distinguishes it from the "induced abortion" in which the pregnancy (which may be either normal or abnormal) is terminated or interrupted by deliberate outside forces; that is, something is done to the woman to relieve (or deprive, as the case may be) her of her pregnancy.

Induced abortions, those abortions performed by a person, are divided into two groups, not so much by the way they are performed, but by the purpose for which they were done. There is the "therapeutic abortion," which a doctor is permitted to perform to save the health and life of the mother. The other is the "criminal abortion" performed by anyone for the sole purpose of getting rid of an unwanted pregnancy. With the meaning of "abortion" as a general term clear, we are ready to seek the meaning, in terms of woman's experience, of spontaneous abortion, therapeutic abortion, and criminal abortion.

SPONTANEOUS ABORTION

It is easy to define spontaneous abortion and to discuss in general terms the symptoms, the probable causes, and what should be done. But when we apply this to an individual case, it may be very difficult to be specific on any of these points. It may be hard to know whether the woman is having or has had an abortion, or why she aborted, and therefore what is really necessary to be done for her welfare. This difficulty arises from the fact that most abortions occur in the early months of pregnancy when a woman is not yet sure that she is pregnant. The fact that she failed to menstruate does not always mean that she is pregnant. On the other hand, bleeding during this time does not mean that a pregnancy, known to exist, is being threatened or has already been lost.

The study of the fertility of a couple and the determination of cause of the seeming sterility require attention to many details; but the questions of paramount importance are: Has the patient ever been pregnant? Has she had any miscarriages?

Jane came in for medical help because she wanted to have a baby. She had been married six years and was still childless. She could not be sure she had ever been pregnant. There was one instance when she had missed her period and was very happy in the thought that she was pregnant. Then she started to bleed, just a slight amount for a few days, and then the flow became somewhat heavier than normal with cramps and clots that lasted a little longer than usual. Had she been pregnant and had a miscarriage? That can never be known. Even if she had gone to a doctor when the bleeding started, it would still have been too late to make a positive diagnosis of a lost pregnancy. This sort of thing happens very frequently to many women. We can be sure that an abortion occurred in these early months only when the diagnosis of pregnancy was established, either by a pregnancy test or by recognition of the fetal parts in the aborted material.

Danger Signals

When the fact that she is pregnant has been established, how can a woman know that she is in danger of aborting? The symptoms vary, but bleeding of any kind should always be considered a danger signal. Sometimes a woman will start with just a small amount of bleeding, no more than spotting. Sometimes it is bright red blood, sometimes dark brown. It may occur even as early as the time of the first missed menstrual period and continue as slight bleeding, off and on, for several weeks. She may also have cramps or heavy discomfort low in her abdomen similar to menstrual discomfort. These symptoms may disappear entirely for a few days or a few weeks only to recur again and be more pronounced. Or the woman may be apparently progressing quite normally for weeks or months and suddenly start to cramp and bleed. In a short time, the pregnancy is without a doubt ended when she passes something that can be recognized as the products of conception. The actual amount of bleeding is also quite variable. In early pregnancy one woman may bleed no more than a normal period and yet have lost her pregnancy, while another may bleed considerably more and still maintain hers.

Bleeding, however, does not always mean an abortion is threatened. The question is often asked: "Can a woman menstruate after she becomes pregnant?" The answer is a qualified yes. There are two types of bleeding during pregnancy that are considered physiological and do not endanger the pregnancy, although they are not true menstrual periods. One is a slight amount of bleeding that occurs only once and lasts only a few days during the first month of pregnancy. This corresponds to the time that the ovum is burrowing into the lining of the uterus and opening blood vessels. Once the placental arrangement is defined, the bleeding stops. The second type is recurrent scanty bleeding at the time of the first two or three missed periods and is due to the fact that the menstrual rhythmicity has not been completely suppressed. There is still another type of bleeding, which appears occasionally, that is not a signal of danger. This is harmless, as far as pregnancy is concerned, because it comes from slight abnormalities of the cervix such as erosion (raw area) or a polyp. Such bleeding is not accompanied by pain, is usually bright red in color, and frequently appears after intercourse.

Complete Abortion

How is a woman to know that she has lost her pregnancy? This is usually not difficult if the pregnancy has progressed for three to six months. The fetus by that time has achieved the recognizable form of a miniature baby. The membranes and placenta are also well developed. Such an abortion is therefore a miniature birth, the typical symptoms of bleeding and labor pains are less regular but still quite severe, and the duration of labor is shorter.

An abortion is also recognizable in the first three months, even in the first few weeks, if a woman knows what to look for. The baby-to-be will probably not be recognizable as such and often cannot be found at all. Usually, death has come to it days or weeks before it was expelled or aborted, and it is therefore not as large as might be expected and has undergone degenerative changes. The membranes, however, are usually quite distinctive. The "abortus," as doctors call the product expelled, will look like a greyish-white puffball filled with fluid if the membranes have not ruptured; or, a flat sheet of tissue of irregular shape if the membranes have split. In either case the glistening, pearly white color will usually distinguish it from the surrounding clots of blood. If it is placed in water the outer surface will appear velvety while the inner surface is smooth and glistening. Occasionally, nothing is recognizable.

It is important for the doctor to know what has been expelled so that

e may decide what is necessary to be done for the safety and comfort of
is patient. If all the products, membranes and fetus, have been passed,
1e abortion is complete. He then does not need to do more than give
ipportive care, which includes precaution against infections, something
>r her pain, and treatment of anemia if she has lost considerable blood.

igns of Incomplete Abortion

Once in a while one hears a woman complain that she had trouble after
miscarriage, sometimes at a much later date, because "I didn't have
roper care—the doctor didn't clean me out." This is probably not true,
>r usually there is no need for "cleaning out," or curettage. Nature does
pretty good job of getting rid of the remains of her failure, just as she
iscards an imperfect product. Sometimes, when she fails and the abortion
, incomplete, the doctor must step in and give her a helping hand.

In an incomplete abortion, the uterus is not completely emptied. In
>me cases only small parts of the placenta and membranes are retained;
1 others, almost the whole product, although it has broken off its con-
ections with the lining of the uterus, is still retained. In either case
1e woman will continue to bleed and is vulnerable to infection. The
octor must clear out the debris by curettage, so that the uterus can
:turn to normal.

Iissed Abortion

There is one kind of abortion that has none of these symptoms—the so-
illed missed abortion. In this instance the woman has the usual signs and
ymptoms of pregnancy for a month or so, then the symptoms disappear.
"he uterus does not grow because the fetus has died. She may have a
ttle bleeding. In most instances abortion occurs weeks later; occasionally
curettage must be performed.

Causes of Spontaneous Abortion

Miscarriage of her pregnancy is a blow to a woman, shattering her hopes and plans. If she is young or has other children, she may accept it philosophically. But to an older, childless woman it spells tragedy and much grief. In either case it indicates to her that she has failed in her ability to have this child, and she looks for the cause within herself, in things that she has done or not done, or some hidden abnormality of her body. She is encouraged in this belief by the widespread misconceptions as to the causes of abortions.

The most common misconception is that falls, physical shocks, or blows are the cause of abortion. Almost every woman who has had a miscarriage can look back and find some instance in which she stumbled or fell or lifted something heavy, and she blames her misfortune on one of these. But these same things happen just as frequently to women who have a full-term pregnancy and pass unnoticed. Nature protects a normal pregnancy to the extent that bodily injuries will not dislodge it.

The truth is that most spontaneous abortions occur because the pregnancy itself is defective. It is therefore usually a blessing in disguise because there would be little hope for a normal baby even if it carried to full term. What do we mean by defective pregnancy and what causes it to be defective? There is no single, simple answer. Rather we may say there are two types of defective pregnancies for which there are many causes.

The first type is the one in which the fault lies in the fetus itself. It just didn't "have what it takes" at the very beginning to grow and differentiate properly. In other words, the germ plasm of either the ovum or the sperm was defective. Why was it defective? So far as we know there is only one reason, heredity—some deficiency in the chromosomes and genes that is incompatible with life. But this need not be frightening for it does not necessarily mean that because one germ cell was defective all will be defective. This is rarely, if ever, the case. But nature is not perfect, she does slip up sometimes. There are many familiar examples of this.

If you have ever planted seeds, you know that all the seeds do not come up even though each is carefully planted. A more vivid example is the kernels on an ear of corn. Most are turgid and juicy because they are mature, ready to germinate. But in almost every ear, there is at least one that did not develop at all. This faulty germplasm is therefore just a random occurrence in all nature and not the fault of the parents. The random defects are just as likely to occur in one pregnancy as another and can still be followed by normal pregnancies.

The second type of defective pregnancy is the result of a faulty environment. Some factor outside the fetus was harmful enough to destroy its life; or the environment did not supply all the necessities for fetal growth and development. What do we mean by "environment"? It includes the structures and physiologic functions of the woman's body that are involved in the establishment and maintenance of pregnancy, such as her reproductive organs, her endocrine glands, her nutrition. It also includes the things that happen to the mother that are injurious to the pregnancy, such as disease, shock, or injury. Environment therefore is a broad term. We can understand it better if we break it down into the various factors and examine them one at a time. We can then see not only how and why each environmental factor may be at fault but also which environmental factors are the most frequent causes of defective pregnancies. In contrast to defective germ plasm, for which the mother is not responsible, environmental factors include many for which she is responsible and which could have been prevented or corrected before pregnancy.

It should not be surprising to find that the deficiency of some endocrine gland is a frequent causative factor in spontaneous abortion, when we consider the enormous role these glands play from the moment of conception to birth. They must be on the job every moment, each one working steadily and efficiently to prepare the bed for the ovum to be implanted, to stay the flow of menstruation, and to foster the changes in the endometrium that will furnish nourishment and protection for the new life. This is a complex mechanism that must be in good order before the pregnancy starts. There is little reason to believe that an endocrine mechanism that was functioning well before conception will break down after the pregnancy is well established. When it is defective at the start of a pregnancy, the ovum is insecurely lodged and is unable to obtain adequate nourishment. As a result the embryo cannot grow and develop, but eventually dies of starvation. Then and only then does nature discard the pregnancy. The ovum or fetus dies early or late, depending on when its needs exceed the available supply. This is usually sometime before the third month.

So much for how deficiency of the endocrine glands in general is a cause of abortion. Now we want to know which glands are most likely to be at fault. Theoretically, it would seem possible that the chances should be about equal for each of the glands concerned. Actually, studies of individual cases of spontaneous abortion do not bear this out. One type of glandular deficiency is far more common than all the rest.

Thyroid deficiency has been found to be the only cause in about one third of the cases and a contributing factor in another third. Thus in roughly 65 per cent of spontaneous abortions due to glandular deficiency, the thyroid is the gland at fault. This is heartening information because thyroid deficiency is easily detected (if one looks for it) and also easily corrected.

Considering the important role that the ovarian hormones, estrogen and especially progesterone, play, it would seem that progesterone deficiency might be a likely cause, but this is hard to prove. Doctors have used both estrogen and progesterone in their efforts to save pregnancies that were threatened, but they are not agreed on the effectiveness of this form of therapy. Other types of glandular dysfunction rarely cause abortion.

The general nutrition of the mother is certainly an important environmental factor of pregnancy. How often and to what extent malnutrition contributes to the loss of a pregnancy, we do not know. We have seen how it may interfere with normal glandular function, leading to amenorrhea and menstrual abnormalities. In times of starvation, such as have occurred in wide-spread famine and in life in concentration camps, sterility, stillbirths, and fetal abnormalities occur more frequently than in a normal population. Certainly pregnancy must be supplied with adequate building materials of proteins, minerals, and vitamins. Which vitamin is more important is a question. Vitamin E had quite a vogue in the treatment of sterility and repeated abortion, but there is insufficient evidence to prove that it is as important in humans as it is in some laboratory animals. It seems more reasonable to suppose that an adequate amount of all the vitamins is more important because each has a specific role, and each is needed for a normal pregnancy. It therefore behooves every woman to maintain a normal nutritional balance, not just during pregnancy but long before she starts a pregnancy.

When a pregnant woman becomes ill, what are the chances that her illness will adversely affect her pregnancy? This will vary with the type of illness. The acute infectious diseases, such as pneumonia and measles, are apt to be more harmful. In rare cases they may cause death of the fetus either by bacterial invasion, in which the fetus contracts the disease, or intoxication, in which the toxic products of the infection circulating in the mother's blood stream pass to that of the fetus. On the other hand, the chronic diseases or illnesses that are slowly progressive, such as tuberculosis, may not affect the pregnancy at all. In some instances the mother's health may seem to improve during pregnancy only to fail rapidly after the birth of her baby. Tuberculosis and cancer do not cause abortions. Syphilis is more likely to cause stillbirths. Gonorrhea leads to sterility.

Some abnormality of the woman's pelvic organs is considered to be a frequent cause of abortion. This is a misconception. The truth is, if the organs are normal enough for a pregnancy to be established, it usually goes to term. Retroversion of the uterus ("tilted womb") has been blamed most frequently for many of woman's ills and for her miscarriages, but it is rarely the cause of any such difficulties. Retroversion is corrected naturally in pregnancy. As the uterus grows, it is gradually raised up from its reclining position in the pelvic cavity in the only direction in which there is room for expansion, which is upward into the abdominal cavity. Only rarely is it entrapped in the pelvis (caught behind the promontory of the sacrum), and then the increasing pressure of growth in confined quarters can cause abortion. The doctor can correct the abnormal position of the uterus if it is recognized early, and no harm need result.

Fibroids of the uterus can cause abortion, for the reason that they consist of hard, gristly material that will not respond with normal growth and elasticity necessary for pregnancy. They may be the cause of faulty implantation when the ovum lodges over one where the endometrial bed is thin and poorly developed. Or, if a single, large fibroid is present or fibroid changes involve a good part of the musculature of the uterus, normal expansion of the uterus may be impeded. But even those do not preclude the possibility of a successful pregnancy. Many times such a pregnancy goes to term without difficulty. A single large fibroid can be removed even during pregnancy, and the woman may go on and have her baby. More frequently, it is discovered too late when abortion is imminent or has already occurred. Removal then makes possible a subsequent normal pregnancy.

Significance of One Spontaneous Abortion

The threat of abortion sometimes hangs heavy over woman's head. She may become anxious at the start of her pregnancy that something may happen to make her lose it. The loss of the first pregnancy may not be a severe blow to a young woman as it often happens before she knows that she is pregnant, but it makes her a little uneasy until nature dispels her doubts with a normal pregnancy. To an older woman who has been trying for years to have a baby and has been studied and treated for her infertility, the loss of a pregnancy confirms her fears that motherhood is never to be hers. How real is this threat of abortion? What are a woman's chances when she becomes pregnant that she will have a successful pregnancy? What are the odds against her having a normal pregnancy after she has had one, two, or even three or more miscarriages? The prospects are better than one might think.

Women are not particularly addicted to betting or adept at evaluating odds. Rather they are interested in what is going to happen in their particular case. Nor are most women interested in statistics, which is sometimes just as well, for they can be quite disturbing. But it all depends on how one looks at statistics, for they can also be quite reassuring. This is true for what we know about the incidence of abortions.

There can never be an accurate count of the number of abortions that occur spontaneously each year. But from studies of large series of women who have sought medical care from their own private physicians or were treated in hospitals or clinics, doctors have arrived at the estimate that about one pregnancy in ten ends in spontaneous abortion. In other words, when a woman becomes pregnant she has nine chances out of ten of a successful termination, which is certainly not too disturbing. They found also that bleeding, which is a threat to pregnancy, does not make abortion inevitable. For every woman who bleeds and loses her pregnancy, there

; one who bleeds and yet goes on to have a normal baby. So even with threatened abortion, a woman still has a fifty-fifty chance.

Furthermore, one abortion does not lessen the woman's chance of having normal pregnancy thereafter. These first abortions, no matter whether hey are the woman's first or fifth pregnancy are due to random causes, vhich just happened to occur in that particular pregnancy and will not ecessarily be present in a subsequent one. Among women whose first regnancy ended in abortion, nine out of ten will have a normal subseuent pregnancy. Even after two abortions the chances are still better han six in ten for success the next time. Of course, when a cause is ound for the abortion and corrected, the chances for a normal subsequent regnancy are greatly improved.

When a woman has had three spontaneous abortions and no normal regnancies, doctors label this "habitual abortion." Even then she still has bout three or four chances in ten of a normal pregnancy. If she is careully studied and treated, her chances are improved according to the eriousness of her problem and how amenable it may be to treatment.

Rarely is any case hopeless. Nature herself effects the cure in many nstances, and women have normal pregnancies after several false starts.
Give nature a helping hand before and during pregnancy rather than mpede her, and she usually does a superb job. These unsuccessful first regnancies are frequently due to immaturity of the reproductive process, glandular imbalance, faulty nutrition, and emotional disturbances in varyng degrees and combinations for each case. Once these are corrected, and the woman has one normal pregnancy, she is not likely to continue o abort. She will return to the normal pattern in subsequent pregnancies. On the other hand, when a woman gets older, has had several children, and then habitually aborts, the situation is different. The causes then are njured reproductive organs (especially the cervix), diseases of these organs, general lowered health, and aging of the reproductive process. Her chances to return to a normal pattern are poor.

THERAPEUTIC ABORTION

Sometimes a pregnancy, which in itself is normal, is terminated in th interest of the welfare of the mother. This, a "therapeutic abortion," performed by a qualified and reputable doctor in a hospital for the purpos of protecting or perhaps saving the life of the mother. It is a legal an above-board procedure, but doctors are very careful in the selection cases in which they consider it is medically and legally justifiable interrupt the pregnancy, for there are no hard and fast rules to guic them.

From a legal standpoint, to induce abortion of a normal pregnancy a crime except in certain circumstances. The laws vary from state state. Most states permit abortion to save the life of the mother. Som states, but not all, also make it legal when the woman's health is en dangered. What constitutes danger to her life or to her health, whic can be mental as well as physical, is nowhere spelled out, so the decisio is left to the doctor. Thus in some states a young girl pregnant as th result of rape could be legally relieved of the pregnancy, but in othe she could not. Actually, doctors run little risk of getting into troub with the law. You have only to read your newspapers to know that court have great difficulty in getting a conviction that will "stick" on th outright "abortionists," people who make criminal abortion their busines What doctors are concerned about is their own integrity and their pr fessional reputation.

What is considered medical justification for abortion has changed witl medical advances through the years. Many conditions, which used t constitute hazards to a woman's life, such as a heart condition and tuber culosis, can now be handled safely through pregnancy in many instance and are therefore no longer indications for interruption of pregnancy. O the other hand, mental illnesses and the probability of the birth of defective child, which have only recently received recognition as medica problems, are now considered "possible indications" for abortion. Thes are "possible" indications, for the interpretation of "justifiable circum stances" varies from place to place, that is, whether the case comes u for decision in one state or another, a large city or a small town, or eve different hospitals in the same city. This may be illustrated by two cases.

Mrs. X had four healthy children before the Rh incompatibility between herself and her husband affected her ability to have normal children. Her fifth baby was born erythroblastotic with monstrous physical deformity and lived only a few hours. When she found that she was again pregnant, her reaction quite naturally was terrible fear that she would have another abnormal child and that it might live. She was told that the local laws, and the doctor's interpretations of them, did not admit the possibility of an abnormal child to be sufficient justification for the termination of her pregnancy. She went to another state, where law and medical opinion were different, and had a therapeutic abortion.

Miss Y had for several years been under the care of a psychiatrist for episodes of profound mental depression in some of which she had tried to commit suicide. When she became pregnant, it was not difficult to find both another psychiatrist to agree that pregnancy was a dire threat to her mental health and possibly her life, and a gynecologist to remove the threat.

The vagueness of the law and the stigma that is attached to induced abortions create a dilemma that most doctors have little taste to try to resolve. Of course in the case of a woman who seeks medical care during her pregnancy and in whom conditions are present or develop that clearly jeopardize her life, most doctors (but not all) would consider her life first and have no hesitation in terminating the pregnancy. Neither are they bothered too much by the demands of those women who just don't want a pregnancy. But not all cases are so clearly defined. There are many instances when the doctor must make the decision. No reputable doctor will perform an abortion that is clearly illegal, nor will he relish having to perform many therapeutic abortions, however justifiable they may be medically. By doing so, he runs the risk of acquiring the reputation among other doctors of being too quick to do an abortion, if not actually labeled an abortionist.

Hospitals, too, are careful of their reputations. Some will not permit any therapeutic abortions to be performed in their operating rooms. Others limit the number allowed within a specified time, as a month or a quarter. Most hospitals have established, both for their own protection and that of their doctors, a clearly defined method of procedure, which must be followed before a therapeutic abortion is allowed. The doctor must have a consultation with at least one, sometimes two or three, other doctors, all must agree after examining the patient that the procedure is necessary, put in writing their findings and recommendations, and sign their names. Some hospitals have a committee to pass on all cases instead of the consultation.

A therapeutic abortion is a surgical procedure done in the hospital under the strictest sterile technique. The risk to the patient is not as great as some believe. The dangers are mostly those of any other pregnancy—hemorrhage and infection. But with blood for transfusions and antibiotics readily available to stave off infection, these dangers are usually quite successfully eliminated or controlled. The medical condition for which the abortion is done may make the procedure more dangerous. The procedure will vary with the duration of the pregnancy. If it is within the first three months, a curettage is done. After the third month, this is more difficult, so the doctor uses the method most appropriate for the specific case to induce premature labor.

CRIMINAL ABORTION

No one knows how many criminal abortions are performed each year. Judging from available data, students of the subject conclude that there are just about as many criminal abortions as there are spontaneous abortions. Thus, of every hundred pregnancies, ten end in spontaneous abortion, ten to twelve are criminally aborted, and less than one per cent are terminated for therapeutic reasons. With the present birth rate, this means that there are more than 300,000 criminal abortions a year in the United States or about 1,000 every day.

Who are these 300,000 women who each year find ways and means of ridding themselves of unwanted pregnancies? Obviously they can't all be unmarried girls. The surprising truth is that only a small percentage are. Nine out of ten or 270,000 are young married women mostly between the ages of 25 to 35, many of whom have two or more children.

Confronted with an unwanted pregnancy, these women attempt to secure an abortion in one of three ways: they try to do it themselves; they go to a lay abortionist; or they go to a medical abortionist.

Most women know very little about their anatomy and physiology and so are incapable of inducing an abortion. They may resort to several ineffectual methods such as exhausting exercises, hot baths, strong purgatives, or they take "medicines" advertised "to regulate" (meaning to abort), which are impotent to harm the pregnancy but may endanger or cost the woman her life. Sometimes they try direct methods. Douches containing strong chemicals are used or vaginal suppositories inserted in hopes of killing the pregnancy. The chemical used is often so caustic that it literally burns holes in the walls of the vagina causing dangerous hemorrhage and opening the way to infection, which the woman has herself introduced. The most direct method—and the most dangerous—is the use of "instruments" to try to physically dislodge the pregnancy. The things that they have employed as "instruments" are appalling to name and unbelievable, such as hat-pins and knitting needles. The results of their use is injury to the woman, not her pregnancy, and such injury is frequently fatal.

"Lay abortionists" are people who know little more than the woman and use much the same methods of douches, packing, pastes, and bougies. They may have induced a few abortions previously, but certainly they do not have the knowledge or the skill to do them safely.

By far the largest number of abortions are done by a few doctors who, in most instances, use some surgical technique that guards against the dangers of infection and hemorrhage. Doctors who make a business of doing abortions are careful to protect themselves not only by seeing that no harm comes to the woman, but by making their services accessible only through channels they can trust not to divulge their actions to the authorities of the law. Since it is strictly a business to make money, their prices are high, and they require cash across the board before the service is rendered.

The fact that a criminal abortion is illegal is really insignificant beside the fact of its dangers to the woman. It may cost her her life, it may injure her health and render future pregnancies impossible, and it is a psychic injury from which she may never completely recover.

The physical dangers to her life and health are those of infection and hemorrhage. Septic abortion causes more maternal deaths than any other single cause. Eight thousand women died in the United States in 1956, one third of the total maternal mortality, as the result of septic abortion—

not necessarily criminally induced. The seriousness and ever-present threat of infection comes from the fact that there is probably no part of a woman's body, at any time in her life, that is anywhere nearly as susceptible, or is such a fertile ground for infection to flourish, as the pregnant uterus. This is especially true when the pregnancy has been disturbed but not completely dislodged, and the uterus is unable to regress to the non-pregnant state. This is also conducive to hemorrhage. Criminal abortions attempted by unskilled persons or the woman herself by the introduction of some instrument frequently result in puncturing the soft thin walls of the uterus and almost always in the introduction of infection. The results are hemorrhage and acute illness, which is like the puerperal sepsis that we have met in the dark days of obstetrics.

The lives of many women are saved by prompt and good medical care, but there are some who, fearful that doctors will not treat them, do not even seek medical care or do so only when it is already too late. For every woman who dies after abortion, there must be ten at least who will pay the price—and it is a large one—the rest of their lives in physical suffering, sterility, or unhappiness. Any abortion may be and often is a psychic trauma to a woman. This is especially true of an induced abortion. The feeling of guilt at having destroyed a life, the shame, and the remorse may so disturb her emotionally that normal adjustments become difficult or impossible. Anything from unhappiness to mental illness may be the result. The abortion, undergone in desperation, was made more of an ordeal because of its clandestine nature, the strange, forbidding, and often squalid place where it was performed, and the type of people she came in contact with, all of which added to her uncertainty and fear. It will forever be a painful memory, difficult to dispel, which comes back to haunt and rebuke her.

There are other cases when the woman thought she was pregnant and did something to get rid of it. These are the women who come in and say "Doctor, I think I am pregnant—can't you give me something to start my period?" They are laboring under the misconception that there is a twilight zone in which a "touch" or "threat of pregnancy" exists, that life itself is not yet involved. These are the women who have had a delayed period and have taken some kind of medication or hot baths, jumped off step-ladders, or exercised themselves to exhaustion to "prevent" an unwanted pregnancy. They do not realize that such efforts are in vain if pregnancy exists, that is, if the ovum is firmly implanted (which is well before the woman starts her efforts to "bring on her period"). Nature is adamant in her desire and determination to assure the perpetuation of the species. If she had good material for the pregnancy, she will hold on to it in spite of all the woman does. The drugs the woman takes will make her sick, she may break her arm in the fall, the baths and the exercise may exhaust her, but she most likely will not dislodge her pregnancy. If her efforts are seemingly crowned with success, they were still useless because she probably was not pregnant in the first place.

A similar misconception is that "shots" will interrupt a pregnancy. These consist of either one or two large doses of progesterone or three doses of prostigmine, and they are used merely to bring on a menstrual period delayed by some cause other than pregnancy. They will in no way affect a pregnancy. For this reason they are sometimes used as a test for pregnancy, but are not very accurate as such. They do not always bring on the period. If they do, you may be sure no pregnancy ever existed.

ECTOPIC PREGNANCY

There is one type of pregnancy that is doomed to failure, with rare exceptions, from the very start. In this, not only is the life of the fetus almost always lost, but the mother's life is greatly endangered in the process. This is ectopic pregnancy—a pregnancy that is implanted in some place other than within the body of the uterus. The ectopic implantation can be anywhere along the route the ovum travels. In rare instances this may be within the ovary or in the abdominal cavity. In the majority of ectopic pregnancies, probably as high as 99 per cent, the fertilized ovum is lodged in the Fallopian tube and becomes implanted there. Hence, this type of ectopic pregnancy is called "tubal pregnancy." Because of the inability of the tube to meet the demands of the growing fetus, sooner or later something has to happen, either the pregnancy is aborted (expelled from the tube into a less confining position, such as the abdominal cavity, where in rare instances it continues to grow) or more frequently the tube ruptures. Both are accompanied by internal bleeding that endangers the life of the mother.

One Friday evening as I was leaving my office, I fell into a casual con-
versation with another doctor and remarked that it was good to reach
the end of the work-a-day week and to go home for a quiet week end.
He started quizzing me about what I meant by a "quiet week end." Didn't
I have office hours on Saturday? Didn't I expect hurried calls on Sunday?
At first I tried to explain that I didn't do surgery, that I didn't deliver
babies, and that the practice of medical gynecology was not primarily one
of emergencies and hurried hospital calls. But as he persisted unimpressed
but seemingly shocked that I did not work twenty-four hours a day
seven days a week, I realized that he was just "taking me for a ride,"
and the implication was: How could a woman have the effrontery to
call herself a doctor and still claim the privilege of a woman's private
and personal life? Being vulnerable, as most women are, to personal slights
and criticisms, and tired too, my rising anger overruled polite restraint.
When he said, with a condescending smile, "Well, doctor, what do you
do about your ruptured ectopic pregnancies? Don't you think they are
emergencies? I find them so," I snapped back, "No, doctor, because I don't
allow my ectopics to go along to rupture." That silenced him, but I could
have bitten my tongue out the moment it was said, not because I was
rude in implying that he was not accurate in his diagnosis and treatment
of ectopic pregnancy and I was sorry for my rudeness, but because no
doctor in his or her right mind should ever make such a claim.

The diagnosis of ectopic pregnancy, before it ruptures and becomes a
threat to the woman's life, is one of the most difficult diagnoses a gynecologist is called on to make. And I am just superstitious enough to
believe that when one brags, one is inviting trouble. Somehow fate
would see to it that I would see the day when I would doubly regret my
insincere boast. That is how ectopic pregnancy has come to be a sword
over my head—some day it may fall. That is why the case of Carmen gave
me such satisfaction. It seemed to be a reprieve if not a release.

Carmen telephoned me (late on Friday afternoon) and said that she
was having severe pains in her lower right side and felt miserable. She
thought it was because she was having an abnormal menstrual period.
It had been late by about three weeks in the first place, which was not
too unusual for her, and the flow just couldn't seem to get started. Rather,
there had been just off-and-on-dribble for the past ten days. Couldn't

I send her some medicine that would start the flow? She was sure that then she would feel better.

I recalled that Carmen had come to me several years previously, as a bride from a foreign country. Her husband's business involved rather frequent trips back and forth. At that time, I had treated her for a pelvic inflammatory condition. I had not seen her since, so at my request she filled in what had happened. On her return to her country, about a year previously, she had again become ill and had been operated on for a "bad ovary." In response to my query, she said she had had no pregnancies, although they wanted a child very badly.

Suspicious that something more than a delayed period was wrong, I told Carmen to call her husband and have him bring her to my office as soon as possible. She was reluctant to do so because she thought she wasn't that sick and that she could just wait until Monday. But she finally agreed. When I examined her, I believed that my first suspicions had been right, that she probably had an ectopic pregnancy. Whether it had ruptured I did not know. Her abdomen was swollen, quite hard, and tender. On pelvic examination, the uterus was somewhat larger and softer than normal, and there was a boggy mass on her right side, which I could not outline very well because it was so very tender. Her blood pressure was low, her pulse rapid but not strong. She had a slight elevation of temperature.

I told her husband what I thought was wrong. They were not particularly impressed and certainly not as concerned as I was, partly because Carmen had been sick before and nothing catastrophic had happened, and partly because ectopic pregnancy did not worry them as much as it did me. However, they finally agreed that Carmen should be hospitalized and seen by a surgeon. But all was not yet clear sailing.

The surgeon agreed with my diagnosis and recommended immediate surgery. But Carmen had other ideas. She had been operated on once, and here she was sick again. Perhaps it was the same thing wrong with the other ovary, and if she had another operation, she could never have a baby. Anyhow, if she had to have another operation, she would fly home to the doctor who had operated on her previously. He would know better what was wrong because he had seen inside. Since she seemed to be in no immediate danger, the surgeon agreed to keep her under observation for a while. He ordered a frog test for pregnancy, which was positive. Her blood pressure dropped some as did her red cell count (which suggested internal bleeding) during the night and early morning, but stabilized by midday. Her abdomen remained tense and swollen, and vaginal bleeding continued.

To make a long story short—and it was a long story because it took more than a week to get Carmen to consent to surgery—an ectopic pregnancy was found in the right tube. Carmen can give thanks for her life to the infinite patience and skill of her surgeon, and even that might not have been enough, had she not been lucky in what had happened. There had been no extensive rupture of the tube, but only a slight tear with leakage of blood into the abdominal cavity. But the doctor would not have been so patient if she had had symptoms of a frank rupture with profuse hemorrhage, and maybe she would not have been so stubborn!

What is the cause of ectopic pregnancy? Why should the ovum settle down in an unsuitable spot before it reaches its normal destination? The answer does not lie in the perversity of the ovum; there is nothing wrong with it. The truth is, the ovum cannot do otherwise, because the way is blocked. When we recall that the passageway of the tube is small and tortuous and that the ovum is completely dependent on forces outside itself for propulsion, it becomes apparent that the tube must be normal both in its structure and function if it is to deliver the ovum safely to its destination. The tube may be unable to afford transit to the ovum because it has been damaged by some previous disease such as infection or because it had never developed to normal size and proportions. Occasionally, the passageway may be rendered too small by pressure on the outside of the tube by such things as tumors or it may be blocked by adhesions. In any event, the ovum is stalled, but it continues to grow and develop.

A tubal pregnancy is hard to diagnose because there are no characteristic symptoms that anything is wrong. In the early weeks, the pregnancy continues along normal lines, the ovum differentiates into the embryo, and its membrane burrows into the wall of the tube as it would had it been in the uterus. While it is still small, this causes no particular trouble. The woman misses her period. The uterus grows in response to the increasing hormone levels, which also hold back menstruation, but not quite as completely as in a normal pregnancy, so there is slight vaginal bleeding or spotting. At this time the woman thinks she has a normal pregnancy or, as Carmen did, that her period is just delayed.

Eventually the tube reaches the limit of its ability to accommodate, and it ruptures. It has been stretched to the limit by the increasing size of the fetus and its membranes, and it has been weakened by the burrowing fingers of the developing placenta, which soon extend through the walls of the tube. Rupture of the tube always causes bleeding. If the rupture or break is sudden and extensive, the bleeding will be profuse. If it is a slow tear, the bleeding may be only a trickle for a while, as in the case of Carmen. But each is bleeding that is internal, cannot be seen, and is recognized only by the symptoms produced. Such bleeding must be stopped because it is a threat to the woman's life. And the only way to stop it is by surgery. The doctor must operate and remove the tube or at least the part involved in the pregnancy and rupture.

UNWANTED PREGNANCY

There is another type of pregnancy that is potentially unsuccessful in that it rarely affords any hope for complete fulfillment of the ideal mother-child relationship. This is the unwanted pregnancy, particularly the illegitimate pregnancy. It is not strictly a medical problem, but it is one that frequently confronts doctors. It may be a pregnancy that is unsuccessful in terms of the life of the mother and baby or it may fall into any of the types of unsuccessful pregnancies, usually of abortion. It is, in our culture, one that is always frought with danger, heartache, and human suffering.

A doctor who has been in practice for any time has had to meet the problem of the unmarried girl who is pregnant. Some shrug it off with, "she got herself into the mess, let her get herself out." Others who would never think of doing an abortion themselves, will help her make contact with a doctor who will. Others will sit down and talk with the girl and try to help her work out the solution that is best for her, and there is certainly no one solution.

Sometimes it seems to pose no problem at all, as in the case related to me by a teacher in one of our schools, where senior and junior high school girls in increasing numbers are being excused from attendance because of pregnancy. Lillie, we shall call her, a tall thin girl of fifteen, was obviously pregnant, and her school advisor was talking to her:

"Lillie, do you know that you are pregnant, that you are going to have a baby?"

"Yes, mam."

"Do you know who the father is?"

"Yes, mam, it's Joe—he's my boy friend."

"Well, don't you think you and Joe should be married right away?"

"Well, no, mam. We thought we would just wait and have the wedding and the christening at the same time—that would be lots less trouble."

Then there was the case of the young woman who came to me some years ago on some feigned complaint, but actually to see whether I would tell her if she was pregnant. I did, and asked her whether she had any plans to be married. She replied that she couldn't do that because the man responsible was already married, and she couldn't marry him if he should ever be divorced. It further developed that she already had one illegitimate child, whom her grandmother was rearing. The only question that seemed to bother her was what excuse she could give to her office for being away a few months so that she would still have her job on her return. She apparently found one and went to a nearby city and placed herself under a doctor's care. But she didn't have to stay long. Fortunately or not, nature interrupted her pregnancy. Certainly it was fortunate that she was under a doctor's care, for she had a placenta praevia, which could have endangered her life had she not had prompt medical care for her premature delivery. She returned to me for her five-week check-up. I asked her why, if she intended to go on with this affair, which had already produced two illegitimate pregnancies, she did not make some effort to protect herself. To which she replied, "I can't do that. If I am carried away by my passions, that is one thing, but to use birth control is a deliberate sin. I could never do that."

These girls were of limited intelligence and education and certainly far from responsible maturity. To them an illegitimate pregnancy was perhaps bad luck, but not a catastrophe. They did not consider what the handicap of illegitimacy would mean in the life of the child. But to other girls and young women who are desperate in their plight, what can a doctor advise?

Marriage, of course, is the first suggestion, but not necessarily the best. Frequently it is out of the question because the man is either already married or has faded from the scene. Such a marriage starts with two strikes against it. First there is the difficult job of learning to live together, which under the best circumstances takes time and considerable effort on the part of both man and woman. This is made more difficult by the physical limitations placed on the woman by the pregnancy and the necessity to put on a bold front and explain to their families and friends the "seven-months baby." Perhaps the greatest obstacle to such a marriage is the feeling of compulsion that hovers over it. A woman usually does not want a husband who had to marry her. Occasionally, there is one who is happy to get her man in any circumstances, will even deliberately so ensnare him, trusting to luck that she can hold him. "Luck" is rarely so obliging. There are difficulties enough when the woman and man have known each other fairly well, have a certain degree of compatibility, and even consider that they are "in love." Too frequently there is only infatuation, and sometimes they are little more than strangers to each other. The story is a familiar one—a party, too much liquor, too little restraint—and pregnancy is the result.

Sometimes the marriage turns out well, as in the case of Eileen. Sometimes it fails completely, as in the case of Amy. Perhaps more often it lumbers along, wrecking the chances of happiness of the mother and father and denying the child its birthright of love and security in a happy home.

Eileen and Tom had been friends for many years. Both were in their thirties, both had been hurt in previous love affairs and were afraid of being hurt again. They had found satisfaction in their purely friendly relationship and truly expected to maintain it as such. A New Year's celebration, too much conviviality—and Eileen was pregnant. Neither blamed the other, both were sorry that it had happened. They were married, to the great satisfaction of their families and friends, but with some misgiving between themselves. However, they had many things in their favor—long acquaintance, similar backgrounds, mutual interests, mutual respect, and a serious determination to do the best they could. Eileen wrote me some years later that they were happier in their marriage and their child than either had ever dreamed they could be and were looking forward to the new baby they would soon welcome to the family.

Amy was the bobby-soxer that we have already met in the section on amenorrhea. She was 15, the boy 16, when she became pregnant. Her mother took them to another state that allowed the necessary dispensations, and they were married. They never lived together, but each returned to their parents' home. After the birth of her baby, Amy finished high school and went to work. Eventually, she got a divorce and married a second time, when her child was ten years old. She had missed her girlhood. In its stead she had soberly met to the best of her ability the responsibility of motherhood. Ironically, or perhaps to be expected, she had great difficulty in having a second baby. She was married several years before she became pregnant again and had two miscarriages before she finally had her second child.

The second alternative is for the woman to have her baby and keep it. This is a choice that should be made with a great deal of thought, for it involves not only the effect it will have on the life of the woman but, more important, the question of whether it is fair to the child. Life is difficult enough when one is born into a home with two parents and has the socially acceptable background of legitimacy. A child needs much more than this in love and security in order to grow to healthy maturity. What chance will it have when it is denied these?

Unfortunately these questions are never asked in that segment of the population where illegitimate pregnancies are most common. Here, low economic status, crowded living conditions, illiteracy, and low cultural and moral standards prevail. Here also is the spawning ground of those things that mar the record of our country's physical and mental health by high maternal and infant mortality rates, high incidence of venereal diseases, septic abortions, problem children, and juvenile delinquency.

But there are women in all other segments of our society, rich or poor, intelligentsia or middle class, who must face this question. Few such women would choose to admit to the world that her child is illegitimate or to have the child grow up in that knowledge. Occasionally, the woman will want her baby so badly that she is willing to resort to any subterfuge and take the involved risks in order to have the child as her very own. M was such a woman.

M was in her late thirties, an intelligent person. I never knew anything about the father or the circumstances; they did not seem to count too

much in M's mind. She just wanted her baby. She went to another city
and worked in one of the homes dedicated to the services of unmarried
mothers during the last few months before the birth of the child. After-
wards she boarded the baby in a private home. She had to save every
penny of her modest salary and every day of her annual leave to support
the baby and make the occasional trips back to the other city to see it.
No one could doubt her love for the baby or question her ability to be
a good mother had she had the opportunity. Her life was enriched in
spite of the heartache and worry, by having another to love and feel
responsible for. She could maintain her illusion of motherhood while
the baby was small. But she had created a situation that would bring
different and more serious problems with each new year of the child's life.
How could she ever claim the child as her own and what effect would
this have on the child? Whatever her life ahead might hold of sorrow,
remorse, and disappointment, it would come as the result of her own
action and choices. The child's future was blighted by circumstances in
which it had no choice and at a time when it was vulnerable—infancy
and childhood.

The third alternative is for the woman to have the baby and give it
for adoption. This is the one usually chosen and on the surface might
seem to be the best. But it too can lead to heartache and misery for
both the mother and the child if we look forward some years in the life
of each.

Mrs. F came to me as a sterility problem. She had been married three
years and as yet had no children. Both she and her husband were carefully examined with appropriate tests made and nothing was found to
account for their infertility. She was an attractive young woman, but
there was something sad and withdrawn as if she were living behind a
protective wall that allowed entrance to no one else, neither her friends,
her doctor, nor her husband. She wanted a baby desperately and when
nothing was found that might be corrected and give her hope, she revealed
why the need was so great. During the war years, long before she met
her husband, she had had a baby. She was unmarried, the father overseas,
and so she gave the baby for adoption, although she wanted very much
to keep it. The years passed, but they brought no surcease in the yearning
for her child, but only the unanswerable questions: Was the child happy?

Did the foster parents truly love and understand it? She had failed to be a mother to her first-born. Perhaps, she reasoned, she could in some way make up for her failure by having another child. She had never told her husband any of this. She eventually did have other children who filled her life with their needs and presence, but there will always be moments when her unknown first-born will make its unseen presence felt.

Miss S was in her late thirties when she became pregnant. It was one of those peculiar affairs of an older woman and a very young man. Marriage was not the answer, so she too gave her baby for adoption. The foster parents adopted her child through the regular social service channels of another state. They certainly gave the child a good home and more cultural advantages than the mother could have given him, and they lavished all their love on him. Even so, an adopted child will have its times of heartache when it questions: Why? They started early for this little fellow when an older cousin taunted him with the fact that he did not have any real mother and father like other children. Children can be cruel. The cousin may be excused on the ground that he got his information from adults, but nothing can erase completely the hurt he inflicted on the adopted child.

Sometimes illegitimacy affords an amusing story, as in the case of Fanny, whom I had known for twenty or more years. She came into my office not so long ago all dressed up and with a broad smile on her face. She exclaimed, "I'm as nervous as a schoolgirl. Pappy and I are going to be married today." She had come to the clinic some twenty years ago a widow of six months and the mother of several half grown children. Her complaints then were obesity and amenorrhea. The obesity we have been struggling with ever since, but the amenorrhea was spontaneously cured within a few months by the birth of twin boys. It seems that Pappy or the "Old Man," as she usually called him when his behavior was not so pleasing, had just moved in to help with the children, and they had lived together all these years without benefit of legal or clerical blessing. The twins were accepted as Pappy's children, although they had no legal right to his name, and they grew up in a not too unhappy home. But now they were coming of age when they would be subject to the military draft and would have to have a birth certificate. This morning Fanny was happy because the district attorney's office had assured her that their papers could be put in order. And also, as all women, whatever their age may be, she was excited at the prospect of being belatedly—but nevertheless really—a bride.

You may think that I have taken the problem of the unmarried mother and her child too seriously. After all, illegitimacy is not a crime a woman has committed against the law. Actually, it is no more than an act that does not have the blessing of the law. She has only followed nature's dictates, and there are many extenuating circumstances. Therefore we should be more tolerant and broadminded and not attach this stigma I have stressed to a woman and her child. Perhaps you may say that society is more tolerant, and the stigma is more fancied than real.

You may cite cases, as every one can, where the family has stepped in and covered up, invented a paternity for the child, and all has seemed to go well. Or you may point out that thousands of babies are adopted each year, and the overwhelming majority of these find happy homes and good parents. Certainly, the lives of these childless couples who adopt them have been enriched. But in any case, it is always no more than second best for the child to the ideal of a happy home with its own mother and father.

You may go back in history and cite examples of times when illegitimacy was accepted in society, or cases of individuals born illegitimately who left their mark on history. Even in the relatively short history of our own country, we find men who have seemingly risen above the stigma of the illegitimacy of their birth and contributed greatly to the history of the country in spite of, or perhaps because of, this burden placed upon them. But few illegitimate children (and few legitimate ones) can hope to have the brains of a Hamilton or the wealth and social status of a Smithson to see them through.

But we are not concerned with the past, or the great, or the rich. We are concerned with the simple, common (or uncommon if you prefer) man and woman in the everyday world of today. Our way of life, which we proclaim to the world as so desirable, is based not only on the legality but also on the morality of its structure. We each must conform to the mores of our culture for our individual happiness and for the health and security of that culture. This is not just social theorizing but practical guidance for everyday living, especially important to woman.

THE SIGNIFICANCE OF UNSUCCESSFUL PREGNANCIES

What has a woman who nearly loses her life from ectopic pregnancy to do with one who escapes motherhood by a criminal abortion or with the mother who lost her baby because it was premature? Why should we group together a woman who dies with sepsis because of her crude attempts at self abortion, a woman who dies of toxemia of pregnancy, and the woman who is denied motherhood by habitual abortion? There is one factor common to all. They each represent failure of the fertilized ovum to achieve its destiny. In most instances it need not have occurred.

It has been found that the incidence of unsuccessful pregnancies varies with the character of the population surveyed. The incidence of unsuccessful pregnancies is high in underprivileged countries where general health conditions are poor, where diseases such as tuberculosis, syphilis, and malaria are rampant, where malnutrition is the rule. When other contributing factors are present, and there is the practice of child marriages with early and frequent pregnancies in which prenatal medical care is unheard of and birth practically unattended, then the picture becomes dark indeed. On the other hand, in the more fortunate countries, which can boast of high health standards and of an enlightened population, the practice of later marriages, child-spacing, application of the principles of good nutrition, and availability of good medical care make the incidence of unsuccessful pregnancies much lower.

What does this have to do with us here in America? These are not just facts of interest to a committee of the United Nations studying problems of world population. The same contributing factors are present in different elements of our own population, and account for the number of unsuccessful pregnancies in America today. The recognition of these facts is of necessity the problem of maternal welfare. It is not only what medical science has to offer, but the physical condition of the women and what use they make of the ever-increasing knowledge and skills that are available to them.

Furthermore all of these factors are important to remember when we look for the cause in any one case. The same causative factors are at work. Poor heritage, poor health and nutrition, poor hygiene, poor planning and guidance, poor medical care of pregnancy are contributory, if not indeed the actual cause, in each unsuccessful pregnancy.

Medical science has used the knowledge from its own and other fields of research with great success in one type of unsuccessful pregnancy. Maternal mortality has been greatly reduced from a once frightfully high rate. Whereas at one time a woman's health and her very life were placed in jeopardy as she entered the child-bearing period, each pregnancy was a hazard, and each succeeding pregnancy took its toll, now it is possible for pregnancy to be a safe and rewarding experience for most women. The percentage of women who die in childbirth has been drastically reduced by better prenatal care for more women, better understanding of the causes, and better methods of handling the complications of pregnancy and delivery.

We can be proud of the fact that fewer mothers are dying each year in the process of giving birth and that more babies are surviving the hazard of birth and the dangerous first month when they must acquire the ability of independent existence. These are facts demonstrated by statistics. For example: In the United States in 1915, 60 women died for every 10,000 live births, whereas in 1954 only 5 women were lost. Of the babies born in 1915, 99 of each 1,000 died in the first year of life, whereas in 1954 only 26 died. Also, in 1915, 45 (of the 99) died in the first month, whereas in 1954, only 19 (of the 26) died during this period. In actual figures, in 1954 there were only 2,107 women who died as the result of pregnancy and 2,050 babies who died in the perinatal period in 4,017,362 live births.

On the other hand, there has been practically no change in the number of fetal deaths. The estimate still stands that 20 per cent of all pregnancies end in fetal death. No one knows, of course, but based on the figure of more than 4 million live births in 1954, the estimate would be that there were close to one million fetal deaths for that year, truly a staggering figure.

Such a death rate from any other cause would produce a great hue and cry that it must be stopped. We would have campaigns to raise money so that the cause and the cure could be found. But there have been no such campaigns to enlighten the public on this fetal wastage, its cause and possible means of prevention. The problem has been recognized and included in the efforts of certain government agencies and medical groups in their attack on maternal mortality. Also certain citizens organizations, which include the various committees on maternal welfare and planned parenthood, have attacked the problem. None has received the recognition and help that the problem deserves. They have had to struggle not only against apathy but also actual hostility. They have found it difficult even to get reports of their work or announcement of their meetings in the newspapers because of the fear that it might offend some powerful group.

There are other aspects of this failure that can never be estimated. There is no criteria for measuring the human suffering that unsuccessful pregnancies cause and that follows in their wake. The financial cost involved, while the least important, would be a staggering figure. We can get some idea of its enormity by considering the cost of medical care to the thousands of women who lose their pregnancy and the financial loss due to the days absent from employment. To this must be added the money that the abortionists take, which is estimated to be at least 50 million dollars a year.

The problem extends through the whole fabric of our culture and, unless it is adequately met and controlled, could mar the pattern completely, for this problem involves not only the number but the quality of our citizens. In seeking the solution, the primary aim should be to reduce the number of deaths—that is, to have more healthy babies born to healthy mothers into healthy happy homes. A strong family unit is the very foundation of our culture. This does not necessarily mean a higher birth rate but a better birth rate. It could some day mean the actual lowering of the birth rate. If we continue to have an increasing birth rate and a decreasing death rate, we too may some day have to face the problem of over-population, when the necessities of life will not be enough to go around. This may seem far-fetched in our land of plenty, and certainly it will not happen in our lifetime. But today it is the source of the difficulties of many other countries less fortunate than ours whose problems have become our problems.

The problem as it exists today, the cause and prevention of fetal wastage, must be approached on three levels: the social, the scientific, and the individual. The social includes higher standards of living with better housing, better education, and better medical care for more people.

The scientific approach to the problem includes two elements: the furthering of research into the problems of human reproduction; and the broad dissemination of this knowledge not only to scientists but to the public at large, so that each individual, not only the specialists, will acquire an interest and have the basic facts on the subject. It is appalling how lacking we are in both today. The need for research is pointed up by one vivid example in contrast—the study of the malignant cell (cancer) versus that of the fertilized ovum. The public is aroused and filled with fear by the mysteries of the cancer cell, which brings suffering and death. As a result, thousands of scientists are devoting their lives, and millions of dollars are spent each year, to find the cause and the cure of this menace. On the other hand, the fertilized ovum, the source of new life, is also mysterious, but comparatively little is being done to ferret out its secrets or even to spread what knowledge we do have to those most concerned, the individuals. The public was not interested and had heard little about this until recently when the dangers of irradiation and atomic fall-out began to be discussed. Here again interest is based on fear, fear of harm to future generations. But in our frantic concern to meet new problems of the atomic age and to stave off the evil consequences, we should not lose sight of the responsibility, which has always been with us, to foster the good that is inherent in us. And this brings us to the crux of the problem, the responsibility of the individual.

Four million babies are born each year and perhaps as many as one million pregnancies fail to attain fruition. The importance of this is not the number but the fact that each pregnancy represents the experience of one individual—the woman. It is to her as an individual we must turn in our efforts to reduce the number of failures. It is the woman who is the deciding factor in achieving the ideal goal of a successful pregnancy—that each will be physically normal, wanted, and limited to the number that can be successfully integrated into a stable healthy family unit.

This aim says nothing about superior offspring. The goal is not the breeding of a superior race. But a woman can do much to assure that her pregnancies will be successful and that her children will be endowed with good health, both physical and mental. In our complex culture she cannot rely on her innate ability to do this. She must be taught.

Such training for successful pregnancy includes the acquisition of knowledge of how her body is made and how it functions. She must learn and apply these facts necessary for good health long before pregnancy starts as well as during it to ensure a healthy pregnancy. Many unsuccessful pregnancies are due to poor physical qualities of the mother that could have been prevented or corrected. She must know how to plan her pregnancies—so that they will be wanted pregnancies. But information on anatomy and physiology in general and on sex in particular is not enough. She must be taught the meaning of her sexuality. It is not just a physical force but a personal responsibility. How she meets it is important not only to herself but it can be a source of great happiness or sorrow to others. This training for successful pregnancy and motherhood is really training for the responsibilities inherent in being a mature woman, which should start early in life and constitute the true goal of sex education.

XIII

WHEN PREGNANCY IS DENIED

"I'VE BROUGHT YOU A PRESENT."

It was an unusual start for a patient speaking to me across my desk—
but then Yvonne was not only a patient. She was by now an old friend
who had just stopped by to let me see how beautifully her little daughter,
four years old, was developing.

As she unwrapped the small package, there was an earnestness and
an eagerness that its contents reveal its special message. The wrapping
off, she handed me a small plate. It was in soft tones of golden brown,
a warm and cheerful color, and in the middle was a design that was
pleasing and well balanced.

"As you can see, I have taken up ceramics. It is loads of fun to do
things with your hands. I like to make my own designs and have them
carry a message for me, and there is one message that I have wanted to
send you for a long time, almost four years really. I have tried to express
that message in this design. I'll read it to you.

"Around the whole is this wishbone. It represents our great desire,
the one great wish of our lives when I came to you—to have a baby.
You remember, Jack and I had been married seven years, and we were
near despair of ever having children of our own. The wish now fulfilled,
it represents our good fortune in finding someone who had the interest,
knowledge, and patience to help us. It is the symbol of happiness, which
surrounds our lives.

"Here, at the bottom, you see me—the tears in my eyes, the sorrow on
my lips; and here are your hands extended in kindly helpfulness."

As she talked, I recalled her first visit to me, so like that of many other

303

childless women. It seemed to me that the hands might well represent their pleading for help for relief of a problem that was dominating their lives, sometimes to the exclusion of all else. Surely this was a plea one could but answer with all that one had to give.

"The middle lines," Yvonne continued, "represent the course you laid out for us to follow. They are straight because you never let us falter, become discouraged, or give up hope. To the left you see my spirits rise, as leaves to the sun, changing from utter despair to a spirit of hopefulness with each passing month as we find, and try to correct, the reasons why I couldn't have a baby. And then, from your hands, here starts my pregnancy, followed by these months of joy and anticipation, and here the fulfillment—the birth of our little girl.

"Here are my lips, which will always smile a thank-you."

I took the lovely gift, and now there were tears in my eyes. I know of no greater happiness than the knowledge that one has been of help, that one has brought happiness to another. And certainly there are no more grateful patients than those who have been relieved of childlessness. As I fondled this gift so rich in spiritual values, happiness and pride were mine but also sadness and humility, for I was acutely conscious of the other cases where I had failed. For every Yvonne with her baby, there were two others whose arms were still empty.

Success in one out of three cases is about the general average today for doctors working with the problem of childlessness. It seems a poor one until we stop to consider what it means. There is now one childless marriage in three being fulfilled where previously there was none. Only in the past few decades have we acquired the knowledge that brings success in that one. Therefore, there is reason to hope that with time, more experience, and more knowledge, our percentage of successes will increase.

There is a great deal of misconception, wrong thinking, and false information about childlessness, sterility, and fertility. We hear that childlessness is the woman's fault, that it can be corrected by operation or by hormones; that virility and fertility in the male are synonymous; that the use of contraceptives leads to sterility; that frigidity in the female is a cause of sterility, and so on. To correct these, we must have a clear concept of the meaning of sterility and fertility.

MEANING OF "FERTILITY" AND "STERILITY"

Involuntary childlessness in a marriage is referred to as "the problem of the infertile couple" and with good reason. "Sterility" is a harsh, hopeless word meaning "sterile, barren, unable to reproduce," as opposed to "fertility," which is "rich, abundant, fruitful." Absolute fertility is a state of physical perfection few women or men possess. On the other hand, there are only a very few who are absolutely sterile. Most childless marriages fall in between these two extremes; that is, they are called cases of "relative infertility" indicating that reproduction may be hard to achieve but not impossible. A degree of "relative fertility" is the maximum that most humans possess, and "relative infertility" is usually the most serious degree of deficiency. The term "infertile couple" is used because childlessness is usually not the result of one big fault in one of the partners, but rather to several minor faults or deficiencies in each of the partners.

This concept of varying degrees of fertility as the basis of childlessness brings hope and optimism to the problem and makes it a challenge. How can relative fertility be measured? The obvious answer is by the number of children per family, but this is not true. How many children a couple may have and when they may have them are a result of so many factors that it is not a measure of a couple's fertility.

Because our grandmothers, perhaps your great-grandmothers had large families does not mean that men and women of their generation were more fertile. They married earlier when, in the life cycle, fertility is highest. They knew less about contraception, and many thought it wicked to practice it even if they knew how. A large family was desirable, and they could afford it because they lived in rural or semirural areas where housing facilities were ample and food largely home-produced. Living was cheaper, and they did not have to consider the expense of rearing and educating their children. In many instances a large family was an economic asset because the children at an early age assumed jobs on the farm, in the store, and even went out to earn wages in the new enterprises and industries that were just beginning. Women at that time had no other career available than homemaking, childbearing, and child care. Having a family was expected of a couple, and those without children were considered queer and to be pitied.

Then came the time, a gradual change to be sure, that a large family became a luxury that few could afford. The increasing complexity and high cost of everyday living, the longer period needed for education, later marriage, the mass movement of women into gainful occupations outside the home, the broader dissemination of information about sex and contraception, all contributed to smaller families.

World War II threw all these repressive factors out the window and allowed nature to assert herself. The young generation, because of the urgency and uncertainty of the times, were intent on crowding into a limited time a lot of living, which basically is to love and be loved. So we have a bumper crop of babies of the war years that are bursting the seams of our schools today. This evaluation of the basic and really important things of life has been carried over to the present younger generation. They are marrying at an earlier age, even though they must still complete their education. They are having their babies earlier, and having more of them. It may be because they value human relations above material advantages and are unwilling to forego the fulfillment of "living" today for the so-called "security" of tomorrow.

This is just a small segment of human life, these few American generations, but the facts are universal for time or place. The American Indians, who occupied this continent for thousands of years, never really populated it as their European successors did. But it was not because they were basically an infertile race. Their relative infertility came as a result of their migratory life, tribal taboos, infanticide, high infant mortality, incessant warfare, and their primitive agriculture with periodic famine and starvation. Remove these factors, and the American Indian is as fertile as any of the other races. So it is with the backward, primitive, or underprivileged countries, as they are called, of today. Their population is held in check by economic and social factors. Remove them, and their basic fertility will assert itself. The resulting increase in population will become a problem of great importance in the world of tomorrow. But that is getting beyond our scope.

Human fertility is basically the same for all races and creeds, the expression of it being determined by factors other than the physiological.

We could look back to any era in history and would always find this situation: fertility of a varying degree the accepted attribute of life for the large majority and barrenness the burden of a few. No facet of life exemplifies so pointedly the unique and fortunate social position that modern American women enjoy as the meaning of a woman's barrenness in days gone by compared to what it means today.

In times long past, a woman's sole importance was to please and serve her husband and bear him children, preferably sons. Should she fail and her marriage prove barren, she alone was blamed. Her barrenness was looked upon as a result of her own willful actions, a curse for her hidden misdeeds. Thus, she was accused of unfaithfulness with another man, or perhaps an evil spirit. Her barrenness became a crime of which she alone was guilty and for which she was punished. The husband was considered justified in casting her aside. No longer was she a wife or a respected member of her community. The divorce was often cruel, for the woman was despised, disgraced, and mistreated. With her very existence thus threatened, it is not surprising that the wife resorted to any means that promised help to avert this dreadful calamity. Thus we find in folklore all kinds of superstitions and myths about the cause and cure of sterility. Charms were worn; nasty and noxious filters were taken; special foods were eaten; prayers to the Gods of Fertility were raised with offering of appropriate gifts and deeds of penance.

This concept of a woman's place and responsibility has not completely disappeared even today. American women are being chided for forsaking their femininity, that is, refusing to have only one purpose in life—to please man—and compared unfavorably with their foreign sisters. From a medical standpoint, also, women who are partners in a childless marriage are too often subjected to arduous diagnostic procedure and prolonged treatment, even surgery, while their husbands' fertility is taken for granted, or at least based on a cursory examination. This is partly woman's fault. Most women want children, and a wife deprived of them is often willing to subject herself to any procedure to attain them. She willingly accepts the blame, to save her husband the necessary exertion and inconvenience, but more often to protect his male ego.

All of this refers to fertility and sterility in general terms. Let us now turn to the problem from the standpoint of the individual case—what constitutes an infertile couple and what can be done about it.

When Is a Marriage Infertile?

Infertility of a marriage does not become an apparent fact at any particular time. Rather, it is a matter of opinion, and the time varies with whether the couple (usually the wife) or the doctor makes the decision. The time at which a woman will seek help for her childlessness will depend on the intensity of her desire to have children and her knowledge and understanding of the physiology of conception. If she is eager, but uninformed, she will be disappointed when she does not conceive the first month that she tries; the second month she becomes anxious, and by the third month she is thoroughly alarmed and rushes to her doctor. If, on the other hand, she is willing but not too concerned about immediately starting a pregnancy, she may let several months, even a year or so, go by before she does anything about it. Many never do anything because they do not know that help is available, or they go on the blind faith that eventually they will have a baby, or, timid and embarrassed, they are reluctant to discuss so personal a problem.

Ida-Lou had no hesitancy in stating why she sought medical aid. She wanted to know whether she could have a baby, and she particularly wanted her tubes tested. One of the first questions asked in an infertility case is, "When were you married?" or, "How long have you been trying to become pregnant?" As it happened, I asked her when she had been married, to which she replied, "Yesterday."

This was feminine concern beyond my previous experience, and my surprise must have been apparent, for she added: "You see, our relationship has been quite intimate for over a year and nothing has happened. Now that we are married I just wonder if we ever will have babies."

Should she and her husband be considered an infertile couple? This is a question difficult to answer. There are doubtless many cases of unmarried girls who have "strayed" just once and were "caught." But is a year of extramarital relations a sufficient trial period? There are many factors such as timing, or the psychological impact of their relationship, that might work against the occurrence of a pregnancy and that would disappear as they settled down to a normal marital relationship. Another case represents the opposite extreme to this eager young woman.

Hannah's complaint was a minor menstrual irregularity. She was thirty-seven years old, had been married nine years, and had never been pregnant. Suspecting that her infertility might be due to some abnormality, perhaps glandular, I asked her about her marital relations. She reluctantly supplied the information that she and her husband were happy together, that they had marital relations once a month or sometimes at two-week intervals, and although they had never practiced any form of contraception, they never had any children. She did not seem to be particularly concerned about her childlessness as she had never sought medical advice about it and was not doing so now. On examination one cause of her infertility, but probably not the only one, was readily apparent. She was still a virgin anatomically. She had never really had complete sexual relations. It is hard to believe a couple could be so naive in this day when sex problems are discussed so freely, but occasionally this is so.

Doctors also vary in their opinions as to when a marriage should be considered infertile and steps taken to determine the cause. There are a few who believe that in a young fertile couple having a normal sexual relationship pregnancy should occur in most instances the first month and surely by the third month. Others, also a few, believe that the couple should try for a pregnancy for two or even three years before a fertility study is undertaken. The majority accept one year as an adequate trial period, after which if no pregnancy has occurred, infertility is presumed to be present and should be investigated.

Factors of Fertility

To understand the causes of infertility, we must first recall the factors of fertility. These we have partially considered in the discussion of the physiology of conception. This is a mechanism of such delicate balance of many factors and of such accuracy of timing that it may at times be hard to achieve. One wonders, in fact, how it ever happens to succeed.

The fertility of a marriage depends on three separate factors—female fertility, male fertility, and effective mating. This may sound rather obvious, but it soon proves to be no simple thing, when the meaning of each is considered.

Female fertility is, of course, the more complicated. Woman not only has to produce fertile germ cells—that is, her ovaries must deliver normal mature ova—but the passageways must be open and hospitable for the separate journeys that the ovum and the sperm must make to their trysting place. This means that there must be no mechanical barriers along the way such as adhesions in the tubes or tumors in the body of the uterus. It also means that the secretions, particularly of the cervix, are not too thick for the sperm to penetrate and have no change from their normal chemistry that would make them harmful to the sperm. But that is not all. She must have healthy well-developed organs to house the pregnancy, and she must have endocrine glands that have functioned normally to prepare for pregnancy and that continue their job in maintaining the pregnancy. Obviously, since there are so many factors necessary to woman's fertility, there is no single test to measure it. The problem of detecting any and all faults that might be present is a complicated, but not impossible, undertaking.

The requisites of male fertility are production of a sufficiency of active fertile germ cells and the ability to deliver them to the cervix. Male fertility is easily evaluated. But the cause of a deficiency or reduced fertility, when it is found, may be difficult to ascertain.

Effective mating means that the sperms are delivered to the proper place at the proper time, that is, to the cervix during the woman's fertile period. You may think it farfetched to consider this a factor of fertility, that adults instinctively know how to mate, and that the urge to do so comes frequently enough to ensure its occurrence at the proper time. But this is not always so. There are cases of childless marriages due entirely to faulty mating.

THE FERTILITY STUDY

What is a fertility study? In general, it is a careful, detailed, intimate study of both husband and wife with the purpose of detecting as many abnormalities as possible in each that might lower their fertility. It is not just a pelvic examination of the wife by which it is found that she has the normal complement of reproductive organs in the right place, after which she is told that she is a normal woman and therefore there is no reason why she should not have children. Neither is it a cursory examination of the man's semen under the microscope, revealing a multitude of moving cells, after which he is told that he is a healthy male. Yet this is what couples may get. Fortunately, there are more and more doctors who are interested in the problem and are not only striving to apply all presently available knowledge, but are continuously seeking new knowledge to help the childless couples.

The study of the infertile couple is a job in detection that often calls for all the knowledge, ingenuity, and perseverance the doctor can bring to the problem, and always requires the co-operation of the two involved, the husband as well as the wife.

Specifically, a fertility study of the woman includes a medical history, complete physical examination, blood studies, urinalysis, BMR, tubal insufflation, endometrial biopsy, and postcoital examination of the vaginal pool and cervical fluid. In the man a medical history, physical examination, and semen analysis will usually suffice, but occasionally additional laboratory procedures and testicular biopsy may be necessary. It is apparent that the woman bears more of the burden, because there is no direct test for her fertility as there is in the male. Let us take each of these and see what they mean and why each is important.

Medical History

Having a baby is a very personal, individual affair. Therefore, finding out why a couple does not have one requires the knowledge of highly personal, intimate details of their lives. A full medical history is one of the most valuable parts of the study. In taking it, the doctor will ask about family background, not because fertility per se is an inherited characteristic, but because familial diseases may affect general health and, in turn, fertility. He will want to know about childhood diseases and previous illnesses, some of which merely lower general health while others occurring at puberty and after may leave damaged sex glands. Surgical operations may have left scars or removed organs that affect fertility. He will want accurate and complete details of the menstrual function. The occurrence of the first menstruation at the usual age followed by the establishment of regular, normal cycles indicates good ovarian function, whereas late onset, irregular and scanty flow are symptoms of ovarian deficiency.

In the marital history, the doctor will want to know the ages of the woman and her husband, and when they were married. After the early twenties, fertility slowly decreases, but not enough to make age alone a particularly important factor of infertility. Women who marry late are frequently fearful that they may be too old to have babies, but this is not necessarily the case. Many women today are able to have their first baby after the age of forty.

The frequency and timing of sexual intercourse is important from two aspects, the woman's fertile period and the recuperative power of the male. Woman's fertile period, as we have seen, occurs about fourteen days before she menstruates and lasts for only about twelve hours. In cases of irregular, infrequent intercourse, such as once a month or less frequently, the chances of it coinciding with the woman's fertile period are remote. This may be an important factor although the woman's cycle is regular if the husband and wife are frequently separated even for short periods of time. It becomes more significant when her periods are irregular and infrequent. Popular opinion is that the male is always potent, only the woman is frigid. This is far from the truth. Infrequent intercourse as a cause of infertility is more apt to be attributable to male inadequacy than female rejection. Frigidity in the woman, her lack of sex response, has little to do with her ability to have children. Even a woman who has been raped may conceive, and there are many women who have never had any great physical satisfaction in sex and yet had a family. On the other hand, too frequent intercourse may also be defeating its own purpose by emptying the reservoir of male cells before the woman's fertile period occurs and not allowing time for adequate refilling.

The contraceptive methods practiced previously are important to know, but not because they may have done damage. The usual type of contraceptives are not harmful and do not lower fertility. More often they are inadequate, and their use has hidden from the couple their relative infertility.

Previous marriages and their fertility may be misleading. Failure of the husband to have children in a previous marriage might suggest that he is at fault in this marriage, but it only suggests, it doesn't prove. Nor does the fact that he has children by a previous marriage necessarily mean that he still has a high degree of fertility. The same is true in most instances for women.

In addition to these particular things that relate directly to fertility, the doctor will ask many searching questions, as to the couple's general health and well-being, their habits of diet, of work, and of recreation, their worries and fears, their burdens of responsibility, their frustrations and achievements. These too are capable of contributing to infertility.

The Physical Examination

There is rarely anything found on the general physical examination that would account for a woman's inability to conceive, but there may be indications such as malnutrition, kidney disease, or high blood pressure that might contribute to an unsuccessful pregnancy. Once in a while an abnormality is discovered that would make pregnancy inadvisable. One such situation was found in the course of the fertility study in a woman who had rheumatic heart disease of which she was unaware. The heart specialist advised that while it was not impossible for her to go through pregnancy and deliver safely, she would probably be much better off if she was not subjected to such stress. She was reconciled and accepted the fact that she had closed tubes that prevented her from becoming pregnant.

In the examination of the pelvic organs, however, the situation is different. Gross abnormalities, such as tumors of the uterus or ovaries or acute infection of the tubes, are important and require attention from the standpoint of the patient's health as well as her fertility. But here it is the minor things that take on greater significance. Search is made especially for any evidence of infection of the passageways that might render them inhospitable to the sperm. Vaginal infections, such as monila and trichomonas, may cause a profuse vaginal discharge that inhibits the progress of the sperm. They cause no permanent damage, however, and can be controlled and eventually cured. Low-grade infection of the cervix acts in the same manner, but may not be so amenable to treatment. The effect of previous or chronic infection of the tubes is usually not detected on a physical examination.

There are two pelvic conditions that women have been led to believe are important but which usually are of little significance. They are the position and the size of the uterus. It is imprudent to tell a young woman who has all her organs, and has once menstruated, that she can't become pregnant. Retroversion, "tilted uterus," "up-side-down womb," or whatever it may be called, is rarely the cause of sterility. A true infantile uterus is rarely found in women whose menstrual function is relatively normal.

The history and physical examination completed, the doctor has considerable important information. This includes minor faults and sometimes more serious ones that are to be corrected. Just as significant are the clues that suggest other lines of investigation by selected tests.

Tubal Insufflation

One requisite of fertility in the woman is open passageways for the journey of the ovum to the tube and of the sperm from the vagina to the tube. The patency of the uterus and cervix is obvious both from the fact that menstruation occurs and on pelvic examination. The tubes, however, are inaccessible, so some indirect method is necessary. This is furnished by injecting a gas into the passageways.

In the tube test, or tubal insufflation, a gas (air or carbon dioxide) is forced into the cervix and through the uterus and escapes through the tubes into the abdominal cavity if the tubes are patent. A machine is necessary to deliver the gas at a measured safe pressure and speed, and there is usually a device by which the pressure used is recorded. If the tubes are open, the gas passes through at the normal pressure (80 to 100 millimeters of mercury). If the pressure rises above this, it indicates the tubes are closed. In addition, the doctor may listen with a stethoscope to the woman's lower abdomen and hear gas bubbling through if the tubes are normally patent. No such sound is heard when the tubes are closed.

When the woman sits up for a few minutes after the test, if the tubes are open, she will experience pain high in her abdomen and in her right shoulder as a result of the gas rising in the abdomen and causing pressure on the diaphragm. This is one instance of pain that we eagerly await, and rejoice at its occurrence. It passes off when the patient lies down. A tubal insufflation is an office procedure causing the woman little discomfort. It is both a diagnostic and a therapeutic measure. It not only reveals whether the tubes are normal, but the gentle pressure exerted by the gas may dilate passages that have been closed.

The test must be done at a specific time in the menstrual cycle—that is, a few days after menstrual bleeding has ceased. This time is selected for two reasons. At that time all the congestion incident to menstruation has subsided and the passageways are at their greatest degree of patency. This time is also before ovulation, and there would be not even a remote possibility of forcing a fertilized ovum back through the tube.

Sometimes the doctor will want an X-ray of the tubes. However, this procedure is usually reserved for cases in which the tubes have remained closed after several inflations with gas. To get a picture, material that is impervious to X-ray must be injected into the tubes so that the passageways, as far as they are open, will be outlined. An X-ray picture serves the purpose of locating the place of obstruction and may give some hint as to the cause.

Tests for Ovarian Function

A second and equally important requirement of female fertility is normal ovarian function, which results in the production of fertile ova and the proper preparation of the endometrium for its reception after fertilization. We have no direct way of recovering and examining the ova or even of determining that ovulation has occurred. But we do have indirect methods that are quite reliable. One of these is the premenstrual endometrial biopsy.

During the menstrual cycle, as you will recall, the structure of the lining of the uterus is constantly changing as the result of the stimulating action of the ovarian hormones. Before ovulation, growth of the endometrium follows one pattern, the follicular phase, and after ovulation the pattern is changed to the progestational phase. These pre-ovulatory and post-ovulatory patterns are quite easily differentiated on microscopic examination. To have material for such an examination a biopsy must be taken.

Obtaining an endometrial biopsy is also an office procedure that causes very little discomfort. A small curette, which will pass through the cervix without stretching or tearing it, is used. With this, a few tiny segments of the endometrium from different areas are scraped off. After proper preparation, these little bits of tissue may be examined microscopically as in any other biopsy.

The endometrial biopsy must also be done at a specific time in the cycle in order to obtain the greatest amount of information. That time is premenstrually, just a day or so before the expected period. Some doctors prefer to take it on the first day of the flow to avoid the danger of disturbing an early pregnancy. This, however is a very remote possibility and has the disadvantage of yielding tissue that is already disintegrated and therefore the pattern is not so well defined as it is at the height of growth just before menstruation. The finding of a normal secreting endometrium indicates that ovulation has occurred and that the lining of the uterus has been made ready to receive a fertilized ovum, should one appear. There are other tests that may supply some of the same information.

All of the reproductive tract undergoes cyclic changes in structure corresponding to varying levels of the ovarian hormones. Thus, examination of the vaginal and cervical fluid offers a method of evaluating the proficiency of ovarian function. Also there is a cyclic excretion of the hormones or their metabolic product in the urine. The presence of the pituitary gonadotropic hormone may be detected by animal tests similar to those of the familiar pregnancy tests. Progesterone, which is produced only in ovulatory cycles is represented by the appearance of pregnandiol in the urine, which is detected by a chemical test. These tests have the shortcomings of being either less exact or definitive or more difficult to perform than the endometrial biopsy and are therefore less frequently used, and then for the purpose of corroboration.

Tests for Thyroid Function

We have already seen how important the thyroid is in every phase of body function and especially in the feminine functions of menstruation and pregnancy. It follows therefore that some estimation of thyroid function is obligatory in every study of fertility and infertility. There are several ways to measure the proficiency of thyroid function.

The basal metabolic rate is a test that measures the amount of oxygen used by a person in a period of time. This must be done under basal conditions, which means after a night of rest and before metabolism has been stimulated by food, smoking, coffee, or physical or mental activity. Oxygen is necessary for the chemical processes that go on in the body, and the rate at which it is used is therefore a measure of the rate of metabolism. The thyroid is responsible for the steady rate that the body maintains in the chemical processes. When the oxygen consumption is more than the expected normal, we may presume that the basal metabolic processes are increased because the thyroid is overactive. By the same token, low oxygen consumption indicates deficiency of thyroid function.

The other tests for thyroid function are becoming well known and widely used. They are the PBI (protein bound iodine) and the radioactive iodine uptake tests.

The PBI is a quantitative chemical test of the blood for protein bound iodine, which presumably measures the amount of the thyroid hormone (which is a protein to which iodine is attached) circulating in the blood stream. Amounts below normal would therefore indicate deficient thyroid function, while an excessive quantity would suggest hyperthyroidism.

The radioactive iodine test is based on the physiological fact of the normal thyroid cells' avidity for iodine. Most of the iodine normally taken into the body by food is quickly removed from the blood stream and stored in the thyroid gland. In the test, a substance containing iodine, which has been made radioactive, is administered to the person tested, and the thyroid is examined at a specified time by a geiger counter for the time of appearance and degree of radioactivity present. When the thyroids cells are subnormal functionally, they cannot take up as much iodine, whereas in hyperthyroidism they take up an excessive quantity. This test can be taken one step further in cases of hypothyroidism to differentiate whether the fault is in the thyroid itself or is secondary to pituitary failure.

The pituitary thyreotropic hormone of a high degree of activity and potency is now available for certain clinical uses (though not a practical method of treating thyroid deficiency). When the test with radioactive iodine indicates low thyroid function by low concentration of radioactive iodine, and the thyreotropic hormone is administered, one of two results will be obtained. If the thyroid has been inefficient because of inadequate stimulation by the pituitary, administration of the thyreotropic hormone will speed it up and more radioactive iodine will be detected in the thyroid gland. On the other hand, if the fault is in the thyroid itself, the thyreotropic hormone has no effect, and there is no increase in radio-active iodine uptake.

Each of these three tests furnishes valuable information about thyroid function but from different angles. The BMR measures total body metabolism in terms of the amount of oxygen necessary to support it. The PBI test measures the ability of the thyroid to produce and deliver to the blood stream its specific iodine-containing hormone. The radioactive iodine uptake test measures the ability of the thyroid to take iodine from the blood for its use in manufacturing its hormone and can be extended to differentiate hypothyroidism due to primary failure from that due to pituitary deficiency.

Doctors vary in the choice of the thyroid test they routinely employ. The BMR test was the first clinical method available and is still a good test and a valuable tool. It has the advantage of being simple and reliable and a test that can be made in the doctor's office. The other tests require special laboratory facilities that are not available in all localities. Which test the doctor uses is not very important. Tests are but tools in a doctor's hand, and the experienced physician will use the one with which he is most familiar and which serves his purpose best. Furthermore, the results of any test must be interpreted in terms of the clinical picture as a whole— the patient. They are neither infallible nor absolute truths that stand alone to direct him.

Male Fertility Tests

It is to be hoped that while the wife is undergoing these tests, which will occupy a month or six weeks, the husband has had a direct semen examination. But even if he is unco-operative, there is still something that can be done to estimate his degree of fertility, and that is by a postcoital examination of the semen. This test, however, is not restricted to a few recalcitrant husbands but should be an adjunct to the semen analysis in all cases studied.

The couple is asked to abstain from intercourse for four days. On the day of the examination, the wife comes in immediately after intercourse, preferably within an hour, and fluids from both the vagina and from the cervix are taken for examination. In normal cases, there will be an abundance of live sperm cells in the vagina and a moderate number in the cervix. If such is the finding, it speaks well for male fertility. The failure, however, to find live sperm does not necessarily place all the blame on the male. The semen, though normal, may have been quickly lost from the vagina, or if dead cells are found, it may indicate that the male cells have found the vaginal and cervical fluids incompatible or even harmful to them.

This test should always be confirmed by a direct semen examination. It does not give an accurate count of the sperm, it merely shows the relative abundance of male cells and their ability to survive in the vaginal fluids and to penetrate the thick cervical mucus.

The direct evaluation of male fertility is not a difficult procedure, neither is it time-consuming or painful. A detailed study of the semen is the most important procedure to determine male fertility, but there are rigid requirements for the technique by which it is carried out.

So frequently the wife will say, "I know my husband is all right, he is a great big man, never been sick a day in his life," or "My husband has been examined and he is OK. I'm sure it is my fault." When pressed for what constituted his examination, too often it was a routine physical examination, with perhaps a cursory look at a drop of semen under the microscope. Just seeing live cells does not indicate fertility. It is impossible to differentiate between a semen of 20 million and 80 million by examining one drop microscopically. For example, if you look in a clear, small pool swarming with minnows, do you think you could state with surety whether there were 20 million or 100 million? Nor can a doctor merely look at a drop of semen under the microscope and make even a good guess as to how many cells are delivered in one ejaculation. The semen must be carefully analyzed.

The semen, that is, the whole amount of one ejaculation, must first be measured. It is usually about 4 cubic centimeters (one teaspoonful). Then an accurate count is made using a technique similar to that used in making a count of the cells of the blood. Normally there are 80 to 100 million per cubic centimeter or 300 to 400 million in each ejaculation. Doctors vary in what they consider the lower limits of normal, some place it as high as 60 million per cubic centimeter, but most agree that any count below 20 million per cubic centimeter is a relatively infertile specimen.

That is one of the mysteries of fertility, why at least 20 million sperm must be present when only one will be used to fertilize the female's single cell.

But sufficiency of number is not all that is required of the sperm. They must also be well developed and normal in size and structure. A normal sperm as we have seen consists of a very small oval head and a long hair-like tail. Abnormal sperm may have large heads, elongated or spear-like heads, or extremely small heads. Or the tail may be doubled, or excessively curled. Every semen will have a few of these sperm cells that do not conform to the normal, but when the number exceeds 20 per cent it indicates that the semen is of reduced fertility.

Finally, the cells are tested for their motility and length of life. Under proper environment in the laboratory (protected from excess heat, cold, light, or drying) at least 80 per cent of the cells should be actively motile, that is, be moving about vigorously immediately after ejaculation and retain a good motility for six to eight hours.

Semen found to be normal in these respects is usually indicative of adequate male fertility. But the finding of some deficiency, or even marked deficiencies, does not necessarily mean that the male is truly infertile. Too frequent intercourse, excessive fatigue, prolonged physical or emotional strain, or physical illness may temporarily lower the count, which will come back to normal when these factors are removed. The male should not be considered fertile by the finding of some live cells in one drop of fluid, nor should he be considered sterile on the basis of one examination, however detailed it may be. There must be repeated tests at varying time intervals. Low counts mean only lowered fertility. Only complete absence of cells on repeated analyses indicates sterility.

Testicular biopsy is used in some cases to determine whether the deficiency of sperm in the ejaculated specimen is due to failure of the testes to produce spermatozoa or to closed passageways that prevent their delivery.

Temperature Charts

We consider normal body temperature 98.6° Fahrenheit, which suggests that it remains the same except in case of illness and fever. But his is not altogether accurate. The body temperature varies one to two degrees every twenty-four hours. It is lowest in the morning, after a night's rest and rises as the body warms up, with the day's activity. Moreover, a woman's body temperature varies from day to day with her menstrual cycle.

To demonstrate this monthly variation, the temperature must be taken at the same time each day, and under basal conditions, before there has been any activity such as muscular exercise, eating, or smoking, or mental or emotional stimulation. To conform to these requirements, the temperature must be taken at the moment of awakening. A special thermometer, which is graded in one-tenth instead of the usual two-tenth degree markings, makes reading easier. If the temperature is taken in this manner and recorded each month as a graph, we have what is called a basal temperature chart.

The basal temperature chart for a normal cycle conforms to a fairly well-defined pattern. During the first two weeks of the cycle (starting from the first day of the flow), the temperature remains low. Then about midway there is a rise, sometimes sudden, of about one degree, which is sustained until the onset of menstruation, when there is a sudden fall. When menstruation fails to occur, due to a pregnancy, the temperature remains elevated.

Theoretically, such a chart should be the source of very valuable information for a fertility study. It would indicate that ovulation has occurred, but, more important, when it occurred; also, it would give the earliest indication that a pregnancy was started. But in actual practice, it does not always give such clear-cut information.

There are things other than ovulation that elevate the temperature, the most frequent being a mild infection such as a cold. Also, the rise, which theoretically indicates ovulation, is usually not as abrupt and marked in an actual case as it is depicted in the explanatory graph. The rise may be gradual and extended over several days. No two women's charts are ever exactly alike, nor are the curves for several months identical in one woman's chart. So in looking at a chart that the woman has completed at the end of the month, about all one can say is that the temperature was low the first part of the cycle and high in the later part, with a transition period of one to three days between the two. The best informa-

tion that can be obtained from this is that the woman is probably ov
lating. This can be "guessed at" with just about as much accurac
because failure to ovulate (anovulatory menstruation) is rare in wome
with normal regular menstrual cycles. The occurrence of ovulation ca
be demonstrated with greater accuracy by the endometrial biopsy. A mo
recent test for vaginal sugar which appears at the time of ovulation presen
more technical difficulties and has the same shortcomings as the temper
ture chart.

In dealing with the problem of infertility, it is most desirable to be ab
to predict when a woman will ovulate, or to have some means of reco;
nizing immediately the occurrence of ovulation. This information is rarel
revealed in a temperature chart, even in women whose cycles are regula
In irregular cycles, it is even less informative.

Too much emphasis has been placed on the use of the temperature cha
in the management of infertility, and this has resulted in more harm t
the couple than good. A case that is fairly typical will illustrate this.

Mary came to me a year or so ago, and I can still recall her woe-begon
expression as she sat and told her story. She and John had been marrie
for several years and had been anxious to have a child but were unsucces
ful. So she had consulted a doctor who examined her and told her tha
she was normal. He gave her a chart on which to record her basal tempera
ture and the necessary instructions on how to keep it and to apply th
information it yielded.

She took a packet of folded papers from her purse and handed thei
to me. Here was the record of her temperature, day after day, month afte
month, for a whole year. There were X's to indicate the occurrence c
intercourse. At first the X's were scattered over the month, indicatin
a spontaneity, but by the third month they fell into a pattern concentrate
on the twelfth, fourteenth, and sixteenth days one month; on the eleventl
thirteenth, and fifteenth days the next, and soon only three times, n
more, month after month.

She said, as I was examining the charts, "We have tried so hard. W
have had intercourse only at the time we thought was my fertile perioc
and nothing has happened. And it wasn't easy. Now we are both s
discouraged and fed up with this—and I'm afraid, with each other." Sh
eagerly and with evident relief accepted the advice that perhaps the

had tried too hard, that there were other ways of obtaining the same information and, more important, that there was much other information that should be sought.

There is still a lot that we do not know about how the emotions affect the body functions, especially that of reproduction. It was observed, long ago, that sometimes shortly after a previously infertile couple adopted a baby the woman would conceive and have her own baby. Also, that conception frequently occurred during a vacation that was filled with interesting, absorbing, but relaxed activities. Doctors who specialize in infertility problems all report cases, it seems with increasing frequency, in which they can find no demonstrative physical cause for sterility. All of this points to emotional stress as a contributory cause of infertility.

Any test that will create this state of emotional stress is therefore of questionable value. Temperature charting, by its demanding, unrelenting repetitiousness, by the incessant self-examination and introspection it engenders, and the reduction in spontaneity of expressed affection to a dull fixed unrewarding routine, is such a stress.

Let's put it another way. John and Mary were married because they loved each other. Their early marital relations were a deeply personal and private way of expressing that love. They wanted a baby as a fulfill-ment of that love. Had that occurred, their marital relations could have retained this spontaneity and increased in emotional richness. By its failure, Mary became involved in a procedure (temperature-taking) that never for a day let her forget her infertility.

This procedure, in addition, reduced their marital relationship to a job, merely physical effort, to be performed whether they had any pleasure in it or not. Eventually, it became not merely unwanted, but actually distasteful, repugnant, repulsive. They were in danger of becoming dis-tasteful to each other. What then would they have attained, even if they eventually had a baby and lost the love and joy they had in each other? Just as important, how could they hope to fulfill their most important responsibility to the child—to give it the security of its parents' mutual love?

Results of a Fertility Study

A fertility study such as we have described is arduous, time-consuming, and not without expense. But these factors are more than counterbalanced by the information obtained. To search out at one time all possible faults and endeavor to correct them simultaneously will in the long run save both time and money and perhaps heartache too. What could be more discouraging than to work for a year or two on the woman's closed tubes, only to discover that the husband, who had not been examined, was not producing adequate germ cells? Yet this has happened many times.

When the study is complete, the doctor will have all the information it is possible to obtain concerning the factors detrimental to fertility in both husband and wife. He will outline what can be done to correct these faults, and he can give a fair estimate of their chances for a pregnancy. In some cases he will have to tell the couple that there is little hope for a pregnancy. Tragic news, yes, but it may be a blessing if the couple can face the truth, which they have suspected for a long time, and adjust their lives accordingly.

In the large majority of infertile couples, abnormalities are rarely found to be of such seriousness that there is no hope for a successful pregnancy. In studying large numbers of cases of relative infertility, doctors have gathered facts that may be quite surprising. In the first place, it is rare that only one fault is found; usually there are two to six for each couple. Second, rarely are these faults in only one partner, but both have some contributory abnormalities, and the man is just as often at fault as the woman.

What are these faults that lower fertility? In general they are conditions that we may hope are amenable to treatment. In the wife the most common cause of infertility is closed tubes, which are found in about 50 per cent of the cases. The second most common finding is endocrine failure, which includes anovulatory menstruation, inadequate female sex hormone production, and thyroid deficiency. The third group consists of abnormalities of the cervix, which constitute a barrier to the migration of the sperm.

In the husband, by far the most common cause of infertility is the inability to produce adequate germ cells. Occasionally, there is some obstruction of the passageways.

These are direct causes of sterility and are sex specific, that is, they are due to abnormalities in the reproduction function of the husband or the wife. But they are not the only kinds of faults. There are many indirect causes, which may be present in either husband or wife, that lower fertility, such as poor general health, anemia, faulty nutrition, overwork, overindulgence, faulty timing, or faulty consummation of marital relations.

TREATMENT OF THE INFERTILE COUPLE

There can be no fixed routine for the treatment of infertility since there are so many possible contributory factors, any combination of which may be present in one married couple. The general plan is to try to correct all the faults that have been found in each partner. This requires the concerted effort of the husband, wife, and doctor and the careful attention to details that might seem unimportant in other circumstances. There are no short-cuts.

The first step in treatment has already been taken as the couple undergoes the fertility study. Here they learn the factors necessary for fertility, and what they have been doing and not doing that contributes to their infertility. It then becomes their responsibility to correct these faults, not only those that pertain to their marital relations but also those of general health such as proper nutrition, adequate rest and relaxation, and avoidance of excessive stress and tension.

Women seeking relief of infertility frequently ask, "Can't we be given hormone shots?" or "Won't an operation make me able to have a baby?" or "Can we try artificial insemination?" Each of these may have a place in the treatment of a few selected cases, but none is a cure-all.

Hormone Therapy

Hormone therapy will be of value only when there is some specific indication for it—some indication of glandular imbalance. Even in those cases of proved glandular deficiency, attention to the general health, nutrition, and habits, as well as the emotional attitude, in an effort to establish a normal internal environment for glandular function, is just as important as specific hormone therapy.

We have no direct means of curing any kind of glandular deficiency. We can only supplement the deficiency, or by various methods change the internal chemical environment or hormone balance with the hope that the gland in question will acquire more efficient function.

Thyroid has proved to be the most helpful form of hormone therapy that has been employed in treating infertility. There are several reasons for this. A low thyroid function is a common contributory factor in infertility. It is relatively easy to diagnose and easy to treat since oral medication is used exclusively, and the cost is within the reach of the most limited budget (which cannot be said of other hormones that require injection and are frequently costly). It has been the experience of many doctors over a period of many years that thyroid medication is helpful even though there is no marked deficiency or there is a normal BMR.

The thyroid by stimulating general metabolic function improves the efficiency of function of all cells of the body, including those of the endocrine glands. We have seen how thyroid medication has been important in the correction of functional menstrual abnormalities and in the threat to a normal pregnancy, abortion. These are of course also contributory factors of infertility.

Thyroid extract is the form in which the thyroid hormone is usually administered. As the name implies, it is not a pure chemical hormone but a concentrated extract of the gland (from which as much extraneous material as possible has been removed), which contains the thyroid hormone in a biologically active form. It should be pointed out that there are several closely related chemical substances, such as thyroxine, di-iodothyronine, tri-iodothyronine, thyreoglobulin, that are involved in thyroid metabolism. They represent the forms in which the hormone is manufactured and stored in the thyroid gland, delivered to the blood stream, and converted for passage through cell walls to where it performs its definitive function. Efforts in the past to use a pure chemical such as thyroxine in hypothyroidism have not been as successful as the use of thyroid extract.

Recently tri-iodothyronine has received considerable favorable publicity, which gives the impression that here is a new wonder drug that will cure a large number of trying symptoms such as fatigue, headaches, muscular weakness, menstrual irregularities, and sterility. (In one week no less than six clippings from different sources were brought to my attention by patients who thought the condition described as hypometabolism fitted their cases and that here was a quick way to cure it.) It has been represented as a new thyroid hormone that can do more than the old reliable thyroid extract. The hypothesis is presented that low metabolic states may be due to either deficiency of production of the thyroid hormone, which is truly hypothyroidism, or inability of the cells to utilize it, which results in hypometabolism. It is suggested that tri-iodothyronine is the chemical form of the thyroid hormone, which can pass through the cell membrane and be useful to the cell.

This undoubtedly emphasizes the intricacies of cell metabolism and endocrine function. It may prove useful in some cases previously not helped by thyroid extract, but it certainly has not relegated thyroid extract to the category of outmoded and no longer useful medication. Tri-iodothyronine is discussed in detail not because a woman will have to know which thyroid medication is being used in her particular case but because it presents a general principle that is true for all endocrine products. Because a new name is added does not necessarily mean a spectacular advance or any great change in concept of hormone action.

Sometimes women are reluctant to take thyroid medication because they have heard that it is harmful to the heart. This idea stems from the fact that before drugs were placed on the restricted lists, it could be bought at any drug store without a doctor's prescription. It was particularly abused in self-medication with large doses for obesity with the result that the heart was greatly speeded up and sometimes overtaxed. The thyroid hormone (and all other hormones) is a normal, necessary component of the body. There is no danger in taking it when prescribed by a physician for a particular need and the dose regulated to meet that need.

Sex Hormone Therapy

Sex hormone therapy must be restricted to serve specific purposes, and even then the results are unpredictable. When endocrine deficiencies are manifested by irregularities in menstruation, they are treated in the manner previously discussed in the chapter on "Disturbances of Feminine Function." It must be remembered that it is usually not difficult to induce periodic bleeding in a woman whose uterus is fairly well developed even when her ovaries have been removed or to establish a regular menstrual cycle by improvement of her own ovarian function. But neither the induction of bleeding or the establishment of regularity are any guarantee that the true significance of menstruation has been attained—that is ovulation and fertility.

Ovulation is of course of paramount importance in fertility. From the beginnings of hormone therapy for infertility, doctors have sought means of detecting and regulating the time of ovulation and to induce its occurrence in what would otherwise be anovulatory cycles. Through the years many techniques have been employed, using different hormones, different dosage, and different timing, but none has been eminently successful. There would be little purpose in recounting even the typical examples or samplings but for the fact that most have been dramatically announced in popular articles as "new hope for the childless" and have resulted in false hope and disappointment. There will be more of these which can be realistically appraised only by the light of knowledge from past experiences.

The first hopes were directed toward obtaining a pituitary hormone (for clinical use in women) that would produce ovulation. The first one available was the chorionic gonadotropic hormone from pregnancy urine (the familiar APL, Antuirin-S, etc.). When first obtained, it was minute in strength; now it is exceedingly potent. This proved to be mainly luteinizing and incapable of inducing ovulation. Then followed the gonadotropic hormone from the serum of a pregnant mare, which was follicle-stimulating in laboratory animals. It was dramatically administered intravenously (and sometimes with unpleasant and even dangerous effects) at what seemed to be the most propitious time for ovulation. It also failed to produce the desired results. The difficulty lies in the fact that ovulation occurs as the result of a delicate timing and balance of the pituitary gonadotropic hormones, which we do not as yet know how to imitate.

The failure in the use of various pituitary hormone preparations to induce ovulation lead to the search for some other method of stimulating the pituitary itself to do a better job or of directly stimulating the ovary. One solution proposed was irradiation (X-ray stimulation) of the pituitary or the ovaries or both simultaneously. This method was employed enthusiastically by some doctors for a while, but met with disapproval from the first by others. No one has ever explained how X-ray, which is usually destructive to cell life, can be stimulating, however small the dose, al though there have been some reports of good results. Irradiation of the pituitary is still advocated by some, but no one would have the temerity to irradiate the ovaries in light of present concepts of the effect of radiation on germ plasm and the inherent danger to future generations.

And there have always been some who turn to the psyche as the source of any and all difficulties. They have suggested that ovulation may be suppressed by neurotic mechanisms. Their contentions were bolstered when evidence accrued of a definite connection (either humoral or neural) between the pituitary and the central nervous system via the hypothalamus where a "sex center" is supposed to be located. Psychoanalysis, hypnosis, autosuggestion, and other psychiatric methods were employed to remove the block—the woman's subconscious desire not to have a baby—and various degrees of frequency of success reported. Even in cases of infertility of long standing, however, pregnancy occasionally occurs with no therapy at all. The report of success in a few cases in a small series treated by whatever method really has little significance.

The ovarian hormones, estrogen and progesterone, have been used in many ways in the effort to improve fertility. Their effectiveness here is limited by one fact—an axiom of endocrinology—that any hormone administered in sufficient amounts (usually above what would be the normal level) depresses the ability of its parent gland to produce it. Thus, estrogen depresses or suppresses the ability of the ovarian follicle to produce estrogen, and progesterone inhibits the corpus luteum in its production of progesterone. How then could their administration ever be helpful in establishing normal ovarian function? Indeed, would they not be more harmful than helpful? Their use has been vindicated on the basis of what we may call "supplementation," "pump-priming," and "shock."

The most clear-cut example of supplementary therapy is the use of progesterone in cases in which ovulation occurs but is followed by inadequate corpus luteum function. The result is lack of preparation of the endometrium for implantation of the ovum and failure in the mechanism that prevents menstruation. This is certainly a valid reason for its use but it is doubtful whether many cases of infertility are the result of this type of failure.

The cyclic administration of estrogen and progesterone (previously described) is a pump-priming procedure the purpose of which is not to affect ovarian function, but rather to bring the uterus up to normal activity which it may have lost if ovarian deficiency has been marked or long lasting, and to establish in it the habit of responding to the ovarian hormones. At the same time, the pituitary is also being stimulated by the varying levels of the ovarian hormones to go through its cycle of gonadotropic hormone production. This is a valid application of the physiology of the sex cycle, but can be expected to help in those cases of mild ovarian or pituitary insufficiency. Its chances of success are increased if abetted by attention to general health and nutrition and thyroid therapy.

Hormone shock therapy has been administered in several ways, although it has rarely been called that. In general, this means giving the hormone in unphysiologic doses that are excessive in quantity or do not conform to the cyclic pattern.

Estrogen has been given in one or two large doses about midperiod in the hope that it would induce or trigger the pituitary to produce the hormones necessary to effect ovulation. There is little proof that it works in that way. A second type of shock therapy is based on the fact that large doses of progesterone will cause the endometrium to bleed if it has been primed by estrogen. Thus one large dose or usually two to four doses given on successive days each month will cause cyclic bleeding. If the woman has been amenorrheic, she may think that she is becoming normal again, but in fact she has gained little if anything in her fertility status. She has not been made to ovulate.

Recently a very potent progesterone-like hormone has become available and used on women for anovulatory menstruation as well as in women in whom no cause for sterility was found. It is given by mouth for twenty to twenty-five days, and bleeding follows within four to five. It completely suppresses ovulation. The reasoning is that ovarian function is "off-center," and by administering a shock to it there will be countershock, and then like a pendulum it will settle down with a more normal center of equibrium—that of fertility. What frequently happens is that the woman's cycle is completely disrupted, the period delayed by several weeks, and several months may elapse before menstruation assumes the woman's usual pattern.

There are two important facts to be remembered in all forms of endocrine therapy, especially as it pertains to the menstrual function. First, the hormones available for clinical use today are very potent. It is very easy therefore to employ excessive amounts, which are apt to be disturbing rather than corrective. The second is that the endocrine regulation of fertility is an intricate dynamic interaction involving many hormones in constantly changing amounts. We do not know how to imitate it, we do not have the keys to regulate it. Therefore, our best chance is to limit our efforts to helping nature with especial care that we do nothing that will impede her.

Surgery

There are two reasons for resorting to surgery in the treatment of infertility, one to remove and the other to repair some abnormality.

Occasionally, in the course of a fertility study, gross pelvic pathology is discovered that may require surgery for the woman's health. A tumor of the ovary, usually a cyst, is one of the more common of such findings in young women and in most instances should be removed. There are several justifications for this. From the standpoint of fertility, such an ovary is nonfunctional, and its removal will not decrease the young woman's chance of becoming pregnant. Rather it increases the possibility of a successful pregnancy, for a large cyst can interfere with the normal progress of pregnancy. It sometimes becomes twisted on its stalk, becoming a surgical emergency, which is a hazard to the pregnancy. And it often increases rather rapidly in size during pregnancy and has to be removed later anyhow. There is also always the remote possibility that it is more than a cyst. For these reasons, the removal of a true ovarian tumor (not transitory swelling) is conservative surgery, which contributes to the woman's health and her fertility.

The case for fibroids of the uterus is not so clear-cut. They do not interfere with the woman's health unless they cause excessive bleeding (by involvement of the endometrium, which is not always the case) or unless they are large enough to cause pelvic pain or pressure symptom such as a feeling of heaviness in the pelvis or disturbance of bladder or bowel function. Small fibroids may have no effect on the woman' fertility and are usually kept under observation rather than removed Large fibroids may so involve the whole uterus that a successful pregnancy is impossible. Either the woman does not conceive, or she loses the pregnancy early due to faulty implantation or in the later months because the uterus cannot expand to meet the normal requirements. The most fortunate type fibroid that is occasionally encountered and may be the cause of sterility is a single discrete mass that can be removed, leaving a uterus that is then capable of housing a pregnancy. It is not believed that fibroids increase the potentiality of a malignancy—that is, they are not cancerous or even precancerous.

Inflammatory masses involving the tubes and ovaries used to be a fairly common occurrence in days gone by. The common practice of removal meant the end of a woman's hope for a pregnancy. Today, with prompt diagnosis and adequate treatment with the wonder drugs (sulfa and the antibiotics) such masses, which practically destroy a woman's fertility need never occur. But even when the infection is neglected and larger inflammatory masses are formed, medical treatment should be tried first before surgery is resorted to.

Endometriosis is a relative newcomer in the field of pelvic pathology and has a very interesting history. The condition is one in which endometrial tissue is found in or on other pelvic organs (and occasionally remote parts of the body). This ectopic endometrial tissue is responsive to the ovarian hormones and undergoes cyclic changes including bleeding just as the normal endometrium does. When it is located in the ovaries, it causes cystic enlargement and interferes with normal function. If masses are formed around the tubes or in the walls of the uterus, it interferes with normal function of these organs.

The occurrence of ectopic endometrium in the pelvis was first discovered about one hundred years ago, but it was not until 1921 that it was recognized as a clinical entity and given the name endometriosis. Since that time, doctors have become more and more alert to look for it, and for this reason more cases are being found. It is difficult if not impossible to diagnose endometriosis by examination alone. Its presence may be strongly suspected, but positive diagnosis depends on direct examination of the tissue. More often it is an incidental finding in the course of surgery for other conditions.

The cause or mode of formation of these masses (small or large) of endometrial tissue around the pelvic organs is not known. The first theory was that it was the result of retrograde menstruation. That is, some particles of endometrial tissues, sloughed off with menstruation, for some unknown reason passed out of the uterus through the tubes (rather than the vagina), became attached to the ovaries and other pelvic organs, and continue to live and grow. The second theory was that the tissue grows from embryonic cells in these areas, which remain undifferentiated and quiescent until stimulated by the ovarian hormones after puberty.

The important thing is that endometriosis is a disease of young women making its appearance between the ages of twenty and forty. And it has been found more frequently among white women and private patients than among ward (charity) cases. This has led to one school of thought that endometriosis is a product or the price that woman pays for her cultural advance because she waits later to have babies and has fewer pregnancies or none at all. This restriction of endometriosis to women of a higher culture level is probably more apparent than real. A large percentage of these young women have problems of infertility. It could just as well be that their infertility is the result of endometriosis rather than that failure to start early to exercise her reproductive function encouraged the development of endometriosis. Whichever it may be, the situation is by no means hopeless.

Many young women are enabled to conceive and have a normal pregnancy if they are treated conservatively. Endometriosis is not a threat to her life, but it may be the source of intractable pain with each menstrual period. It can be "cured" promptly and completely by removal of the ovaries, for then the periodic growth ceases and symptoms disappear. Such treatment is far too drastic for women in the childbearing age (except in rare instances) and is therefore reserved for older women. In young women, good results can be obtained by the administration of hormones— either estrogen or the male hormone, which suppresses the growth of the ectopic endometrial tissue. The symptoms of pain and pelvic discomfort may be relieved and fertility restored. In some of the more severe cases, surgery to remove the masses and release adhesions, which interfere with normal function, increases the woman's chances of a pregnancy.

These are the more typical and common forms of pelvic pathology encountered in a fertility study that require surgery. There remains one surgical procedure that has played a conspicuous part in the treatment of problems of infertility in the years gone by, and that is dilatation and curettage.

Before the advent of endocrinology, the D & C was used to treat almost any and all functional feminine problems from amenorrhea and bleeding to backache and sterility. Today most of these problems are amenable to medical treatment, and a curettage is resorted to for diagnostic purposes. But sometimes in cases of infertility when nothing else is found to do, doctors in desperation resort to curettage. Perhaps we should call this pelvic shock therapy, for occasionally it works! This is not so far-fetched as one might imagine. In certain laboratory animals, the rabbit for instance, ovulation occurs only when the cervix is stimulated. Such stimulation is normally provided by copulation but can be artifically produced by electric shock or mechanical dilatation. Presumably this occurs by a reflex arc via nerves from the cervix to the central nervous system, through the hypothalamus to the pituitary gland. No one knows whether this ever occurs in women, but there is some evidence that it may.

Plastic surgery has a small place in the treatment of relative infertility. In the past, it has caused more sterility than it has cured. The one condition that might appear to be amenable to surgery is closed tubes. Because it is one of the most common causes of sterility or infertility, many types of operations have been devised and tried, but only rarely is patency restored. There is one exception when the possibility of success is greater— when the obstruction is confined to the ends of the tubes where the fimbriae or finger-like projections have become glued together. Plastic surgery here has a fair chance of success.

In the past, tilted womb or retroversion of the uterus was considered a cause of infertility, and many women were operated on to correct it. The various suspension operations are rarely performed today with the hope of relieving infertility.

Artificial Insemination

Artificial insemination as a means of relieving sterility has received a great deal of publicity of late for two reasons. First, intriguing possibilities have been raised by the term "test-tube babies"; and second, legal aspects of the procedure have brought such cases into court.

Of course there is no such thing as a test-tube baby. No one has devised any means of by-passing any of nature's steps in procreation, with the exception of the one element—insemination. The father still has to produce adequate male cells. The mother still has to produce the ovum and provide a suitable environment for its fertilization and growth. The only "improvement" science can offer is the placing of the male cells within the woman's body by artificial means rather than by natural intercourse. That is artificial insemination—an "improvement" of questionable value or acceptability, to say the least.

What is done is this. The doctor tries to determine the fertile period in the woman's cycle. Because he can't be sure, he usually uses insemination two or three times in one month. The procedure consists of taking up the semen into a syringe and injecting it either on the cervix, into the cervix, or into the uterine cavity. The first two methods are just an imitation of nature, the cells are no further along on their journey than they would be in natural circumstances. In the third, the cells are only one inch nearer their goal in a journey of six inches—not much of a boost.

What can one hope to accomplish by this? It is quite obvious that it is not a technique that can be of value to most infertile couples. There are three reasons that limit its value—medical, psychological, and legal. Let's examine each of these.

The prerequisites of success, from the medical standpoint, are that the woman must be normally fertile, the cause of sterility residing completely in the male. This at the outset limits the cases in which it might be used, for we have seen that infertility is a fifty-fifty proposition. If the husband's cell count is low, would anything be gained by reducing their necessary journey by less than 20 per cent? Most likely not, because distance is not the only factor. His cells must have vitality—the ability to fertilize, which has already been demonstrated as lacking. There are few, if any, such cases in which artificial insemination has been successful.

This brings us to the use of a donor. The semen used is from a healthy male, other than the husband, whose cells are normal. The chances of starting a pregnancy by this procedure are fair. Success, however, raises the other two questions.

Proponents of artificial insemination seek to reduce the psychological hazards by selecting a donor who resembles the husband so that the child's appearance will not clash with the physical characteristics of the parents. Also, great pains are taken to ensure that the parents (and usually the presiding doctor) and the donor are unknown to each other. Some have gone so far as to propose semen banks, where cells can be held and sent out on call, just as they are for artificial insemination of cattle.

The proponents of artificial insemination give many reasons why it is preferable to adoption or childlessness. They say that the wife will have a baby that is her own flesh and blood; the couple will at least know the maternal half of the child's heritage; no one but themselves need ever know that the husband is not the father; the wife will love her husband more because of his generosity in accepting the child as his own; and the husband will love the child more than an adopted child because it is the child of his wife. It might, however, produce just the opposite effect and be a means of separating husband and wife.

It might happen that the wife and mother would consider the baby as hers alone and refuse the husband the privilege of assuming the role of father. It is not hard to imagine the many common family disagreements when the mother sides with the child, in which this might occur. Or the "father" might not accept the child as his own but might see in it the constant symbol of his inadequacy. All these arguments and many others fade into insignificance when we consider the other important person in this procedure—the child.

Having a baby is not just for the purpose of elevating a man and woman to parenthood—the state of possessing an offspring for their own self-satisfaction. They must also assume the responsibility of bringing a new and helpless individual into the world, cherishing, guiding, and protecting it until it is able to be independent.

I do not believe any thinking person would relish the idea of never knowing anything about his ancestors—to have a background of nothingness on his father's side. Certainly, we are not a people of ancestor worshippers, but recognition of family ties give a stability to life. That they have been less strong in the past generation is a misfortune, not a sign of progress. We hear much today of security. But security must have a basis of more than material possessions. There must be the spiritual element as well, which derives its strength from love. The family ties, the mutual love of mother, father, and child, are essential and fundamental.

Finally, there is the legal aspect. Some courts have ruled that artificial insemination makes the child a bastard and the mother guilty of adultery. The proponents of artificial insemination have ways of getting around this also. They suggest that one doctor do the artificial insemination, and then send the woman to an obstetrician who knows nothing of what has gone before. He, the obstetrician, then signs the birth certificate that will make the child the legitimate offspring of the husband. This condemns the couple to a lifetime of concealing a fraud—not a very happy prospect.

Looking back over the past twenty-five years, which have seen such advances in our knowledge of fertility and in our concept of how to deal with infertility, two basic facts stand out to guide us and inspire confidence for continued and further advances.

The first is that many if not most cases of childlessness are not hopeless. The problem resolves itself in our determination to apply infinite care to all details. Such efforts will be rewarded by success with increasing frequency as our knowledge increases. In some cases we are unable to demonstrate any valid reason for sterility, but as we learn more about the mysteries of sex physiology and procreation, many cases will be removed from the ethereal psychosomatic category where they now find themselves.

The second fact is to have children, to be fruitful, is not an inalienable right. Fertility is a privilege, which must be guarded and cherished. Many of the cases of sterility we now see are the result of conditions that could have been avoided. This places on doctors and parents a double responsibility to the next generation. They must be alert to detect abnormalities of physical development as they first become apparent in adolescence and correct them, for the chances are children will not outgrow them. The children of the next generation must also be helped to acquire an adequate knowledge and appreciation of themselves so that they may attain maturity of body, mind, and heart.

THE AGE OF THE UNBORN

XIV

THE JOURNEY TO BABYHOOD

"WHAT ARE little girls made of? Sugar and spice and everything nice?"

"Where do babies come from? From heaven or does the stork bring them?"

Even toddlers are too sophisticated today to accept such answers, and you would never dream of telling them such stories lest they get an inferiority complex or come to feel rejected and insecure! And so you try to tell them the truth. But how much do you know of this first age of woman? You know where her home is, how she comes to enter it, how and when she leaves it. But do you have any idea what happens to her and how it happens while she is there? Do you know, for instance, that she is a female when she is a tiny speck of only one cell and that she has attained her human female body form when she is still so small that she could be fitted quite comfortably into a golf ball? Perhaps not, for the Age of the Unborn is the age of mystery, and when it is complete, it is the age of a miracle—nature's miracle of creation.

The mystery of how a new life comes into being has always intrigued mankind. Indeed, man has always felt a great need to have an answer that he could not only accept but also one that would afford him guidance. We would find, if we paged through history, many answers ranging from the myths, superstitions, and taboos of ancient people and even primitive people of recent times, through the half-truths of early scientific groping to the real answers in the scientific truths of today. The answers are varied because they have been dictated both by the extent of man's knowledge of himself and by his beliefs concerning himself and his relationship to the world about him—real and spiritual.

341

Among primitive people, the answer to the mystery of a new life was found in spirits because man did not recognize that there was any relationship between his sexual act and a baby born to the woman nine months later. They thought that the woman became fruitful, that is, pregnant, because a spirit had entered her body. According to some myths, the spirit came from the body of one who had recently died and found entrance to the woman's body through her navel. Other myths related that spirits lived in trees—girl spirits in one particular kind and boy spirits in another. Woman, therefore, was careful how she approached such trees lest she find herself possessed of child.

In the early beginnings of science, "humors" were substituted for spirits, but these were scarcely less mysterious forces. The early scientists— more philosophers than scientists—believed that humors or fluids were carried in channels from all parts of the body of both male and female and accumulated as semen in their reproductive organs. When the semen of the male united with the semen of the female in the uterus, it coagulated to form the body of the baby. The humor that had been brought from the head developed into the head of the baby. The humor from other parts of the body was the origin of the corresponding parts of the baby's body.

The early scientists became familiar with the changes in form the human body undergoes before birth and were intrigued and mystified by the force that guided these changes. For a solution they, too, fell back on the spirits. Life came to the body, they believed, when the soul entered it. Some thought there was a succession of souls—the "nutritive" came first, to be followed by the "sensitive," which was finally displaced by the "rational" soul.

The science of embryology, which had its beginnings in these gropings of the ever-inquisitive human mind, has solved many of the mysteries of the Age of the Unborn. From it we can learn what happens and when it happens, and we can speculate why it happens. But how nature does it is still her secret. Scientists are seeking the answers in chromosomes, genes, and electrical and chemical changes within the most minute particles of living matter. But the mystery of life persists.

The Age of the Unborn is perhaps the most eventful of all ages from the physical standpoint because within it are crowded the series of tremendous changes that not only must take place at the proper time in proper order but also must be completed within a definite time limit. This new life must not only grow to look like a baby—it must learn to act like a baby in just 280 days! Yet, we rarely think of this first age as that of an individual. We are more apt to think of it in terms of the mother—the changes in her body, her comfort and health, what she should do and not do so that her baby will be normal. Age One as far as the new individual is concerned is only anticipation. The " expected " is due to make her first appearance as a finished product at a calculated date.

It may be difficult to attribute the reality of an individual to one unborn, for most people have never seen anything but the finished product. You may have visited a medical museum and seen models and specimens in jars representing the stages of development of the human. They may have seemed grotesque to you, so repulsive that you turned your face away, or they may not have interested you enough to stop and look at them. Or you may have had some experience with an unsuccessful pregnancy. Here too, the interest is directed solely to the mother. The aborted new life is only something to be hidden from sight and quickly disposed of. This life that failed may be regretted, but its image in memory is forever characterless and nameless.

Put all of these pictures out of your mind. The wax models are cold and rigid, fixed in size, shape, and posture. The charts and pictures are mere caricatures. The specimens are limp masses of tissue that will retain their form only as long as they float in their preservative. The first have never possessed the magic spark of life while the others have lost it. Try, instead to visualize the unborn as it really is—a living, growing, ever-changing bit of life. It does not matter whether it is a single cell or a baby waiting to be born—it has the same attributes of life that you have.

NATURE'S TIMETABLE

The Age of the Unborn is a dynamic age, full of life and accomplishment. The rate of growth is prodigious—from one cell to an estimated 26 trillion, and from a length of 1/200 of an inch to 20 inches or 4,000 times greater at birth than at conception. The change in form is little short of magic, from a tiny speck of one cell to a well-formed baby. The accomplishments acquired by the unborn as an individual are things we take for granted, but they are the foundations on which all its future accomplishments must depend. The heart learns to beat, the muscles to contract, the nerves to carry messages to the brain, which is learning to assume its directive powers. And the unborn is getting ready to perform the most significant act of its life—to take its first breath of air, the breath of life itself. This ability it will fight to maintain through all the years, for with it goes life itself. On this seemingly simple ability to breathe, it will learn to express itself in the human voice, with all the myriads of meaning this has for a human being.

To accomplish such a tremendous task in such a short period, nature has a perfect plan—a timetable that specifies just how far along she must be with each minute detail each succeeding day. She is exceedingly proficient in adhering to this. Her timing is perfect, her accomplishments rapid, accurate, and purposefully correlated. We cannot follow her day by day as she accomplishes this but will have to content ourselves with spot checking at regular intervals. Scientists divide the 280 days into 10 lunar months of 28 days each. We shall use these as the stops in nature's timetable.

A single cell, rounded like a ball, is all that nature has to start with. Its appearance gives no indication that it holds the potentials necessary for the creation of a human being. The changes that take place during the first two weeks of life we have already followed in the story of pregnancy. We saw how the ovum and sperm unite to form a new cell, and with that union comes a property that neither possessed alone—the power of growth and transformation. We saw how this new cell divided and redivided until it was a solid ball of cells. This was quickly transformed into a hollow ball filled with fluid with a thin plate of cells across the middle. This plate of cells becomes the embryo, while the shell takes on the function of housing the new life and maintaining communication with the mother, who supplies it with the vital necessities.

From the beginning, when the first cell divides, nature uses two guiding or directing forces to achieve her purpose of growth and maturation. One force directs the cells as they multiply to specific changes in structure whereby each cell or group of cells becomes specialized to assume a specific duty. By the second force, the cells are held together as a unit, each in its proper place, increasing at the proper speed toward an optimum limit of growth, and each cell contributing to the welfare of the whole. These are the same forces that nature employs throughout life to maintain the integrity of body structure and function. Growth continues as long as there is life, new cells replacing old cells every moment of life. When nature loses these directive powers over the growth process, distortions and sometimes disaster occur.

The unborn at eighteen days of age is still a flat, pear-shaped disc. Its structure appears quite simple, for it consists of only three layers of cells that still look much alike. But appearances are deceiving, because the cells of each layer have already received their orders, and each has a different responsibility for providing some specific structure of the body. They will divide and redivide many thousands of times, and with each division they take on a new form and arrange themselves in clusters of different configurations until the final form has been achieved.

The ectoderm or outside cell layer (at this time the upper layer of the plate) must provide the physical structures related to the external environment. Some of these cells will differentiate to form the skin, the sheath that will serve the body in many ways in relation to the outside environment. Other cells of the ectoderm are the forerunners of the nervous system, which provides the means of recognition of and action within the external environment, for it includes the brain, spinal cord, and nerves as well as the special sense organs—the eyes, the ears, and those of taste and smell.

The endoderm, or the innermost layer of cells (now the under layer) has as its destiny the means of providing the body with the necessities of life, food and oxygen. From this layer will be developed the digestive system, with all its glands, and the respiratory system.

The mesoderm or middle layer of cells must supply the framework and supportive structures such as bone and muscle as well as the structures devoted to the internal functions such as the circulatory, urinary, and reproductive systems.

By the end of the first month in the life of the unborn, significant changes have already taken place. (This corresponds to fifteen days according to the mother's reckoning from her failure to menstruate, when she cannot even be sure she is pregnant.) The unborn is no longer a pear-shaped disc or flat plate. The disc has already become separated from the walls of the hollow sphere that enclosed it, in all except one small area. This connection will persist to form the umbilical cord and life line. Moreover, the margins of the disc have folded inward and partly fused so that the unborn is now a rounded solid body, having the shape of an oversized comma. The free end has grown most rapidly and bulges out to form the head. Even the eyes, nose, and ears are represented, although they bear little resemblance as yet to definitive organs. Behind the expanded head is a long neck with slits on each side somewhat like the gills of a fish. Thereafter the body tapers off into a tail. Just behind the gill slits, one on each side, are buds which will be the arms, and a little further back are the two leg buds. Nestled in front between the bent-down head and the two arm buds is a little tube which will be the heart. It is so tiny that hardly more than one blood cell can pass through at a time, but a heart it is, already busily at work pumping blood to the rest of the body. If we could peer inside this body of the unborn, which is only one tenth to one eighth of an inch long, and understand what we would see, we would find traces or precursors of all the internal organs in their proper places.

By the end of the second month, this tiny living creature is about one inch long. It is different in shape and proportion from that of a month ago, but it does not look quite human yet. It still has a tremendous head, which seems to constitute about one half of the total body length. The neck is shorter, and the gill slits have almost disappeared. The limb buds are beginning to look a little like arms and legs. The hands and feet have the appearance of paddles. The fingers and toes are indicated only by creases, as they are on a rag doll. The tail is much shorter.

In three months the unborn has acquired human form. True, it still looks a little peculiar, because the head is still disproportionately large and consists of a large dome-shaped crown and forehead and small face. The fingers and toes are separate now and have soft nails, the external sex organs are distinctly male or female, and the unborn begins to make feeble movements. It is a tiny human being only three inches long and weighing only one ounce.

These first three months are eventful and crucial in the life of the unborn. Yet, they pass almost before others know of this new individual-in-the-making. This is the time when the body acquires human form, a human face with eyes, ears, and nose, arms with hands and fingers, legs with feet and toes, and all the internal organs developed in miniature. The completion of the third month of life of the unborn marks an important milestone in the journey to babyhood, because certain dangers have passed that will not be encountered again. During the first three months, when structure and form are evolving, the body is quite vulnerable. Mishaps and harmful influences brought to bear during this period may result in distortion of body form or deformity of internal structure. After the third month the body has only to grow and mature. Any mishaps that befall it will only impede growth and maturation but cannot change the form.

During the next three months, the fourth through the sixth, the fetus is occupied with increase in size and perfection of the functions of the body. In the fourth month, downy hair covers the body, most of which will disappear before birth and the rest soon after. In the fifth month the muscles are strong enough for the fetus to kick its legs, so the mother "feels life." The heart beats with sufficient vigor for the doctor to hear it. But the fetus is still less than twelve inches long and weighs only about nine ounces. Since it is all curled up, its head down, knees drawn up and arms folded on the chest, it is no more than a soft little ball that would fit in the palm of your hand.

The completion of the sixth month marks another important milepost, for when the fetus is safely through this month, should it perchance be thrust into the world of independent existence, it has a chance, although a slim one, of living. But if birth occurs in the sixth month or any time before, the fetus may move and even cry feebly, but death is almost inevitable. Its organs just haven't reached the point of development for them to function adequately to maintain life. A six-months baby is about one foot long and weighs one and a half pounds. The skin is wrinkled because it has no fat under it. The face has the appearance of a wizened little old person.

The seventh month marks the beginning of the home-stretch. The fetus, if born now, is a premature baby with a chance to live. The chance becomes greater with each succeeding day. This is contrary to the old saying that a seven-month baby has a greater chance of survival than an eight-month baby. Each month it gains in strength and ability to survive. In the seventh month, when it is 13 to 15 inches long and weighs two and a half pounds, life would be precarious. In the eighth month, it has gained another two inches in length and another pound. Its skin is red and covered with a thick cheesy material, but it is still wrinkled. In the ninth month these wrinkles disappear because paddings of fat under the skin have been added, and it would have a good chance to live if born. In the tenth month the task is complete. It has grown to look like a baby.

No two newborns look exactly alike. Each has its own particular characteristics, but in general conforms to a pattern. The newborn is about twenty inches long and usually weighs six to nine pounds. Its head is still proportionately large, constituting one quarter of the length, and it is as broad as the shoulders. The head may be perfectly shaped, but more often the crown is elongated because of the part it has played in the birth process. The new mother, unprepared for this appearance, may think that she has given birth to a Hottentot. She need not be disturbed, for the head will go back to normal shape in a few weeks. The head seems to be attached almost directly to the narrow sloping shoulders because the neck is very short, little more than a crease. The hips are narrower than the shoulders and are made to appear even smaller by the protrusion of the rounded little belly. The short arms and legs stay folded in much the same position they have been forced to assume in the close confines of their previous quarters. The skin is soft pink or red and sometimes blotchy on the head and face. The newborn may be chubby due to pads of baby fat, and there may be hair on the head, back, and chest. The eyes are usually gray.

This is nature's timetable by which the unborn comes to look like a baby, but this is only half of the story. The unborn has been acquiring skills that will enable it to assume its individual existence.

LEARNING TO ACT LIKE A BABY

The newborn, snug in her crib, seems oblivious to the world about her. She opens her eyes occasionally, but she doesn't seem to look at anything.

Sounds seem not to affect her in one way or another. But she is acting, nevertheless. She holds her head to one side, her arms across her chest or up to her face. She keeps her fists closed, but she will grasp your finger. She cries insistently and kicks vigorously for one of her size, when she wishes to express her displeasure with the world about her and to demand attention to her comfort.

Rather far-fetched, you say, to call this helpless little being, whose repertoire is so limited as compared to her mother or even her two-year-old sister, an actress. But actress she is and of no mean accomplishment for one of her age. In the few months since the day life began for her until birth thrust her on the stage of life to act as a human being, she has become a complete individual. She has not only the correct number of fingers and toes, a body of human form, and the necessary organs to take care of the processes of living, but much more. These simple acts of behavior that she displays represent the foundation of all behavior and foreshadow all the abilities she will ever have as an adult. From these will develop not only the ability to maintain harmony and efficiency in the internal functions of her feminine body, and the skills in physical activities, but also the ability to act the part of a mature woman, maintaining her identity and expressing her individuality as she adjusts to the ever-changing, unpredictable world that will be her stage.

Perhaps she will be a great opera singer. Her career was launched when she took her first breath of air. Later her ears, her mind, and her heart will open to the wonderful world of sound. Perhaps she will be an artist. That manual skill is foreshadowed in the clutching of her tiny hand, and her eyes will open to the beauty and meaning of the world about her. Her feeble cry represents her desire for comfort. What is comfort to her as an infant is simple in comparison to what comfort will signify to her as an adult, but the basic needs are the same. The means for satisfying these needs are present at birth. She must learn by experience how to use them.

This ability of behaving like a baby is not some sudden endowment that comes with birth. Just as the unborn had to grow and develop to achieve its goal of looking like a baby, it had to learn to act like a baby. The learning process, the development of the pattern of behavior, has a timetable. We can follow this timetable more easily if we first define more specifically what we mean by "behaving like a baby." What are the abilities that a baby is born with? She breathes; she takes in food; she rids herself of waste material; she moves, and her body has a characteristic posture. She is sensitive and responsive to the physical world about her of heat and cold, darkness and light, sound and touch, and she is sensitive and responsive to the new world of people and things. Hidden in the structure of her body, she has the ability to reproduce, ready to be called into action at the appropriate time many years hence.

She has all these abilities at birth, and they are all she will ever have. She will modify, expand, and perfect them as life advances, but no new ones will be added. These abilities are inherent in the first cell, and as the body develops they too are perfected as the need for each arises. During the Age of the Unborn some are perfected and in full use; some are near completion ready to be put into operation at a moment's notice, and some are only foreshadowed and will require years of maturing and experience before any degree of proficiency is acquired.

The first needs of the unborn are food and oxygen. When it is only a cluster of cells, these necessities may be obtained from the surrounding fluids. When growth has proceeded to the embryonic stage, other means must be provided. Among the first cells of the body to be differentiated are the red blood cells. The heart is the first organ and the circulatory system the first system to be called into use and to attain definitive form. The heart learns to beat just as it will for the rest of life. This is demonstrated by the fact that the electrocardiogram of an unborn only nine and a half weeks old is similar to that of an adult.

The digestive system is complete and begins to function even before birth. The intestines have learned motility. The unborn even swallows or drinks some of the fluid in which it is immersed. The same degree of behavior has also been attained by the kidneys and the urinary system.

While the systems of the body are evolving to take care of specific needs as they arise, nature is already beginning to provide for their overall control. Their functions must be co-ordinated so that they work in harmony with each other and with efficiency for the welfare of the whole. So, nature begins mapping out the three levels of control that, as we learned in "The Age of Maturity," will dominate and control all the activities as a human being. These levels are the central nervous system, the autonomic nervous system, and the endocrine glandular system.

The Nervous System

From the earliest days of the embryo, nature seems to be preoccupied with the development of the nervous system. She has the task of providing the millions of cells that constitute the brain and connecting these by nerve fibers to every part, even the remotest cell of the body. All of these must be in place and properly connected at birth. The brain cells will be her masterpiece of specialization, for they, in their mysterious way, are the physical basis of the mind and emotions. By their action, behavior of the body as a whole is controlled. All the brain cells that a human being will ever have are present at birth, although it will take many years after birth before the individual has learned to use them. If any are destroyed, they cannot be replaced. Nature does provide some margin of safety, however, in that other cells may take on the function of the cells destroyed, but only to a limited extent. If many cells are destroyed, the ability inherent in those cells is lost forever.

The nervous system is started in the first few days of the embryo by an enfolding at the midline of the ectoderm. This soon forms a rod of cells extending the whole length of the embryo. The head end expands to form the brain; the remainder becomes the spinal cord and nerve fibers. The head is the most rapidly growing part of the embryo and fetus. In the embryonic stage, the head constitutes three-fourths of the total length of the body. In the fetus in the early months, it comprises one-half of the body length. In the newborn it is one-fourth, compared to one-eighth to one-tenth in the adult.

The nervous system acquires its ability to control in the sequence in which the needs for control arise. The first areas of the brain to function are those that throughout life will regulate and maintain harmony in the automatic functions of the body, such as the heart beat and the blood pressure. It is here in the old brain, or hypothalamus, that the cluster of cells that will regulate breathing (the respiratory center) is located, ready to start functioning at the proper time. Just what holds this center in check, when the others are all functioning smoothly, is a mystery.

Next, the nervous system learns to control the movements of the body. The unborn moves its arms and legs. This ability will be very limited even at birth, for the newborn has little bodily control, but the mechanism—the physical basis and the pattern for behavior—is there. She has to learn by experience how to make full use of it. In time, physical movements too become not only automatic but rapid and efficiently coordinated.

Consciousness is the last function of the nervous system to be called into action. The newborn arrives in the twilight zone of consciousness. It has to learn to go to sleep. It has to learn to wake up. It must learn to renew its strength by deep refreshing sleep so that it may awake to an intense awareness of itself, its wants and desires, as well as awareness of the world about it with its dangers and rewards.

The brain, the seat of consciousness, is the first organ to be started, as we have seen. It increases faster in size, but it is the last to be completed. The cells that are to serve a lifetime are all there long before birth, but they are still far too immature even at birth to go to work. They have to be shaped by experience and learning before they can function. The acquisition of knowledge does not come from any increase in brain cells. No one has any more gray matter than another. Some are just able to make better use of what they have.

The Endocrine Glands

The Age of the Unborn is an age of tremendous metabolic activity. And metabolic activity needs hormones to stimulate, guide, and keep in balance these physical and chemical changes. Nature has made abundant provision for these needs, for the unborn has not one, but three, sources of supply of hormones. First, there are hormones from the mother's endocrine glands. Circulating as they do in her blood stream, they may pass through the placenta to the fetal blood stream. Second, the placenta itself is an endocrine gland that secretes hormones we know are necessary for the protection and maintenance of pregnancy and perhaps have other functions in the body of the unborn. Last, the unborn's own endocrine glands develop early and undoubtedly begin to function long before birth. Just how nature uses these hormones, and which source she depends on at the varying stages of development, we do not know.

It is quite obvious that we cannot make tests in the unborn to determine the degree of hormone production by its endocrine glands. We can only observe the changing structure of the glands and surmise from this what their degree of activity might be. The possible exceptions are those pertaining to sex, which we shall consider in a later chapter.

Some general observations as to the origin of the cells that are to become endocrine glands, the time that each gland begins to emerge, and the size that they have attained at birth are interesting and suggestive of both the character and importance of the role they are to play in later life.

The pituitary, the master gland, as might be expected, is the first endocrine gland to develop. It is to be, we might say, the " brain " of the endocrine system. It is also to be the " go-between," or connecting link, between the endocrine glandular system and the nervous system. This peculiar or specific function of the pituitary seems to be foreshadowed by its origin in the embryo. The cells that make up the anterior pituitary are derived from the ectoderm, the outer layer of primitive cells, which is also the origin of the nervous system. These prepituitary cells migrate to a position at the base of the developing brain and become attached to it by a stem or stalk, thus connecting the two great systems of body control. Just when the pituitary of the unborn begins to function we do not know, but it is ready to take on responsibility at birth. Its full maturity of function is not established until the Age of Maturity.

The thyroid, as we have seen, is second only to the pituitary in its importance to the welfare of the body as a whole, but it is concerned more with the nutritive aspects. This importance and function is foreshadowed in the fact that the prethyroid cells appear in the third week of life and are derived from the endoderm, just as the digestive tract and its glands and the respiratory system are.

The adrenal cortex and the ovaries are derived not only from the same primitive cell layer, the mesoderm, but also from the same area of this primitive tissue, which could account for the close functional relationship between the two. The adrenal cortex produces not only its own hormones, but the sex hormones as well.

THE MEANING OF BIRTH DAY

Birthdays are something special for each of us. Why are they celebrated as an anniversary of the event of our birth? Why shouldn't the actual day we are born be designated the first birthday? The obvious reason is that events of birth are never repeated in the life of a person. The more significant reason is that birth is the one experience in life common to everyone. What is the meaning of this experience of being transformed from the unborn to the newborn? There have been many diverse answers.

Birth has been called "the greatest catastrophe" in the life of an individual. Life in utero is represented as utopia for the unborn. It lives a life of perfect ease. There is no change in its environment—no stormy blasts of winter winds, no blistering heat of summer suns, but always the constant warmth and gentle pressure of the fluid world in which it lives. The unborn has no struggle for existence, for food comes to each cell of its body automatically. It does not even have to attend to bodily excretory functions, for there is an automatic disposal system also. In this world of aloneness, there is no sound of people going about the noisy business of living or even of nature's wind through the trees or thunder from the clouds, only utter stillness and silence.

Birth, it is said, abruptly changes all this. Utopia is destroyed. The newborn is thrust into a world filled with people—big people, with blaring noises and blazing lights. Her body needs are no longer automatically attended to. She must do these things for herself, and, to make matters worse, she doesn't know how. She is completely at the mercy of the big people. So begins her struggle to maintain her identity and establish her independence, but always with nostalgia for the good old days—a longing "to return to the womb." She learns the meaning of conflict and frustration, love and hate, little of joy and much of sorrow in this hurley-burley world in which she has become a citizen by no choice of her own. In later years, she will not know why she is unhappy, ill at ease, or neurotic, because the memory of these struggles has slipped down into her subconscious mind. But she is a "crazy, mixed-up kid" until she learns to recall these early experiences and to see that in her immaturity she had misjudged things, and it is not such a bad world after all!

Some years ago a cult that called their theory "dianetics" went a step further and searched their memories for happenings not only in infancy and childhood but back into the Age of the Unborn. They professed to find that it was not such a utopia after all; unpleasant and weird things had happened to them that they could remember with just a little of the right kind of trying. Recently the fad of Bridey Murphys has caught the public's fancy, and we hear of people who can remember when they were someone else a hundred years or more ago. So we have completed a cycle but in reverse. We are back with primitive man and his world of spirits.

We do not have to accept any of these concepts of the meaning of birth. The science of physiology of the human body and of the human mind has given us concrete facts, based on objective findings, rather than unsubstantiated theories. It would be queer indeed if nature in her infinite wisdom had laid such perfect plans for the Age of the Unborn and neglected completely to provide for the transition to being a newborn. Her plans are complete and protect her handiwork. The new environment does not come as a shock to the baby for the reason that its nervous system is not yet tuned to receive all these shocking messages at once, or indeed to recognize them as shocking. They come in faintly and a few at a time. The eyes see dimly, the objects are blurred. The ears do not at first transmit sound. This lack of sensitivity to the world about her after birth has been proved by controlled scientific investigation, and therefore it seems most unlikely that she could have reveled in the comfort of her previous environment. She does not remember the shocking experience of birth, again for the reason that the physical basis of memory, the brain cells, are not developed to the point that these events have any meaning. They are not connected up to receive the messages (sensations) or mature enough to interpret and record them if they did. Thus, nature allows the perception of the world about her to come gradually and in divided doses. She can, and must, take her time in making up her mind whether she likes it or not. Her knowledge of the world can grow only as the brain cells mature.

So much for birth as a catastrophe. Let us explore some of the other meanings that have been ascribed to it.

Birth, it is said, is a natural phenomenon that should be a soul-lifting experience for the mother and that engenders a deep and abiding love for her baby. Why should a mother pick out just one day to glorify above all others that contribute to the creation of her baby? It is the whole 280 days that are important. The fact that the miracle of creation is taking place within her body should have as much if not more meaning to her than the fact that she was conscious of the pain of her labor. As for mother-love, we can't go back a thousand years or even a few generations to see what mother-love was like when woman did not understand the mechanism of her labor, but doubtless she loved her baby just the same.

Birth is described as the most hazardous experience of all life. But if nature's plan has gone smoothly for both the unborn's development and for the mother's physical adaptations to meet the needs of pregnancy and delivery, and most important if her timetable has proceeded to full maturity, birth itself is not a hazard.

These interpretations of the significance of birth day, and many others that could be related, are interesting hypotheses not to be taken too seriously. There is however, one positive, objective, undeniable meaning of birth in the life history of each of us which is crucial. Birth marks the transition from life in an environment of fluid to a life of breathing air, and this is accomplished by a dramatic change in the method by which we obtain oxygen.

THE BREATH OF LIFE

The unborn, surrounded as it is by fluid, has its own particular way of getting oxygen. The newborn discards this mechanism and calls into use an entirely different system. This switch-over must be accomplished quickly and completely if life is to continue. The need for oxygen is continuous, and the supply must be constant since the body cannot store it.

Starvation from lack of food is a long drawn-out process. A person can go without taking food for days and even weeks and still live and return to health. Death from thirst comes more quickly but still is a matter of days. Death from lack of oxygen is a matter of minutes. There are many familiar examples of this need for oxygen. A person drowns when subnerged in water for only a few minutes and deprived of oxygen. Artificial espiration can be effective only if applied while the blood still contains nough oxygen to support life processes in the vital centers of the brain. Many of our lifesaving procedures are in reality attempts to keep sufficient xygen flowing through the blood stream. A person suffering from a heart ttack is placed in an oxygen tent so that the injured heart will not have o work so hard to maintain the flow. In cases of pneumonia, in which reas of lung cells are put out of commission, the remaining normal cells an better compensate when the supply of oxygen is more bountiful. Whole blood for transfusion is far more valuable for treatment of hemor-hage after an accident or surgery than plasma or other fluids, because it lone can supply the oxygen-carrying elements of the blood, the red lood cells.

The unborn has this same critical need for oxygen during the months before birth, and during birth itself, that it will experience through all the years that are to follow. Only the amount of oxygen needed and the method of obtaining it are different. This has recently been recognized by scientists, who have determined that many of the accidents fatal to the newborn are due to lack of oxygen and that many of the mishaps along the journey are due to oxygen deficiency at some crucial time or to some vulnerable area.

In the first few weeks of life, the early embryo can obtain sufficient oxygen from the surrounding fluids just as it gets its food, but this soon becomes inadequate. However, by this time the unborn's organ for breathing, the placenta, has begun to take shape. Here the unborn's red blood cells absorb through the walls of its tiny blood vessels (in the villi) the oxygen that the mother's red blood cells have brought and released into the surrounding fluid.

By the time the unborn has reached the stage of a fetus its supply line for oxygen has become quite long, and it continues to increase until birth. It starts or has its origin with the air in the mother's lungs, extends through her circulatory system, then through the placenta and umbilical cord to the baby's body or blood vessels, and finally to each remote cell of its body. In any long line of communication or transportation there is some loss along the way and in the depots of transfer. So it is with the unborn's oxygen supply line. The unborn's blood never contains anywhere near as much oxygen as the mother's blood. Fortunately it does not require the same amount for its comfort or its safety. We can understand how great this difference is if we first recall some familiar facts about an adult's need for oxygen.

When a person goes from a low altitude to a relatively high altitude as from the seashore to a high mountain resort, there are rather uncomfortable symptoms for a few days or weeks. The person will find herself quite lackadaisical, tiring easily, and made breathless on the slightest exertion. She may become dizzy and experience fainting spells or blackouts. These are all due to oxygen deficiency. But soon she becomes acclimated, which means that the body has adjusted not to need less but to make the most of what is available. This it does by increasing the number of red blood cells to carry more oxygen. Mountain climbers who aspire to scale the highest peaks make provision for this body need of oxygen in several ways. They climb slowly, rest frequently to conserve oxygen, and carry extra oxygen with them. Modern airplanes are pressurized, which means that when they are closed they are really like oxygen tents that keep the oxygen pressure at the level needed for safety and comfort at high altitudes. Aviators black-out when deprived of this extra source of oxygen even for a few moments and cannot survive for very long without it. Yet the unborn lives with ease and comfort at an internal oxygen pressure much less than the atmospheric oxygen of the highest mountain. As a matter of fact, that would be too much oxygen for comfort or safety for the unborn. Its available oxygen is about the same that jet pilots encounter as they rise to six miles above the earth. The amount of oxygen the unborn needs, therefore, seems quite small in comparison with an adult. But the necessity of a constant level and continuing supply is more crucial.

While the unborn is "breathing" through the placenta, it is preparing to make the transfer to breathing air. The lungs are growing and developing a system of branchings, which starts with a single trunk or large tube just behind or below the throat and continues in the ever-increasing number of smaller and smaller tubes to end in the air sacs. Of course this system contains only fluid. But the fluid in the lungs serves a useful purpose. It helps to train the structures to maintain a continuous, clear passageway. Even the little sacs are distended with fluid, which gives them a rounded, patent posture, all thus ready to serve as a passageway for air when the fluid is expelled. In the unborn, even as early as the fourth month, the chest muscles begin having feeble contractions, which move the chest walls, thus warming up for the time when they must work vigorously to effect the expansion of the chest wall and suck in the vital air. They will be ready for action when the signal is given. What holds the mechanism of this true breathing in check until the proper moment at birth we do not know.

There is one great difference between the lungs of the unborn and those of the newborn, and that is the amount of blood circulating through each. You will recall that blood returning from all parts of the body enters the right side of the heart, is pumped from there through the lungs, and then is returned to the left side of the heart to be pumped to all parts of the body. In the unborn there is no need for this large volume of blood to go to the lungs, so it is shunted from the right side of the heart to the left, thus by-passing the lungs. At birth this by-pass is quickly closed, and the full volume of blood passes into the pulmonary vessels, where it takes on the needed load of oxygen and also expands the lungs.

Birth then is the discarding of an old and taking on of a new way of breathing. It is an abrupt change to be sure, but nature has provided aids that make the transfer easier and safer as we have seen in the mechanism of birth.

This account of the journey to babyhood is only an outline of nature's plan for her greatest creative work. The details of all phases, which are efficiently planned and executed constitute a story too long and intricate to be told here. But the outline is sufficient to impress us with the magnitude and speed of nature's accomplishments. Nature, of course, is never perfect. It is no wonder that her plans go awry, at times, and a baby is born with a physical abnormality. Rather, it is a marvel that such mishaps occur as infrequently as they do. This is especially true because we humans are too often guilty of not trying to understand and help nature, but are always doing things that actually interfere with her work.

XV

MISHAPS ALONG THE WAY

WAITING FOR the newborn at the end of the journey are the welcoming
arms of the mother. And like mothers everywhere, she has had her
moments of anxiety for the safety of the traveler. Unlike most other
people who welcome a traveler the mother does not know what her new
arrival will look like. She doesn't even know whether she is welcoming a
son or a daughter. But these are of no consequence. Her greatest concern
is that her child be normal, her greatest fear that it will not be perfect.
She has tried to do what she could to ensure the safety of the journey,
taking care that no act of hers would mark her baby or interfere with its
growth and development. Actually, most of her fears are ungrounded.
She cannot mark her baby, and the chances that it will have a physical
abnormality are remote.

Only one baby in two hundred, as an average, has some apparent
physical abnormality at birth. Even this incidence is not as bad as it
might seem at first, for it includes minor defects that will not mar the
child's appearance or interfere with its normal life. It also includes defects
that, while serious in nature, can be corrected surgically so that the baby
need not be handicapped for life. Only a few will be hopelessly defective.
Truly, nature has conducted well these journeys of the unborn.

One of the reasons for nature's success in producing normal babies in
such a high percentage of births is that she rejects a seriously faulty
product long before it has reached completion. Investigators have examined babies (embryo or fetus) aborted in the early months of pregnancy
and found that the vast majority were abnormal. If these babies had
survived, they would have been tragically deformed. Nature did not let
that happen.

Why do abnormalities have to occur at all? If nature can do so nearly a perfect job in 199, why does she fail in the 200th baby? This question haunts and torments the parents of an abnormal child. They ask themselves over and over again: " Is there something so wrong with us that we cannot have normal children? " This suspicion of themselves as the cause of the child's abnormality, either by physical inadequacies or faulty heritage, makes the parents afraid to have another child.

Until quite recently, there was not much that a doctor could tell such parents that was either consoling or encouraging. Doctors themselves believed that congenital abnormalities, with the exception of birth injuries, were due to faulty germ plasm, that is, that hidden in either the ovum or the sperm was some defect or deficiency that resulted in the abnormality. We have learned that abnormalities need not be due to faulty material at the start, but may be due to something that happens to the fetus that disturbs the normal pattern of growth and development. This means that such abnormalities were not inevitable from the start, but are the results of some particular circumstance during that one particular pregnancy.

This is a much more optimistic viewpoint both for parents who have had one abnormal child and for all " expecting " parents. When we can identify what constitutes a peculiar circumstance, there is hope of finding means of guarding against it and preventing it happening again in other pregnancies. The story of German measles, and how it came to be recognized as a cause of congenital abnormalities, is an excellent example of this.

A PARTICULAR CIRCUMSTANCE

Some years ago a noted eye specialist of Australia observed that an extraordinarily large number of youngsters were being brought to him for defects they were born with, particularly cataracts. Some were also deaf, mentally deficient, or had heart abnormalities. He further noted that they were almost all of the same age. Suspecting that this was more than coincidence, he inquired of other doctors in the area and found that they too were having the same experience. Then he and others started the search for some common factor, some particular circumstance that had been present during the months before these children were born. They found the common factor to be German measles. Almost all of the mothers of these abnormal children had had German measles during the epidemic that swept over the country in 1941. Searching further, the doctors found that only the mothers who contracted measles during the first three months of their pregnancy had abnormal babies. Those who had the disease later in their pregnancy had normal babies.

This was the first scientific demonstration of a specific cause of a particular kind of congenital abnormality in the human. It corresponded to the findings of scientists who, for years previously, had been working with animals. They had demonstrated in breeding experiments with many different kinds of animals that stressors, such as X-ray, pin-pricks or chemicals, applied to the embryo resulted in abnormalities. Now it was proved that the human embryo or fetus is also vulnerable to stress.

The information that German measles could cause congenital abnormalities proved to be news that traveled fast. Soon American doctors knew and were on the lookout for examples. And just about as soon, women knew and were frightened. It was sensational news, which was exploited to the fullest for their consumption. The possibility of a blind baby, a deaf baby, or one hopelessly deficient mentally haunted the woman who had even a mild rash during her pregnancy. Doctors were confronted with the problem of whether a pregnancy complicated by measles should be terminated immediately to prevent such a catastrophe.

But time tempers emotions and judgments, adds facts, and illuminates the truth for our guidance. Not every woman who has German measles, even during the first three months is going to have an abnormal baby. Recent reports from American clinics indicate that in not more than one in four cases, 25 per cent, is the baby abnormal, and these cases are usually limited to the type of measles occurring as an epidemic when the infecting organism is especially virulent.

The significance of this finding is not that German measles alone is the cause of any great number of abnormal babies. Of the total number born defective each year, only a few are due to that disease. The significance lies in the insight it has given us about how such abnormalities may be produced. The study has proved beyond doubt one cause for congenital abnormalities that has nothing to do with heredity or faulty germ plasm. Here is a concrete example of one destructive force, or stress, delivered to the unborn from the outside that interferes with nature's plan for normal development. If there is one such cause, it is logical to assume that there may be others, even of an entirely different nature from that of infection. Such things as chemicals (drugs administered to the mother), X-ray, irradiation, vitamin deficiencies, or hormone imbalances become possible sources of danger (stress) to the unborn. If we can identify these causes, we may be able to control or prevent their harmful action on the unborn. Thus cerebral palsy, mongolian idiocy, epilepsy, and other dreaded afflictions may be removed from the category of " acts of God " or tainted heritage and become accidents that can be prevented.

There is another significant fact that the study of German measles has emphasized—that most fetal abnormalities are induced during the first three months after conception. If we re-examine nature's timetable, we see that this is the period in which not only are organs and systems taking form but growth and differentiation are proceeding at a very rapid pace. It is therefore at this period of rapid change, before it has attained its form, that an organ or part of the body is most vulnerable. The one possible exception is the nervous system, particularly the brain. Because it is still very immature even at birth, it is the most vulnerable of all organs during the whole Age of the Unborn and during birth itself.

With this concept of fetal abnormalities, let us examine some specific examples that are familiar to all. Almost everyone has seen a child or adult with a hair lip or cleft palate. Perhaps you have read of a baby born with its heart outside its chest wall. To explain these, we must go back to the time that the embryo was an oval-shaped flat plate. The face is formed by the two edges being folded inward to be the cheeks and the top edge folded downward to be the nose. A failure of the cheek folds to grow together with that of the nose results in a cleft palate. The heart is a functional organ before the two edges come together to form the anterior chest wall, and failure of fusion in this region leaves the heart exposed.

So we see that fetal abnormalities occur not because nature's plans have been discarded and growth allowed to proceed along some freakish line; they are merely arrests at some particular stage of development. Nature got so far in her plans and could go no further. All fetal abnormalities are just this—arrest in development and failure of the part or organ to acquire the ability to function.

This brings us to the third reason the findings of the relationship of measles to abnormalities are important. It demonstrated that the type of abnormality depends on the time at which the particular circumstance happened to occur and its duration and severity in the Age of the Unborn, not on the actual nature of the stress. In other words, different kinds of harmful agents may produce the same kind of abnormality because they hit the unborn at precisely the same time, when specific organs are particularly vulnerable. These harmful agents have been called " stressors," " catastrophes," " insults," " accidents."

We have not as yet proved the identity of stressors in specific cases but we do know what circumstances are suspect. The first includes those things that, administered to the unborn, are harmful to it. Most of them can be delivered to the unborn by its only connection with the outside world, its own and its mother's blood streams. These include the toxic substances, which are part of infection in the mother or drugs administered to her. The one exception is X-ray or irradiation, which passes directly to the unborn. But stressors are not always positive harmful agents. They may also be a deficiency of some substance of which the unborn stands in vital need, such as hormones, vitamins, and nutrients. Most important of all as a stressor in the life of the unborn is deficiency of oxygen.

Even localized infectious diseases may harm the unborn by toxic products thrown into the blood stream of the mother, although the unborn does not acquire the disease. We know little about this at present. As in the case of measles, we do not know whether the embryo harbored the infection or was injured by its products.

Today, however, infections are not so great a potential danger to mothers or their unborn. Most of the serious infectious diseases such as typhoid, diphtheria, scarlet fever, and poliomyelitis are well prevented by vaccines, and others such as pneumonia are usually controlled by the antibiotics. Localized infections such as in teeth, tonsils, or appendix can be removed surgically.

The harmful effect of radiation on humans is a new and frightening possibility. Scientists have found in laboratory animals that radiation to either potential parent, before a pregnancy is established, can affect the germ plasm to the point of causing sterility or abnormal offspring. Radiation during pregnancy may cause abnormalities or death of the fetus (or embryo). The case for the human is not yet clear. We do know that excessive exposure to radiation may cause sterility, but we do not know just what lesser effect it has on succeeding generations. There is sufficient evidence that it may be harmful so that potential mothers should have as little exposure as possible.

There is one type of peculiar circumstance that happens to the mother during pregnancy that we can remove from the category of being a stressor. Her mental and emotional experiences, whatever their nature, cannot exert direct stress on her baby. Yet, strangely enough, women in the past have feared this most. They accepted the gross abnormalities as "acts of God" and therefore beyond their comprehension, right to question, or power to prevent. At the same time, they earnestly believed that by their own acts, thoughts, or experience they could mark the unborn.

Fear of marking the baby led to many superstitions and taboos. Birthmarks were attributed to some mental experience during pregnancy. A woman craved strawberries, so the baby was marked with a strawberry on its cheek. She was frightened by a dog, so the baby had a dark brown blemish shaped like a dog on its thigh. She must listen to good music if she wanted her child to be musical. She must never lose her temper, lest she bear a tyrant. A very casual look at the mother-baby relationship during pregnancy makes it quite obvious that marking is impossible. There are no nerves in the umbilical cord. Therefore, there is no possible means of transferring her nervous, mental, or emotional experiences to the child. She certainly will not mark her baby by unhappy thoughts or unfortunate experiences. Nor can she predestine a serene disposition by listening to soft music.

Birthmarks are abnormalities in the development of the skin. They consist of an overproduction, in one limited area, of normal elements of the skin. The red or purplish ones are made up of many tiny blood vessels. Others may have an excess of pigment, hair and the corny layer of the skin, giving them a brown wart-like appearance. Why they occur we do not know specifically. They represent a few cells that went wild and overproduced themselves for a very short interval at the time the skin was taking form.

ANOXIA

There are times when the unborn travels the whole journey, seemingly without mishaps, only to meet disaster at the very end. It is born dead or dies shortly after birth. Inability to survive birth or to assume an independent role is understandable when the baby is malformed. It is indeed a blessing, for life could never be more than mere existence for it and a sorrowful burden to all concerned. But when a baby, perfectly formed, does not survive, this is tragic for the parents, and they find it hard to understand or accept. Why does a seemingly normal baby die at birth?

Stillbirths, until just a few short years ago, were generally attributed to birth injury, particularly injury to the head, which caused hemorrhage into the brain. When such babies were carefully examined, in only a small percentage was such evidence found to account for death. In the majority of babies born dead, there was no apparent injury at all, and the cause of death was stated to be "congenital atelectasis, unknown etiology." This was just a technical way of saying that the lungs did not expand and the baby did not breathe for some unknown reason. There were some doctors who were not satisfied with this diagnosis. They wanted to know why the babies did not breathe. They realized that only by knowing the cause or causes of death could they hope to prevent death and save more babies. They began their search and have found the causes for a large percentage of stillbirths.

The answer was found by studying the case histories of a large number of babies who were unable to survive. This included those who were born dead (stillbirths) and those who died in the first month after birth (neonatal deaths). The doctors re-examined all the available facts pertaining to the mother's pregnancy, the duration and kind of labor she had, what medication she had received, and the presentation by which the baby was born. They examined the babies for any clues and hidden abnormalities. They found that most of the mothers had had normal pregnancies, and labor had been of all types, long and short, difficult and easy, normal and abnormal. Could there be just one cause of death of the infant that was applicable to all? The answer was "yes." The solution was found in the physiologic significance of birth—the necessity of a continuous and adequate supply of oxygen to the baby and the means by which this vital need is attained before, during, and after birth. The newborn lives because it learns to breathe. Or, it dies because of insufficient oxygen. In practically every case, something had happened that had cut down the baby's supply of oxygen. It died because of *anoxia*.

The unborn requires a relatively small amount of oxygen, as we have seen, but its margin of safety is small. The reduction of that needed amount, even by just a little or for a very short time, may be fatal. There are many ways this may come about, and therefore many possible causes of anoxia.

Anoxia may occur before or during birth if something happens to the baby's life line—the placenta and cord. It thus may be the result of the placenta being separated (breaking connection with the walls of the uterus) before the baby is born or of pressure on the cord. Even prolonged hard labor pains can cause anoxia by constricting the blood vessels of the uterus, whereby less blood goes to the placenta and thus less oxygen is available to the baby.

The baby may have had adequate oxygen up to and during birth but was unable to take on the responsibility of breathing. There are many possible reasons for this. You will recall that, early in the Age of the Unborn, certain centers of the brain assume control of all the automatic functions of the body except one, that of respiration. By some unknown force the respiratory center is held in check. It does not function until the very moment of birth. Then like a switch it is turned on, the current (of nerve impulses) flows, and the whole mechanism of breathing starts operation. Sometimes the switch doesn't work.

The switch, that is, the respiratory center, may fail if it is not quite finished. This is the situation in many premature infants. Or, the switch may be developed sufficiently but has been put out of commission and is unable to transmit the current. Certain drugs administered to the mother may so depress the respiratory center that it cannot function. Toxemia of the mother may also have this damaging effect on the unborn.

Another reason that may account for the baby's inability to start breathing is found in the lungs themselves. Cells of the tiny air sacs may be covered with a thin membrane, which makes it impossible for them to absorb oxygen from the air within the air sacs.

Thus, many other seemingly unrelated conditions are really basically anoxia. Even in babies who die because of the RH factor anoxia is the largest factor. Anoxia then is the killer of babies. It kills because the vital centers of the brain must have a constant and adequate supply of oxygen to sustain life. Deprived of this, they fail and death ensues. The study of anoxia has thus revealed the cause of stillbirths and neonatal deaths. But it has done much more than that. Mishaps and in many instances tragedies worse than death in terms of human suffering, which are hidden at birth, are also the result of anoxia. There may be instances in which anoxia is less severe and/or of shorter duration than that which deals the death blow, yet it may do irreparable harm to the vulnerable immature brain and its related sense organs. Such anoxia may thus be the cause of babies being born blind or deaf, or mentally deficient or with cerebral palsy.

The doctor can now tell parents why babies are born with imperfections and why normal babies die at birth. To a particular mother and father who have experienced this misfortune, he may not be able to point to the specific cause in their case, but what he can tell them will relieve them of their anxiety and fear as to their faulty heritage and give them hope for a normal baby. These facts are equally important and helpful to all prospective parents as a guide in achieving what they want most— a normal baby.

RULES FOR A SAFE JOURNEY

These facts have enabled doctors to formulate rules for the conduct of pregnancy for the safety of the baby. The rules, which include both what the mother must do and the doctor's responsibility, have already been outlined in the chapter on pregnancy. Their importance to the welfare of the unborn is emphasized by this knowledge of the causes of fetal abnormalities.

During pregnancy the doctor seeks to protect the unborn against stress, by supervising and guiding the mother; protecting her against infections with vaccines as indicated; detecting early and treating promptly the first signs of complications; avoiding exposure of the mother to excessive X-ray, and guiding the mother, not only telling her what she should do and what she should not do but encouraging her to know the physiology of pregnancy and labor.

When we read of the recent advances in obstetrics, how these are reducing the number of mothers and babies lost each year, and of this new concept of how abnormalities of the baby occur, we may get the impression that normal babies or abnormal babies are the result exclusively of what happened during the pregnancy—what the doctor did or did not do, what the mother did or did not experience. We must never lose sight of the fact that pregnancy is a natural process, and the Age of the Unborn is a normal part of life. The need for expert medical care is to prevent circumstances that will impede nature, to supply her with the necessary building materials, and to aid her when she has a faulty mechanism to operate. In other words, care is directed toward maintaining a normal environment for the unborn.

The most important factor contributing to the birth of a normal baby is not what the woman does or does not do during pregnancy, but what has been her physical background before she became pregnant. This goes back to the early years of adolescence and includes both her physical growth and development as preparation for pregnancy and the physical circumstances that may have impeded or distorted this preparation. It is the familiar story of good seed, good soil, a healthy plant. Most couples have this potential heritage to pass on. But however good the seed may be, it must have fertile soil and a favorable environment if it is to flourish.

A woman who has grown and matured normally, is in good health, has normal nutrition (and normal means the usual, not some unattainable degree of perfection), and spaces and limits the number of pregnancies, can with normal care expect to have a normal pregnancy and a normal baby.

XVI

BOY OR GIRL?

"DOCTOR, will our baby be a boy or girl? This is one question that a doctor is asked over and over again. How can you answer this?" Our professor of obstetrics was speaking to us as medical students many years ago. What he said was correct then, for he spoke from years of experience, and his way of answering the parents, facetious as it was, is as good as any we have today. This was his solution:

"Of course neither you nor I nor anyone else can tell a woman what the sex of her baby will be—and I'm not so sure it would be particularly desirable anyhow. But you must tell her something. You have one of three choices.

"You may tell her the simple truth—that you don't know. When you start out in practice that may prove a difficult admission for you to make, maybe it will always be so. But with a few years of experience it won't come so hard. At any rate it has the decided advantage that you won't ever have to retract your word.

"If you think that you have to tell her something, you can flip a coin and make a guess. You have a fifty-fifty chance of being right. The ratio of boys to girls is 106 to 100.

"Perhaps a better way is to counter—and ask her what she wants. This has a very definite advantage. If she answers 'girl' shake your head sadly and tell her that you think she will have a boy. On the other hand, if she wants a boy, you prepare her for the worst and predict that she will have to settle for a girl. In this way you will save your pride—if she hasn't changed her mind in the meantime, which is a chance you will have to take. When the baby arrives and your prediction proves to be correct, you can say that you are sorry but you told her so. If the baby is the desired sex, your wrong prediction will be forgotten in her joy and satisfaction of getting what she wanted. But it really doesn't make any difference. Right or wrong, two days of possession of her own newborn is enough to convince her that she got just what she really wanted."

Prediction of the sex of the unborn has always been an intriguing problem to prospective parents, and their ingenuity in finding a solution has been limited only by the extent of their imagination. Primitive people, living close to nature, sought their answer in the elements and came up with many solutions. Babies conceived in the full of the moon would reflect the majestic splendor of that august body and therefore would be males. A waning moon could do no better than produce a girl. When man moved indoors, the elements became less important, and early folklore transferred the responsibility to the parents themselves. If the mother most wanted the baby, it would be a girl, but if it was the father who was most eager for an offspring, it would be a boy. Or, if the father was masterful and the mother shy, they would have mostly sons. If the reverse were true, they could look forward to a house full of girls.

More recently, the answer was sought in signs that the mother could see or feel in her own body. So we still hear that if the mother "carries" the baby low it will be a boy. Or, the baby that starts moving early and kicks vigorously will be a boy. Or, if the doctor hears a faster, stronger heart beat it will be a boy. There is no truth in any of these assertions.

The question is just as lively today as it ever was, and the answer is being sought in some laboratory test that will accurately reveal the sex of the unborn. Perhaps you have read the exciting news: "Now you can know. Doctors can do a simple test and relieve you of the anxious months of not knowing whether your baby will be a boy or a girl." If so, don't take it too seriously. Scientists have investigated the hormone levels in the mother's body, her blood, her secretions of urine and saliva to see if there was any significant difference attributable to the sex of the unborn. Most of this research is directed toward the understanding of the physiology of the unborn and not as a means of predicting sex. The saliva test for sex determination, which received considerable publicity, was a by-product of the search for a simple and rapid test for pregnancy. Its accuracy is about 50 per cent—no more than a good guess. Another test, the examination of the cells of the amniotic fluid, has greater possibility of accuracy, but is one that few doctors would care to use because of its inherent dangers.

Is it really important, or even desirable, to be able to predict the sex of the unborn? Probably not. In most instances, such knowledge would not add to the parents' happiness and would deprive them of the pleasure of anticipation. It would be like opening that very special Christmas present in September and having to wrap it up and put it away until December.

Humans in their concern with the sex of the unborn have not limited their aspirations to mere ability to foretell the sex. They have hoped to find a way of attaining the sex desired. There have been many theories as to what determines the sex of the unborn based on the knowledge— more often superstitions and taboos—of the times. But there has always been only one scapegoat to bear the guilt for the failure when these theories did not produce the desired results. In a male-worshipping society from time immemorial woman has always been held responsible for the sex of her offspring. Often she had been cast aside because she did not produce male offspring. Even in modern times, newspapers have carried stories of royal potentates who divorced their wives because their children were all girls.

Going back in time, we find that women wore charms, drank magic potions, and made offerings on special altars of the gods to ensure the birth of a male baby. In other instances she sought to influence the sex of the unborn by the kind of food she ate. Thus to ensure the birth of a son, she relied on a strong diet of meat. If she wanted a daughter, she confined it to the mild sweet foods such as fruits and vegetables.

Even after some knowledge had been attained of the basic physiology of fertility and conception, woman was still held responsible. There was once a widespread belief, even among doctors, that boys developed from ova coming from the right ovary and girls from the left. Modern surgery has dispelled this. Many women have had one ovary removed and continue to have babies of both sexes. Another theory held that a child conceived in the early part of the menstrual cycle would be male while one late in the cycle would be female. This is, of course, false for a woman is fertile at only one time in the cycle.

More recently, since it has been recognized that the sperms carry the sex determiner, it has been said that woman's secretions determined which male cells would survive. If her vaginal fluids were acid, they would kill off the female-producing cells, and the result would be a male child. If her secretions were alkaline, the male cells could not survive, and a girl would be the result. This theory went so far as to advise certain kinds of douches to predetermine sex.

Nature, however, seems to have known best and put the power of decision out of reach of human meddling. She has devised a system that in the long run will result in about an equal number of each sex. It would be quite a different and unfortunate state of affairs if humans had their way. There have been many times in history when all babies would have been boys, and a few short intervals in which the opposite would have been true—either situation a quick way to exterminate the human race. Even today, when prospective parents have been polled, 70 per cent stated that they would like to have a boy.

HOW SEX IS DETERMINED

Sex is no secret that nature withholds during a part of the Age of the Unborn. Scientists will learn to predict sometime during pregnancy what birth will disclose, but nature determines what sex is to be at the moment of mating of the male and female germ cells. The first single cell formed by this union is destined not only to be a human being, but also to be a specific sex. Whether this destiny will be maleness or femaleness depends entirely on the contribution that the sperm cell, not the ovum, makes to the new individual.

The human body is made up of some 26 billion cells of thousands of different kinds, each living and contributing in its own way to the welfare of the whole. The difference in size, shape, and structure of the various kinds of body cells is due to difference in the cytoplasm, which is modified to enable each cell to perform its particular function. The nuclear material is the same in all.

The two kinds of germ cells afford an interesting example of this specialization of the cytoplasm. The ovum is one of the largest cells of the body due to the amount of cytoplasm, which will be its food supply for many days should it be fertilized. The sperm is the smallest cell, and its cytoplasm is specialized to form the long whiplike tail for locomotion. It is a mystery where it gets all the energy it must use in its quest for the ovum. These two germ cells also demonstrate the constancy of nuclear structure. Their nuclei are of the same size and appearance and have a comparable amount of vital nuclear material but an important difference in kind.

We live and grow because the cells of our body are constantly undergoing division. When a cell divides to form two new cells, each requires an equal share of nuclear material—equal as to amount and kind. To assure the equal division, the nuclear material is arranged in separate packages called chromosomes. The formation of chromosomes is an exact procedure, with a particular kind of nuclear material going to a particular place in each chromosome, and always results in the formation of a specific number of chromosomes in the species. Cells divide by chromosomes splitting down the middle, half of each chromosome going to each new cell. The result is that each new cell is just like the parent cell.

In the human body all cells in the process of dividing have 48 chromosomes regardless of whether they are liver cells, blood cells, or any other kind of cells. The ovum and the sperm before they "mature" also have 48 chromosomes. This poses a problem, for if they should fuse in this condition the new individual would have 96 chromosomes, and the next generation twice that number—a situation that is not allowed to happen. Each germ cell undergoes a maturing process that involves a different kind of division of chromosomes and results in reducing the number of chromosomes by half. In this division of maturation the chromosomes do not split but line up in pairs, and one chromosome of each pair goes to the new mature cell. Thus the mature ovum has 24 chromosomes, and the mature sperm a like number. When they mate, the new individual will have the normal number of 48 chromosomes. It is in this reduction of the number of chromosomes in the mature germ cells that we find the physical basis for the determination of sex.

In the germ cells, 46 of the chromosomes are somatic, that is, they are concerned with transmitting characteristics of general body structure, and are alike in the ovum and the sperm. The two remaining chromosomes are concerned with sex. There are two kinds of sex chromosomes, a large one called the X-chromosome and a small one called the Y-chromosome. In the ovum before maturation and in all the cells of the female body, the two sex chromosomes are always alike and always X-chromosomes. The sperm cell, before it matures, and all the cells of the male body have one X-chromosome and one Y-chromosome.

When the ovum is maturing, the two X-chromosomes pair, and in the divisions that follow one chromosome goes to each new cell. Thus a mature ovum will always contain an X-chromosome. When the sperm cell matures, it may contain either an X-chromosome or a Y-chromosome. This production of fertile germ cells is going on daily by the millions in the adult male. Thus in the aggregate of mature sperm (the semen) approximately one-half bear X-chromosomes and the other half Y-chromosomes.

If by chance, and as far as we know it is only by chance, the sperm with the X-chromosome fertilizes the ovum, the new cell will have two X-chromosomes, and a female is thus determined. If the sperm contained a Y-chromosome, the new cell will have an X-Y combination, and the new individual is destined to be a male.

Chromosomes are transient bodies in the life of the cell. They are merely packages of nuclear material made up at the time the cell is dividing for the purpose of facilitating the process of division and assuring an equal division. It is the material within the chromosome that is really significant. These particles of nuclear material contained within the chromosomes are called "genes." Once the division is complete, the chromosome form disappears. The package is open, and the genes are released to go to work.

Genes have been called the "architects," the "master-planners," or the "master-workers." They carry the hereditary plans of the body from one generation to the next. They are the "forces of nature," which control the direction and speed of cell growth and differentiation and by which the fertilized ovum is transformed into a living baby within the specified time.

Genes are physical realities, not simply a hypothetical force. They are protein molecules about 5/1,000,000 of an inch in diameter. There are about 30,000 genes in a fertilized ovum or 15,000 in each mature ovum and sperm cell. They are chemical catalysts, that is, they will direct chemical changes but will not themselves be changed. They are copied over and over again as the cells multiply, each new cell containing an exact replica of the genes of its predecessor, and every cell of the body will have a complete set of genes.

Genes are not autonomous forces. They work together and are dependent on each other as they proceed to carry out the master plan. Also, the kind of work they do, the part of the structure they will build, is dependent on the material supplied them by the cytoplasm. Thus the thousands of genes form a huge symphony in which each is producing growth and maturation of cells in its own peculiar way while conforming in harmony and sequence to the general theme—the maturation of the body.

PATTERNS FOR SEX DEVELOPMENT

When sex is involved, almost any story is considered interesting enough to merit headlines. So we frequently find newspapers and magazines carrying the story of an individual who has lived as a male even to adult life when something reveals the fact that "he" is not male at all, and suddenly "he" becomes "she." One such case aroused general interest and speculation several years ago when a young man went to a foreign clinic for a mysterious operation and returned in all the glory of feminine trappings—hair-do, lipstick, fur coat, and high heels. What did it mean? Was it some hoax or could doctors really change the sex of a person? To find the answers, we must go back to the very beginning of life.

Nature does a peculiar thing as she first lays out her pattern for the development of the unborn's sexual organs. It would seem that she is at first not quite sure which sex it will be. During the first six weeks in the life of the unborn, the internal sex organs are developing but not even by the most careful and minute examination can the sex be discovered. This is not because they have not yet developed sufficiently to be recognizable as either male or female. Rather, it is because nature first lays out the pattern for both male and female organs. After six weeks she begins to divulge whether she plans a boy or a girl and starts her molding and sculpturing accordingly. That is, the inherent forces within the embryo—the genes of the sex chromosomes, perhaps abetted by hormones—become sufficiently active to direct further development according to the pattern for one sex.

Nature's first pattern is quite simple and can be effectively represented by two small round beads placed on a surface a short distance apart and four equal lengths of soft cord extending straight backward from the line between them—a pair for each bead. The beads represent the gonads (which may be either ovaries or testes). The two outer cords represent the male reproductive system and the two inner cords the female.

How does nature transform this simple pattern into the finished product of ovaries, tubes, uterus, and vagina with the distinctive characteristics they possess in the Age of Maturity? This is not so hard to understand if we reduce the finished structure to its basic pattern. It is a T-shaped tubular structure, the top or horizontal bar formed by the two oviducts, which join in the midline to form the vertical uterus. It has rounded walls of varying thickness and a lumen that is open and continuous throughout. Situated at each end of the horizontal bar, but unconnected, are the ovaries. The vagina is a soft thin-walled pouch that connects the system to the exterior of the body. Nature molds this finished product from her basic pattern quite readily by bending, moving, and shaping the tubes as she adds to them.

In an embryo of six weeks there is a little cluster of cells on each side of the midline (which will become the backbone) about one-third of the way back from the head end. These are the precursors of the gonads. Extending backward are the two sets of "cords," the male tubes and the female tubes. By the eighth week we begin to get a glimmer of what the sex is to be. If the unborn is female, the gonads begin to contain cells that we can identify as ovarian, and one pair of tubes is larger than the other. These changes become more characteristically feminine as the weeks go by.

As the fetus grows, the female tubes change not only in size but in shape and position. The portions toward the lower part of the body move over closer together. A little later they touch and finally grow together to form one tube. This fusion of the lower portion of the tubes becomes the uterus. The two upper ends not only remain separate, but as the fetus grows, they bend away from each other and thus reach their horizontal position. These are the Fallopian tubes. Muscle develops around each of the parts, a small amount in the tubes, and a much greater amount around the uterus.

The vagina is not derived from these tubes but from the ectoderm. It starts as a solid cord of cells growing inward to meet the lower end of the tubes. The solid cord of cells opens up to form a tube, but some cells remain at the opening to form a membrane, which is the hymen. From this we can understand the variations in the structure of the hymen. If there is almost a complete opening of the cord, the hymen will be only a crescent fold. Occasionally, it does not open at all but remains as a completely occlusive membrane.

During this period of growth and differentiation of the female system, the male ducts are completely outdistanced. They do not grow or differentiate at all. But neither do they disappear entirely. Vestiges of them remain alongside the tubes and uterus into adult life.

While the ducts are undergoing these changes, the gonads also have developed so that they are easily identified as ovaries by the appearance of the typical ovarian follicles. But even the ovary is not completely and exclusively female. Embedded deep in the ovaries are little clusters of cells that have the appearance of male sex cells. Here they remain through adult life, quiescent and of no significance. But occasionally these clusters of cells increase in size to form a tumor. Then they show their true character by secreting the male sex hormone, which may have some masculinizing effect on the woman's body.

How does it happen that the external genitalia does not proclaim the sex in the early embryo? Nature has a different method here from the one she used for the internal organs. She doesn't lay out two systems. Rather she has one simple pattern that she molds in one direction, either maleness or femaleness. The primitive pattern appears when the fetus is five to six weeks old and consists of a little rounded knob called the genital tubercle, with gently curved mounds of tissue extending back from each side, called the genital folds. Behind the tubercle and between the folds are the openings of both the urinary system and the genital ducts.

In the female there is little change in this plan, only growth and development. The tubercle remains small and becomes the clitoris. And the folds become the lips or labia between which are the openings of the urethra and vagina. In the male, considerable modification has to take place. The tubercle grows, and as it does, it enfolds the urinary opening and the two male ducts (which do not fuse as in the female) and becomes the penis. The genital folds become sacs, which come together and fuse behind the penis to form the scrotum. The male gonads (testes) move downward carrying their tubes with them, just as in the female but to a much greater extent, for the testes pass through the abdominal wall and descend into the scrotum. Thus, the male and female external genitalia start off looking very much alike. The female doesn't change much from that of the basic fetal pattern, but the male does. If for some reason the fetal male organs do not go through this change, they would continue to have the appearance of female organs.

SEX ORGANS OF THE NEWBORN

By the third month the female reproductive system is formed in miniature. Thereafter it has only to grow during the remainder of the Age of the Unborn. It will not be called upon to mature until some ten to twelve years later. So it is that the reproductive organs at birth are immature and quite different from what they will be in the Age of Maturity.

The ovaries show the most remarkable difference. It would seem that nature is greatly concerned about providing adequate germ cells to assure a next generation. She provides a seemingly overabundance of them. The ovary at maturity contains many follicles, each with its germ cell or ovum, in all stages of growth and maturity. At birth the follicles are all primitive or immature, but there are many of them, more in fact than there will ever be again. The number has been estimated to be 100,000 to 400,000. Whether these primitive immature follicles present at birth represent the total number that the ovary will ever have or produce is a question. Scientists used to believe they did, but there is now considerable evidence that after puberty new follicles continue to be formed. The number of follicles progressively decreases through life. At puberty there are 15,000 to 35,000 follicles in the two ovaries. Only 300 to 400 of these will attain full maturity during the whole life of the woman, one at a time with each menstrual period.

The uterus at birth is larger in proportion to the rest of the body than it will be again until many years later when at puberty it begins to develop its mature characteristics. Immediately after birth the uterus shrinks about one-third in size. The reason for this change is that it was stimulated to increased size by the estrogenic hormones that are produced in such abundance by the placenta during pregnancy. After the hormone supply is cut off at birth, it cannot maintain this growth. Even at this early age it has learned to act like a uterus, so much so that the endometrium sometimes goes through enough change to produce a slight amount of bleeding when estrogen is withdrawn.

ENDOCRINE GLANDS AND THE SEX OF THE UNBORN

Do the endocrine glands play any role in the Age of the Unborn? Do they contribute to the differentiation of sex? We do not know the complete answer to these questions. We do know that the sex of the individual is determined at conception by genetic factors. We also know that the maturation of sexual characters at puberty is an endocrine function. But what the factor is in the embryonic stage, when both male and female reproductive systems are present, that guides and directs the differentiation of the female reproductive system and suppresses the male is a question we cannot answer. It is the type of action that we might expect hormones to perform, and there are some suggestive findings. There has been considerable research in this field using many kinds of animals, but as the reproductive systems of animals are so different in many ways from that of the human, it is difficult to apply the findings to the human.

The pituitary gland is the first to appear and probably starts to function before birth. There are several facts that suggest that the adrenal glands play some part in the differentiation of sex. The adrenal cortex in the Age of Maturity besides producing its own specific hormones also produces both the male and female sex hormones. In the Age of the Unborn we do not know when the adrenals become functional, that is, when they start producing hormones, or how much of each kind is secreted. But we do know that the adrenals appear early in embryonic life and grow and develop rapidly. They are actually much larger during the later part of the Age of the Unborn and at birth than they are in infancy and childhood. They shrink quite rapidly immediately after birth. This suggests that they are of considerable importance to the welfare of the unborn. Another suggestive fact is that when the adrenals remain large after birth, the infant frequently has some type of structural abnormality of its sex organs.

We cannot assume that the ovaries have anything at all to do with sex differentiation in the unborn. They still have eight to ten years to go before they start contributing in any significant way to female hormonology. There is no evidence that during the Age of the Unborn they produce any hormones.

What significance does sex in the unborn have to woman in her Age of Maturity? She was born to be a woman, she may think, so why should she try to understand this involved and complicated mechanism that nature has contrived and executes usually quite accurately long before the baby girl sees the light of day? There are two reasons besides the satisfaction that comes with knowledge. This knowledge of the origin of the basis of her female personality reveals the fact that bi-sexuality is a fundamental part of her make-up. And second, it explains how physical abnormalities of the sex organs come about. They are not something mysterious, some prank of fate, but are readily explained as failures in normal development.

BISEXUALITY

"Just like a woman!" Be a man!" How often one hears these expressions, implying that "femaleness" and "maleness" are two absolute and distinct sets of human traits that have little or nothing in common. In reality, the terms are only relative. So much of what we consider to be purely feminine and purely masculine traits are matters of culture and are not due to innate interests and skills of each sex. These traits of maturity on the mental and emotional level are of course modified by the sex of the individual, and there are numerous gradations and mixtures between what we think of as essentially masculine and purely feminine—a bisexuality—in both sexes.

We are familiar with the petite, apparently ultrafeminine woman and her opposite, the large muscular heavy-boned woman, who may appear quite masculine. When it comes to the true test of femininity, which is fertility, many of the ultrafeminine-appearing women are unable to conceive, and some of the large masculine women have children quite readily. The same is true for men. It is not always the virile athlete who has the highest degree of fertility. He is frequently outdistanced by one of mild manners and small physique.

Perhaps the most obvious example of a woman's physical bisexuality is the amount of hair on her body. Some women have very little that is apparent except in the areas normal to her sex, that is, under the arms and in the pubic region. Others have a heavy growth on the arms and legs, some on the chest and around the nipples of the breast, and some have hair on the chin and above the lips. All of these are normal points of male distribution. Yet she is no less feminine for these. All women have the potentiality of this male distribution of hair, and if they are given enough of the male sex hormone, it becomes a reality, much to their horror.

There is bisexuality on the chemical level. The male sex hormone is a normal component of woman's body tissues and fluids just as are her own sex hormones. A normal balance, which nature maintains, keeps her "normally feminine." Should this balance be upset, the feminine body traits will suffer.

These factors of bisexuality thus explain the physical variations in femininity. They need not intrude on her life as a mature woman. She lives with her bisexuality without ever being conscious of its existence. It is only when something goes wrong that it is brought to her attention. There is a time when the significance of these facts of sex differentiation have a tremendous impact on a woman's life. That is when nature fails somewhere in the execution of her plans and congenital abnormalities result.

FAILURES

Everyone is familiar with the fact that congenital heart abnormalities and external defects of the body occur and that they are now being corrected by surgery. Few know that congenital defects in the female reproductive system occur, although they are just as common. These defects are brought about in the same manner as other mishaps that we have already discussed. They usually represent a cessation of growth and differentiation at some stage in prenatal life. They differ from other mishaps in two important ways. They are usually not apparent at birth but remain concealed until puberty or even years later when the woman is studied for the problem of sterility or some other functional condition. They do not affect her physical health or even her longevity. They may have a terrific impact on her feminine personality and her ability to function as a mature woman. We need not go into all the details of possible defects, but a few actual cases will demonstrate their significance.

Julia, age forty-six, was short in stature and somewhat overweight. Although she did not have a nice figure, she had feminine curves, fairly well-developed breasts, and the adult female distribution of hair. Even though she had never menstruated in her life, she was complaining of all the symptoms of the menopause as well as many other bizarre symptoms. It was soon apparent that she was an unhappy misfit, considering herself different. She had been unable to get along with others, women or men.

She was so persistent in her complaint of a pain in her right side that an operation for possible appendicitis was performed. The surgeon explored the pelvis also and found that the female reproductive organs were practically nonexistent. Where the ovaries should have been were only small masses of fibrous tissue. The tubes and uterus were represented by long thin bands of undeveloped tissue. These findings signified that the internal sex organs had stopped developing in the first month of prenatal life. Why, then, did she have some of the external features of an adult female, such as breast development, hair distribution, and feminine curves? The answer lies in the ability of the adrenal glands to produce enough estrogen to induce these changes. Her failure to make a happy adjustment in life was due in part to the life-long deficiency of female hormones and to her inability to cope with the fact that she was physically different from other women.

Mary Ellen demonstrates that social maladjustments do not always accompany such physical abnormalities. She was a petite and very feminine girl of nineteen. She too had never menstruated. When Mary Ellen was sixteen she had been taken to a doctor because she had not yet started to menstruate and had been assured that development was only delayed and that "everything would be all right." With this reassurance she participated in schoolgirl activities. When she became engaged, she came for premarital consultation. She was examined, and it was found that while her external sex characteristics were well developed, she had very little development of her internal organs. Her uterus (palpated through the rectum) seemed to be smaller than a little finger. She had only a slight depression where the vagina should have been. This abnormality represented cessation of development at a slightly later time in prenatal life than was the case in Julia.

This physical abnormality presented quite a serious problem as to whether or not she should be married. It was fully explained to all concerned that she could never have children, but the suggestion was offered that it was not too difficult for a plastic surgeon to create a vagina. This was done successfully, and sometime later she was married. Several years later she reported that she enjoyed a satisfactory marital relationship and a happy family life with two adopted children.

Elaine sought medical help because she had been married six years and had not been able to conceive. Her menstrual history was normal, and she had the appearance of being a normal healthy woman. Pelvic examination revealed that she had a double uterus, and this finding was confirmed by appropriate X-ray studies. This meant that during prenatal life, the two primitive cords had not fused as is normal, but had developed independently. There are many variations in this type of abnormality in size and shape of the uterus. They do not always result in sterility.

These are all examples of failure of the female reproductive organs to grow and develop. The differences among them are the result of the time at which differentiation came to a standstill. Nature had got safely past her period of indecision, of bisexuality, and had started molding according to the female pattern. Something stopped her before she was finished. But by this time the pattern for male organs had just about disappeared.

There are still other sexual abnormalities that occur when nature fails to make a decision in favor of one or the other sex patterns but works on the development of both. The result is that such individuals have reproductive organs of both sexes, neither of which is ever completely developed. These are the hermaphrodites.

The name "hermaphrodite" expresses the union of Hermes (the mythical messenger of the gods) with Aphrodite (the goddess of love). It implies that both sexes are complete in one individual who could therefore function as either male or female in the process of reproduction. Hermaphroditism is the normal state of affairs in some of the lower forms of animal life. When it occurs in humans, it never completely conforms to the meaning implied in the name.

Hermaphrodites are really medical curiosities and have no particular significance to normal women. But because they are rare and freakish, such an unhappy individual when discovered becomes newsworthy. To satisfy the curiosity aroused as to the anatomy of these unfortunate freaks of nature, we will briefly outline what is meant by human hermaphroditism.

In the first place, no human is ever a complete hermaphrodite, able to function as either male or female. They are all sterile. As a matter of fact, there have been only a small number of cases reported in all medical literature of an individual having both ovaries and testes and some semblance of the internal reproductive organs of both sexes.

The vast majority of cases are what doctors call pseudohermaphrodites, and there are not many of these. These individuals have only some of the sex characteristics that are male and some that are female. It may be quite difficult to determine their true sex, for one must decide which character to use as the definitive one for maleness or femaleness. Is it the type of gonad, ovary or testes? How well are the internal reproductive organs developed? What is the appearance of the external genitalia? What does the person consider his or her sex to be? Physicians use the character of the gonads, whether they are ovaries or testes, as the basis of their scientific diagnosis. However, they use all of the criteria in deciding what, if anything, should be done about the condition.

There are, in general, two types of individuals of mixed sex. The male pseudohermaphrodite has male gonads and what may appear to be female external genitalia. The female pseudohermaphrodite is one whose gonads are ovaries but whose external genitalia have the appearance of the male.

The mechanism by which the male pseudohermaphrodite is produced is not hard to understand. The primitive (fetal) external genitalia are alike in both sexes. If in the male they were not stimulated to grow and develop, they would continue to look like the female, which is what happens. In the case of the female pseudohermaphrodite, the situation is different. Something has to be added to make the primitive organs develop along male lines. The something which is in excess of normal is the male sex hormone. It may be produced in excessive amounts before birth by the adrenal glands or anytime later in life by tumors capable of producing the male sex hormones, such as the adrenal or testicular cells in the ovary. In other words, male pseudohermaphroditism is really failure of mature sex characters to differentiate. Female pseudohermaphroditism is partial sex-reversal in which female characters are suppressed and male overdeveloped.

What is the fate of these victims of nature's failure or misbehavior whose sex characters are mixed? What can be done to give them some chance of being one sex or the other? The answer depends on many factors, but especially the time at which the situation is discovered.

Occasionally, the condition is recognized at birth or in early childhood. Then doctors may undertake such forms of therapy, usually surgical, followed by hormone therapy, which have some promise of giving the individual the status of one sex or the other, the choice depending on what the physiological findings are. There is little hope of rendering them normal.

The sexual abnormality, far more frequently, is not recognized until puberty or adult life, when the problem is more difficult of solution. "Boys" may have been reared as "girls" or vice versa. Then the doctor must respect the individual's self-identification of sex.

A woman we might call Pauline is illustrative of the problem. She was 24 when she sought medical advice because she had never menstruated. "She" was of normal height, but had few of the feminine curves to her body and little breast development. There was, however, adult distribution of hair on her body. The external genitalia were poorly developed and defined. That is, the labia were small, the clitoris enlarged, and the vagina represented only by a dimple. Further examination revealed that "she" had no internal female organs, and it was suspected that her gonads were testes rather than ovaries. "She" was therefore a vastly underdeveloped male but considered herself to be female and wanted to remain so. Hence the gonads, which proved to be testes on operation, were removed to prevent any further masculinization. Estrogen was given to stimulate whatever female characters would prove to be responsive. No further surgical procedure was carried out in this case. But sometimes doctors will go further removing the clitoris and constructing a vagina in the effort to make some sort of sex life possible. Such modifications can be done only when the sex chosen is female.

Many of the cases in which the individual takes it upon "himself" or "herself" to assume the role of the opposite sex are not cases of hermaphroditism of any type in the physical sense. They are psychological abnormalities in which the individual is physically one sex but wants to be of the opposite sex. To this end they assume the dress and all the external characteristics of the chosen sex. The appropriate name for such cases is transvestitism.

Looking back over this origin and differentiation of sex, we see that nature has a plan, which as a rule she is able to execute effectively. Baby girls are born with the inherent ability to mature to normal womanhood physically. In only a few cases does nature fail to do her job well, and congenital abnormalities result. Very rarely does she produce a freak. All these we can understand with the knowledge of the genetic basis of sex, the bisexuality of the embryo, and differentiation of sex in the unborn, probably guided if not completely controlled by sex hormones.

Nature sometimes outdoes herself and produces an individual superabundantly endowed with all the physical attributes of feminine charm and beauty. Who can say how she did it? Was it by a fortuitous combination of genes of such compatibility and strength of directive powers that she achieved near perfection? Was it the perfect hormonal environment in the Age of the Unborn? Or, was it by perfection of the molding of infancy and childhood? Whatever factors or group of factors she used to produce her masterpiece, it really does not matter so long as she continues to furnish us with this source of pleasure and wonder—the beautiful mature woman. We can only hope that such a woman will also find happiness with her rich physical endowments by attaining equal maturity on the other, and to her more vital, aspects of her feminine personality.

THE AGE OF INFANCY AND CHILDHOOD

XVII

PATTERNS OF DEVELOPMENT

SOME YEARS AGO I went to a carnival. A few days previously the resident
physician of one of our hospitals had called and said they had a baby in
the ward that he thought I would be interested in seeing, the child of
the Bearded Lady and the Alligator Man of the carnival then showing in
town. Of course, I was interested. The baby was about normal in size
and physical development. The most startling thing about it was an
excessive amount of hair. The head was covered with heavy long hair,
which extended low down almost to the eyebrows on a markedly receding
forehead and in front of the ears to the cheeks to make heavy sideburns.
The eyebrows were bushy, thick, and long. The baby also had thick
long hair on the outer surfaces of its arms and legs and good sized patches
on its back and chest. Truly it looked like a little fur-bearing animal.

I was curious to see what its parents were like, so I went to the carnival.
Among the side shows I found the Bearded Lady. She was a normally
developed female, of average height and the usual feminine curves, but
she had as much of a beard as a man who had not shaved for months
and more hair on her arms, thighs, and chest than many men. She and
her baby were not glandular problems. The fact that she was able to
have a child indicated normal sex-glandular function. Nor was the Alligator Man an example of glandular disturbance. He was the victim of
a disease that leads to a peculiar thickening and scaliness of the skin.

I wandered down the midway to see what else the show had to offer.
There were giants, midgets, and dwarfs, and the inevitable fat lady. What
a diabolical joke nature had played on these poor creatures that they
should grow to be monstrosities, misfits in society, and able to earn a

living only by submitting themselves to the wondering and sometime pitying gaze of the crowd.

My attention was then drawn to a pair of onlookers—a handsome young woman and a vivacious little girl of about six whom I took to be he daughter. They presented a perfect contrast of the beauty of the normal which we are so likely to take for granted, to the unattractiveness of the abnormal, which we inconsiderately label as queer and unrelated to our selves. They also brought into clear focus the wonder of growth and development of the human body.

The little girl was exquisite, feminine to the tips of her fingers just as her mother was. But she was not a miniature of her mother because the proportions of her body were entirely different. Her head, with its covering of lustrous curls, was almost as large as her mother's; but her face with its delicate undeveloped features was small, and her sparkling eyes, eagerly searching new wonders, seemed to be in the middle of her face. He arms and legs were shorter in proportion to her body size, her shoulders were narrower, her hips flat, and her abdomen rounded out in front like a Kewpie doll. By nature's guidance, she would one day achieve the graceful proportions of her mother. I marveled that this transformation of the body from normal child to normal woman is the usual, expected sequence of events and that slip-ups and failures, which produce the freaks of the side shows, are so rare.

How does nature bring about this transformation? What patterns o plans does she follow? You might say, "that's simple, we just grow." But growth means merely increase in size, and if we "just grew," the adult would be the same proportions as the baby, and that would be a monstrosity indeed. We would have a head larger than a pumpkin and a rounded body at least twice as large as that of the normal adult, and we would toddle along on short bow legs, with short arms flapping ineffectually to help maintain a precarious balance.

You say, "Well, we mature." But that also is not the answer, for the process of maturing means change in structure so that each particular part or organ of the body can perform its function adequately and efficiently. So maturity would bring no great increase in size, but merely change in proportions. "But," you say, "this is just a play on words." It is not, because "growing" and "maturing" are two distinct processes and nature uses them according to a definite master plan to bring about the transformation. She has " patterns of growth " and " patterns of maturation " for each part of the body, as well as for the body as a whole, and for the mind and personality. Thus, the mature woman achieves her peak of development on the physical, the sexual, the mental, and the emotional levels by these two processes of growth and maturation.

RHYTHM OF GROWTH AND MATURATION

Nature uses these patterns of development with great dexterity, in rhythm, first one and then the other. Sometimes the tempo is slow, sometimes fast, but always in complete harmony.

The pattern of growth for the body as a whole has many phases. There are times when growth is rapid, others when it is slow. There are also patterns of growth for each part of the body, for growth is not of the same uniform intensity in all parts of the body at all times. There are times at which certain parts of the body are growing faster than others. A familiar example is the pre-teen age when the extremities are growing faster than the trunk, and the girl seems to be all arms and legs.

There are also patterns of maturation. Each organ or system of the body matures at the time the body needs that part to mature for the efficient function of the whole. For instance, the heart is the first organ to attain maturity of function. This is because the first need of the body is for food and oxygen. Thus we find a tiny heart pumping away early in the Age of the Unborn when the baby is little more than a mass of undifferentiated cells. It continues its growth and maturation through the prenatal age so that after birth it has achieved adult form and function. It increases in size thereafter, as the body grows, but there is never any change in the way it functions.

The digestive tract, on the other hand, is not needed during the first age, but it is growing and maturing to be ready when called upon. When the food supply from the mother is cut off at birth, the infant's stomach and intestines must be ready to assume the task of supplying the body with nourishment in a form that can be used. That is, food must be eaten and digested. It takes a little time for the digestive tract to get started and to learn to do its work effectively. So we find that the new born baby loses weight for a few days until digestion becomes more efficient. Then the baby starts to gain weight. At first she can digest only the simplest foods, but as the months go by the digestive tract matures in function, and gradually the infant is able to take care of any kind of food.

The muscles also follow a pattern of maturation. At birth, they are immature, weak, and uncontrolled. The baby is a completely helpless individual partly because of the immaturity of its muscles. There is a definite sequence in which the muscles mature and begin to function with purpose and efficiency. The baby learns first to control the movement of its eyes, then to hold its head erect, to sit, to crawl, and then to stand alone and walk.

The baby born before the usual nine months is called a premature baby and rightly so, because its organs are not mature enough to carry on the functions necessary for life. It may look like a baby of nine months, but its heart is not strong, it does not breathe deeply and regularly, and it cannot adjust readily to changes in temperature or resist infection, so its life is precarious. It must have special care until maturity of these functions is attained, and then it can grow and develop just as any other normal baby can.

Thus nature works out her master plan of transformation. The vital forces of growth and maturation she uses in her own way, and there is little we can do to change her patterns. We can only provide her proper building material and shield her work from harmful forces such as infection and injury. For the internal function of the body, which must be continuous and co-ordinated, she provides an automatic system of controls, the autonomic nervous system and the endocrine glands. But early in life she begins to place on the individual the responsibility of learning to use and control the actions of the body as a whole. Learning and maturing go hand in hand, each dependent on the other. This is true whether applied to the use of muscles or the acquisition of knowledge. A child left alone will assume an upright position and walk, but can profit by training in posture and gait.

The changing rhythm of growth and maturation results in definite stages of development: The newborn period, extending through the first

w weeks after birth, is the time required for the baby to adjust to a new
ode of life. Abruptly removed from a life of complete protection where
very need is met without any exertion on its part, it must take on the
sponsibility of independent existence. Babyhood, the first two years of
fe, is the time required for the gradual development in control of the
ody. Complete helplessness gives way to physical independence. The
aby learns to walk, feed itself, talk, and make its wants known.

In childhood growth proceeds at a slow, steady pace. More perfect con-
ol of the body is attained, and the child revels in full and sometimes
oisterous exercise. Adolescence is the final period of body growth and
aturation and the one most intense and rapid change. But another
ctor makes its appearance, the maturation of sexuality. Heretofore, the
attern is the same for both sexes—that of a baby growing and maturing
ward adulthood. Now it changes. It becomes that of a girl maturing
womanhood. This period of growth and maturation, so eventful and
nportant, will have a designation and consideration as a separate age.

ATTERNS OF GROWTH

" Is my child normal? " What does a mother mean, what information
r reassurance does she seek when she asks this question? It varies with
he age of the child. When a mother asks this question about her new-
orn baby, she means, " Does it have its five fingers, and toes, a rosebud
outh and all the other attributes of a healthy well-formed new baby? " But
vhen the child is two or three or six or ten, she is really asking, " is my
hild growing and developing normally? " Perhaps she has tried to find
he answer herself by comparing the height, weight, and other measure-
ents of her child to tables of " ideal height " and " ideal weight," and
as become quite alarmed to find that her child does not conform to
he " average." Does that mean that her child is " abnormal "? Not at all.
There is really no such thing as an " average child " any more than there
s an " average woman."

Children have different rates of growth. Some proceed at a very rapid
ace, others take growth more leisurely. If we look over the children in a
indergarten, we find a few quite tall for their age, a few quite small, and

the majority ranging between the two extremes. All are normal children The parents of the large child have no reason to congratulate themselve on having a healthier child. Neither should the parents of the small chil be concerned that their child is retarded. A child derives no health ac vantage from being the largest in her group, and the small child is not at disadvantage.

Pediatricians long ago recognized the fallacy of the " average child " an sought other methods by which the growth process could be measured They found that by keeping individual records of each child's measure ments taken at regular intervals over a period of years, a pattern of growtl emerges. The rate and intensity of growth may vary from child to child but the general pattern is the same for all. In infancy and early childhood growth is rapid. The baby doubles its weight the first three months o life and triples it in six. Growth is slow and fairly steady during child hood until shortly before puberty. Then there is a marked speeding up of growth, which reaches its maximum at about the time of the firs menstruation. Thereafter the rate of growth slows down and ceases en tirely in a few years. This then is the normal pattern of growth—a perioc of rapid growth, then one of slow growth, and again a period of rapi growth, always in this sequence. The reason children vary is because these periods do not occur at a specific age, and the intensity and duration of the accelerated growth are quite variable.

HOW GROWTH IS ACCOMPLISHED

Growth, that is, increase in size of the body, depends primarily on the increase in size of the bony skeleton. It is easy to understand how sof tissue such as the skin and muscle can increase in size just by multiplying the number of the same kind of cells. But how can a structure such as bone, which is rigid and has a definite shape, increase in size and yet maintain its shape? We know that a drumstick of a chicken looks like a drumstick, although it varies in size, whether it comes from a tender young broiler or a tough old hen. The same is true of all the bones of the human body. How does a bone grow?

To begin with, nature lays out a model for the skeleton very early in the first age. This is not of hard bone but of soft tissue, which can grow as long as it needs to and then can be transformed into bone. This model may be made of a mass of gristle (cartilage), which is the forerunner of the long bones, such as those of the arms and legs. Or it may be a sheet of fibrous material (membrane), which will be transformed into flat bones, such as those of the top of the head. As the individual grows, these fore-runners of bone are transformed into true bone by a process called ossification. The most important part of ossification is the deposition of calcium, which makes the structure rigid and hard.

Some bones become ossified very early. The collar bone (clavicle) has calcium in it by the third week of embryonic life. Other bones do not become completely ossified until the individual is at least twenty years old. This delay in ossification is the way nature provides for increase in size of the bones, particularly those of the legs and arms. When a bone is completely ossified, growth is no longer possible or possible only to a very limited extent.

Ossification starts at one point or center and spreads out through the model. All bones have at least one center of ossification, and most bones have more than one. For instance, the bone of the thigh has a center for the shaft of the bone and centers for each of the ends. The place where the shaft and the end are joined together is called the epiphyseal line. When this line becomes ossified or closed, the bone cannot grow any longer and the person cannot become any taller.

Each center of ossification occurs at a definite time in the growth pattern of the individual. Of the more than eight hundred such centers in the body, half have developed by the time of birth. Also, the time that each bone will become ossified and each epiphyseal line closed has a specific place in the growth pattern.

This information has a practical value. By X-ray we can see whether certain centers of ossification have appeared or certain epiphyseal lines have closed, and this will tell us how far the processes of growth and maturation of the skeleton have advanced. Frequently, such information is very important to the girl and her parents, as it was in the cases of Mercedes and Kitty.

Mercedes was twenty years old. She was less than five feet tall and very anxious to add a few inches to her height. " Can't you give me some growth hormones or vitamins that will make me grow just a little bit more,' she asked? X-ray pictures of her wrists and knees showed that her epiphyses were closed, so she had to be told that there was no hope for further change in her height.

Kitty, on the other hand, was only twelve years old but was already five feet six inches tall. Her mother was concerned that Kitty would be a giantess by the time she was twenty. X-ray of her joints showed that her epiphyses too were closed, indicating that she had already achieved almost full maturity and growth of her skeleton. We could therefore reassure the mother that Kitty had just about attained her full growth and would certainly be of normal height at maturity.

So far, we have seen how the body grows and how patterns of growth and maturation account for variations in size of children and for the transformation of proportions of the body as the child changes to a mature woman. There are still two questions to be answered. What is the force that causes growth? What is the force that brings about cessation of growth at the proper time? There is no simple answer to either of these questions.

Growth is an inherent property of that mysterious force we call life. It starts at the moment of conception and continues to some degree until death. In the first cell of a new life is the force that immutably determines the form, proportions, and body characteristics of a human or an animal, male or female, whether tall or short, small or large, and the thousands of other body characteristics that vary so that no two people are ever just alike. These are the hereditary factors of growth.

Growth, in order to proceed normally, is dependent also on proper and adequate nutrition. What nature needs as building material, when and in what amounts she must have each of the various elements of food (proteins, which are the sturdy building blocks, vitamins, the vitalizers, and minerals for strength and stability), and how she uses them for promoting growth and maintaining health is a fascinating story in itself. It is as new to medical science as the story of the endocrine glands. We can do no more here than stress the importance of that story and hope it will kindle your interest to seek and use more detailed information.

Life, heredity, and nutrition are the fundamental forces of growth, over which there must be a controlling mechanism that keeps order and balance.

This nature has provided in the endocrine glands, which speed up and slow down growth resulting in the patterns of growth and maturation. It is also these glands that are responsible for the cessation of growth. Let us see how they work.

ENDOCRINE MECHANISM OF GROWTH

The growth hormone, as we have seen in our first consideration of the endocrine glands, is secreted by the anterior pituitary gland and is essential for normal growth and development. This means that it must be produced in the right amounts and at the right times for growth to proceed in an orderly, normal fashion. If the pituitary gland falters in its function and does not produce enough hormone, growth is retarded or ceases. If the pituitary is overzealous and produces too much growth hormone, overgrowth may result.

The pituitary does not pour out the same amount of the growth hormone day after day and year after year. The amount varies with the different phases of growth. The slow, steady growth of childhood represents response to a slow, steady secretion of the growth hormone at this time. In late childhood or prepuberty the marked speeding up of growth is the response of the body to a corresponding increased output of the pituitary gland.

But the growth hormone of the pituitary cannot do this job of growth promoting by itself. It needs the help of other hormones of the pituitary and of other glands, particularly the thyroid and the ovaries.

The thyroid hormone is a very important factor for growth. We have seen how necessary it is in the Age of Maturity to produce the vitality, the spark of good health. It is just as important in the earlier ages. Each cell of the body, each organ is " warmed up " by the thyroid hormone so that it can perform its particular functions, one of which is growth, most harmoniously and efficiently.

The ovaries serve a double purpose in control of growth. They provide a specific growth hormone, estrogen, for the reproductive system. And it is estrogen that calls a halt to the growth of the long bones. The ovaries do not begin to function effectively until late in childhood when they introduce two new factors in the pattern of growth, sexual maturation and the slowing down and finally halting of the increase in height. The mechanism and significance of these changes are reserved for discussion in "The Age of Youth."

When growth is completed, the vast majority of individuals conform, with minor variations, to the general pattern that is called the normal because nature had the plan in the hereditary factors, the building material in proper nutrition, and the labor force and supervision in the endocrine glands.

Of course nature is not always able to follow her master plan for growth and maturation. At any time in this age, disease or accident may interfere with, or nutritional deficiencies impede, her progress. Some stress may have occurred in the Age of the Unborn with the resultant congenital defects. On rare occasions, her plans are not perfect. Some wrong detail is passed on from one generation to another, producing individuals with inherited abnormalities such as extra fingers and toes, excessive height, or peculiar body proportions.

Finally, there are instances when nature falters in the execution of her plans. The endocrine mechanism of growth and maturation does not function in perfect balance, and we have the giants and the dwarfs. Giantism, resulting in an individual (usually male) of excessive height, may be due to excessive production of the growth hormone. Dwarfism, causing individuals of small stature of either sex, may be due to a deficiency of the growth hormone. But it may also be due to the failure of any of the other factors necessary for growth and maturation. Hence there are many kinds of dwarfs. These are the little people, who have an appealing and interesting story of their own.

XVIII

THE LITTLE PEOPLE

WHEN THE WORD "dwarf" is mentioned, we are apt to seek a pleasant meaning and visualize those enchanting characters of fairyland, jaunty little men (rarely women) who go about their work with speed and skill and a happy heart, usually doing good, sometimes mischievous, but rarely with sinister motives. Only giants are bad! But those of us who have met dwarfs in real life know that their lot is not such a happy one. They must not only carry the burden of being small, but many have deformities of the body as well and some also have mental deficiencies, which make life difficult for themselves and for those who love and must care for them.

There are many kinds of dwarfism, that is, stunted growth. This should not be surprising in view of the multiplicity of factors necessary for normal growth. Should any one of the factors or forces fail or be ineffective, there would result a specific pattern of stunted growth, a particular kind of dwarf. Failure of two or more factors would produce still other types of dwarfs.

It is not necessary, for our purpose, to review all the types of growth abnormalities. We need consider only a few of the more common ones to remove the stigma that is frequently attached to these unfortunates and their parents to make us more tolerant and sympathetic toward them and to demonstrate that they are not always "acts of God." Some can be prevented. Some can be helped.

When the pituitary gland fails to produce the necessary growth hormone, "pituitary dwarfism" results. This failure usually occurs late in childhood. It is really not a complete failure, but an inability of the pituitary to speed up the production of the growth hormone and to add the gonadotropic hormones, which are necessary for the prepuberty spurt of growth and for maturation. As a result, these individuals do not grow and do not mature sexually but remain childlike both in size and body proportions. They are not unattractive, for the face is small and pretty, the skin and hair soft. They are physically active and mentally alert.

The ultimate height of each will depend on the time in childhood at which the pituitary growth mechanism slowed down. Some few will be truly dwarfs, when failure occurred at an early age. Others will appear to be small adults, when the failure occurred late. We shall meet some of these cases in "The Age of Youth," for this condition is usually not recognized in childhood but becomes apparent only when puberty fails to occur.

Doctors are learning how to detect these failures early, and each year new knowledge brings methods of treating such cases. Some can be helped to a certain degree, that is, some growth and the outward appearance of sexual maturity can be induced. But true sexual maturity we cannot give them; they will be forever sterile.

The cause of this particular type of pituitary failure is unknown. Usually there is nothing to account for it. Occasionally, a disease of early life such as an acute infectious disease seems to have been responsible. Rarely, a tumor of the gland or a nearby structure may inhibit normal functioning of the gland.

Thyroid dwarfism is another matter, for here not only growth but all body processes are slowed down. There are two types of thyroid dwarfs; both are pathetic creatures of stunted growth and deficient mentality.

Cretins are born with a nonfunctioning thyroid or no thyroid gland at all. Their condition may not be apparent at birth or for some time thereafter if the nursing mother is normal and supplies the infant with the thyroid hormone. But soon the effects of the deficiency of the thyroid hormone become apparent. Cretins become the most grotesque of nature's human creatures. Besides being stunted, the body is misshapened. The face is repulsive, with a nose sunken at the bridge and flared nostrils, thick, blubbering lips, which remain open, drooling saliva and allowing a thick tongue to protrude. The skin is pale, grey, thick, and puffy. There are practically no eyebrows. The face shows no animation, no change in expression. The eyes, dull and lifeless, are small and half closed by swollen eyelids. The body, with a pot belly, is so swollen and pudgy that it seems almost to have no shape at all. The muscles are weak and flabby and result in the child being slow in learning to hold itself up, and it never acquires any proficiency in control of itself. Many are deaf mutes. Surely this is a cruel caricature of a human being.

This picture, however, has a bright side in that cretinism is rare in this country and there is much that can be done to ameliorate these symptoms. We say " in this country " because the incidence of cretinism varies in differents parts of the world. In some regions, such as the Swiss Alps, which are called goiter belts because thyroid problems are prevalent, cretinism may be common. Goiter belts result from an environmental factor, usually a deficiency of iodine in the water and food. Correction of this deficiency by the addition of iodine to food and water can do much to prevent thyroid deficiency. As a result, cretinism has become rare even in the goiter areas.

Not all cretins are confined to goiter belts, however. Isolated cases occur without apparent reason in nongoiterous areas and to normal parents. Fortunately, these are quite rare and usually the affliction strikes a family just once. Normal children may precede and follow it. Such cretinism is thought to be due to some defect in embryonic development of the thyroid gland. That is, some chance stress in the mother strikes the unborn just at the precise time that the cells destined to develop into the thyroid gland are being differentiated and are the most susceptible to injury, and they never develop.

Cretins are usually short-lived, when not treated, because of the poor efficiency of total body function and their increased susceptibility to infection. When cretinism is treated, it is like the good fairy waving her magic wand to change the ugly beast to Prince Charming. Sir William Osler, the dean of American Medicine, has said of this: " Not the magic wand of Prospero or the brave kiss of the daughter of Hippocrates ever effected such a change as that which we are enabled to make in these unfortunate victims, doomed heretofore to live in hopeless imbecility, an unspeakable affliction to their parents and to their relatives." The treatment is simple, just the addition of thyroid extract to the usual routine of normal nutrition. But the condition must be recognized early and treated adequately before irreparable damage has been done to mind and body.

The second type of thyroid dwarfism is due to thyroid failure that occurs in early childhood. Such children appear normal at birth and develop normally for perhaps a year or two. Then growth slows down or ceases entirely. The child becomes mentally sluggish, slow, and awkward in its movements. The soft tissues of the body become puffy, the skin coarse and dry. The hair is also coarse and dry, drops out, and becomes quite sparse. Unaided, their fate is imbecility and dwarfism, a modified version of cretinism. But these unattractive, pathetic dwarfs have the brightest prospect of all the little people. Proper medical treatment can restore them to their full potentialities as normal human beings.

This marked degree of thyroid deficiency, which results in dwarfism, is rare, but moderate degrees of hypothyroidism are fairly frequent. In fact, hypothyroidism is the most common endocrine problem of childhood. It is the first thing that doctors think of when a child previously alert and growing normally, becomes dull and inactive, stops growing, and begins to have difficulty in school work. Here again, thyroid medication works wonders.

Ovarian dwarfism is the result of not too little and too late, as in thyroid and pituitary dwarfism, but too much too soon. There is too much estrogen too early in life, which causes precocious sexual maturation and stops growth. Such girls become little women when they should be passing from infancy to childhood. Their body fills out to the normal feminine curves of the adult, the breasts develop, and menstruation begins. But they remain short and stumpy, with short arms and legs.

Here again there are two types of dwarfs, which differ not in appearance or the resulting dwarfism, but in the cause. There are two sources of this excessive estrogen. In one instance, for some unknown reason, the normal mechanism of maturation is speeded up. The ovaries start functioning in a normal way, and maturity comes to the child of two, six, or eight years of age. The unfortunate aspect is that these changes are permanent. There is nothing that can be done to slow nature down in her mad rush for maturity that would not also be harmful to the girl. These really are little women, for they are fertile, and pregnancy can occur. Such precocity has been described as starting as early as the first year of life. The case of Lina Medina, of Lima, Peru, who at the age of five years and seven months was delivered of a son by Caesarean section in

1939 was undoubtedly an example of this phenomenon. The speeding up process in older girls, so that menstruation occurs one to three or four years earlier than normal, is not uncommon. It is significant only in that the girl is cheated out of a good part of her childhood.

When the sex function is introduced early in these cases, there is also a speeding up of the maturation of the skeletal system. This does not mean that there is excessive growth, but rather a cessation of increase in height. Estrogen hastens the closure of the epiphyses, and further growth becomes impossible. If this is accomplished early and quickly, the result will be dwarfism. Even if it happens later and more slowly, the girl will still be relatively short in stature.

The problems that arise in ovarian dwarfism, as it occurs early or late, are illustrated in the case histories of Charlotte and Shirley. When Charlotte was two years old her parents noticed that her breasts were beginning to enlarge, some hair had appeared in the pubic region and mons veneris, and the labia were beginning to fill out. By the time she was four she was menstruating regularly. Except for the fact that she was large for her age, she was a healthy bright child. A thorough examination, including measures to exclude an ovarian tumor (which causes the other type of dwarfism, as we shall see), revealed no other abnormality. The prospects for life and health were good, but she had undoubtedly nearly achieved her maximum height. There was nothing that could be done but reassure her parents that she had no dread disease. Their great problem was to keep her from feeling that she was different from other children and not to have her childhood spoiled by this occurrence.

Shirley was only nine years old when she first came to the clinic, but she was a miniature woman. She was four feet, six inches tall, with a rather long trunk and short arms and legs. She had the body contour of an adult female and well-developed axillary and pubic hair. Her breasts were large and pendulous, with a large dark-brown areola around well-developed nipples. She had been menstruating since she was seven. The problem with Shirley, as we observed her during the following few years, was not only that her body was maturing sexually, but also that she was awakening psychologically to her sexuality. She was intensely interested in the opposite sex. Unfortunately, her judgment and reason were not precociously developed also. She was a child trying to handle a woman's problems. She was always in grave danger of being imposed on by an unthinking boy or an unscrupulous adult.

The second type of dwarfism associated with sexual precocity is due to excessive estrogen produced by a tumor. The result is a false maturation—that is the external sex characteristics develop, but fertility does not ensue. When the offending tumor is removed, the signs of maturation fade, and the girl returns to childish form and resumes the normal pattern of growth and development. Such tumors are usually located in the ovary. Occasionally, adrenal tumors cause precocity. We have seen that tumors and overgrowths of the adrenals occurring in the unborn were often associated with some degree of pseudohermaphroditism. When they occur in infancy and childhood, more commonly between the ages of two and four years, there is a combination of maturation and masculinization.

These dwarfs are some examples of what happens when the endocrine glands do not perform properly for normal growth. But there are other causes of dwarfism.

We grow and mature according to an inherited pattern. Our ultimate possible size and proportions are predetermined by our inheritance. There are some individuals whose inheritance differs from the usual or normal. They are born to be small. They are the midgets and pygmies.

Midgets are normally proportioned. They are adults in miniature, who are physically (except for size), sexually, and mentally mature. Tom Thumb was such a dwarf. Such are the little people we sometimes see in everyday life, particularly in the entertainment world. Perhaps we are wrong in attributing their condition to an inherited factor, because they do not necessarily pass the trait of small stature on to the succeeding generation. They often have children who grow to normal size.

There is another type of dwarf that we may see going about his (or her) business in spite of the affliction. One sold newspapers in front of the hospital where I interned. His head, actually of normal adult size, seemed extraordinarily large. Seated he appeared to be a normal-sized man for his trunk was large, his shoulders broad. But he had difficulty holding the newspapers under his arms. The reason for this became apparent when he held out a paper. His arms were very short and small. When he rose, his short legs added very little to his sitting height. He was an achondroplastic dwarf. These particular little people, with man-sized body and head and arms and legs like a child, are the result of a defect in the growth mechanism of their long bones. Something happened in embryonic life to the cartilage that is the model for these bones and prevented them from developing according to the normal pattern.

Nutritional deficiencies may also result in dwarfism. Dwarfs may have normal endocrine glands and normal inheritance. In fact, they may be normal in every respect as babies, yet not grow because nature has not been provided with the building material necessary to carry out her plans of growth.

Nutritional dwarfism is fortunately very rare in our country today. Not only the abundance of food, but the wider dissemination of information about what constitutes good nutrition have prevented such severe nutritional deficiencies. The use of cod liver oil is an example. Rickets, the result of calcium and vitamin D deficiency, was quite common a few score years ago. The bones, lacking in calcium, are too soft to support the weight of the body. So, the spine may become excessively curved, and the legs bowed, giving them the appearance of short stature. The addition of cod liver oil, because of the vitamin D content, enables the bones to harden normally, and the rachitic dwarf has disappeared from the scene.

The last type of dwarfism that we shall consider is the one that probably has been and still is the cause of the most heartbreak and sorrow because it is born to normal parents and can be recognized at birth. It is the mongoloid dwarf.

Mongoloids all look like brothers and sisters in one large family rather than sons and daughters of their own parents. They are called mongoloids because of their short slanting eyelids and the folds of skin at the base of the nose, which are also the facial characteristics of the Mongolian race. On first sight of their newborn, parents may know that this baby can never grow to physical maturity and will be mentally deficient. And they know that there is nothing that they or anyone else can do about it. Surely they have just cause for despair.

The mongoloid and the cretin are sometimes confused because both have physical abnormalities, retarded growth, and mental deficiencies. They are really quite different. While the future for the mongoloid is bleak, there are some compensations. It is the more lovable child. Even as a baby it is more active. Its skin is soft and rosy. It eats and grows as other babies do. But growth is slow and ceases entirely in childhood. Its mental growth does not keep pace even with its retarded physical development. While its mentality rarely goes beyond that of a normal two-year-old child, it may be quite an amiable little person. It enjoys rhythmic play and other simple activities. It is mother's perennial baby.

The cause of mongolism is not known. It apparently is not a glandular deficiency, for, among other reasons, it does not respond to any kind of glandular therapy. It also does not appear to be an inherited abnormality, for mongoloids do not "run in families." Rather they occur in isolated instances in normal families. It is most likely that mongolism is due to an embryonic defect resulting from faulty germ cells or some injury inflicted during early development.

The great tragedy of the mongoloid is the effect such a child has on its parents, particularly the mother. She may feel that she is in some way responsible and devote all her time and energy to the child. In her preoccupation with it, she may neglect the rest of her family, her friends, and her own physical and emotional health. Because she is plagued with the thought that her heritage is tainted, she may be afraid to have another child lest it too be abnormal.

We once had an exhibit at a medical meeting of pictures demonstrating abnormalities in body growth and development. The newspapers reported it, and among others described the case of a mongoloid girl of sixteen who was the size of a six-year-old and had the mentality of a two-year-old. The next day my phone rang, and the irate mother of one of our clinic patients demanded, "Was that my Elissa that awful newspaper called an idiot? I'll have you know Elissa is no idiot." I had to assure her that it was not her child. Two weeks later I met her on the street with a handsome boy of eighteen. She introduced him as her son and then ignored him. She started chatting about Elissa, and her face lit up with pride as she told me of Elissa's accomplishments. She said that she had left her hat upstairs on the bed and had asked Elissa to get it for her, and she added: "Do you know, Elissa went upstairs, got my hat, and brought it down to me all by herself! Now wasn't that smart?" I looked at her and her son and realized that never in the two years I had known her had she voluntarily told me anything about her other children.

The problem of what to do with a mentally deficient child is a very difficult one that has no one answer. The child's welfare of course must be considered. The physical needs must be met. Patience and skill must be exercised to develop its feeble abilities to assume even a very limited role among others. Its presence in the home, especially when there are other children, poses many problems. For these reasons parents are often advised at the birth of a mongoloid to place the baby in an institution where it will have proper training and care, and the family will be relieved of the stress. But this baby, restricted in its potentialities through no fault of its own, needs love; and stress can be good for a family if they have what it takes, the stamina to meet it. My casual contact with such a family was a heart-warming experience, which emphasized what the qualities of love, responsibility, tolerance, loyalty, and compassion can contribute to the meaning of life in the family and to each of its members.

The mother, whom we shall call Florence, was in her early forties when her last child, Teeny, was born. Her husband occupied a relatively important position in the business world, and they had enjoyed an active social life. They had three normal healthy children, two sons age twelve and fourteen and a daughter of eight years. It was quite apparent at birth that Teeny was a mongoloid, and the parents were advised to place her in a private institution devoted to the care of such children. Florence could not accept that as the proper solution, but neither did she assume alone the responsibility of Teeny. Rather, she was determined that Teeny should live as a wanted and loved (albeit " different ") member of a family group, and her husband fully agreed with her.

The children, who were delighted to have a new sister, were told that Teeny would always be " different," a fact that they had no reason to be ashamed of and must never try to conceal. Instead, it was to be their responsibility to help and to protect one who had the misfortune of not being able to take care of herself. Teeny in her own way made a tremendous contribution to the family, and especially to the lives of her brothers and sister. As the years passed and she grew and developed slowly, she was the healthy, happy baby of the family. Her brothers and sister learned the meaning of family unity—the strength and security it could give, of compassion for one less fortunate than they, of tolerance for differences and deficiencies in others, and of responsibility for contributing to the welfare of others. Of course, it was not always clear sailing. There were times of doubt and trouble. But when Teeny died at the age of fourteen, she left as a heritage many happy and tender memories, stronger family ties in a family of more mature individuals.

These then are the little people. They vary among themselves in appearance and personality, in mental and physical abilities. They have one thing in common—their smallness. So, when we see one of these little people, we should not look down on them from our height of normal growth or turn away from them in horror or disgust. We should remember that nature failed them while she favored us. They are not to blame for their affliction, just as we have no cause to preen ourselves for our normalcy. There should be only compassion and humble thankfulness in our hearts.

XIX

CHILDHOOD PROBLEMS STRICTLY FEMININE

LITTLE GIRLS AND LITTLE BOYS seem much alike. They grow from infancy into childhood according to the same pattern and learn about themselves and the world about them in the same characteristic way at each age. They enjoy boisterous play together, and measles and mumps may strike either without discrimination. Sex may seem to be dormant. In fact, with appropriate clothes the little girl would usually have no trouble passing for a boy. She may prefer a short hair cut and blue jeans to curls and ruffled dresses, and playing baseball to dressing her doll. Even so, she is learning the meaning of sex and laying the foundation for her sexual maturity as a woman, and she sometimes has physical problems that are strictly feminine.

These feminine problems of the little girl are not frequent, and are rarely of serious consequence, but they are quite different from those of the adult. When they do arise, they should have prompt and careful medical attention for the little girl's comfort and well-being. Their seriousness lies almost entirely in the way they are handled and the effect this may have on her future welfare. Very few of the problems can result in permanent damage to her sex organs, but overemphasis and wrong interpretation of them may distort the girl's attitude toward and concept of her sexuality. Such a trauma may seriously affect her ability to achieve maturity in this phase of her personality.

Mothers are likely either to ignore a condition completely or worry about it out of all proportion to its significance. In seeking medical care for her little girl's gynecological problem, a mother should feel no more hesitancy than she would if the child had infected tonsils, a skin rash, or any other illness. She should choose a doctor who is interested and experienced in these problems, who may be the family doctor, her pediatrician, or her own gynecologist.

The physical examination need not be an ordeal to the child, although the external genitalia, especially the hymen and clitoris, are exquisitely sensitive even in the very young. The baby does not mind being touched, but after the age of three or four, the child becomes fearful of another touching these organs, and even gentle pressure may be painful to her. However, simple inspection and sometimes gentle manipulation are usually all that will be necessary. On rare occasions when further measures of internal examination are necessary, small and specially made instruments are used. Shame and embarrassment are not the normal reaction of a child to the examination, but they are very easily implanted in a little girl's mind by an overanxious mother. She may not only overemphasize the problem to the child, but if her own concepts of sex are immature—those of guilt, fear, and shame—she may transmit these to her daughter.

THE LITTLE GIRL'S VULNERABILITY

The most common feminine problems of childhood are trauma, irritation, and infection. They may be illustrated in the experiences of three young girls—Joan, Becky, and Gerda.

Joan, age six, had several days previous to her examination tumbled on her brother's bicycle and had been struck between her thighs by one of the metal bars. The accident had caused her considerable pain and a little bleeding at the time, and now there was marked swelling and discoloration and still some discomfort. One labia (which is usually hardly a perceptible elevation in a little girl) was a hard mass twice the size of an adult's thumb and about the same shape, dark purplish in color, and quite tender to pressure. Joan was made unhappy by the discomfort and the inability to pursue her usual activities. Her mother was apprehensive that some internal injury had occurred or that permanent impairment might result. The condition responded to the usual treatment of a bruise, and Joan was active again in a few days and none the worse for the experience.

Trauma is one of the common feminine problems of childhood. The little girl's external sex organs are less well protected than those of the adult. The pads of fat covered with hair are not yet developed, so the hymen, clitoris, and entrance to the vagina are more exposed. The physical activities of childhood, such as bicycle-riding, sliding, vigorous rocking and swinging fairly often result in minor irritation or injury. Because these parts are very vascular, that is, they have many small fragile blood vessels, and the tissue is loose, a blow such as Joan sustained by falling astride an object may result in considerable swelling and bleeding under the skin. Occasionally, when a large blood clot forms, it may require surgical removal. In such falls, the hymen may be broken causing a slight amount of bleeding, which requires no treatment other than cleanliness.

Our second little girl, Becky, age four, seemed quite young for even a slight vaginal discharge, and her mother, who was quite meticulous, was at a loss to account for it until she chanced upon Becky and an older companion in what seemed to her horrible abnormal sex activity. On examination, there was some irritation, redness, and swelling around the vaginal orifice, and a small twig was removed from within the vagina.

Redness and swelling of the external genitalia with a slight amount of discharge are usually only a sign of irritation, which may be caused by such things as uncleanliness, too tight clothing, or pinworms. Rarely is there a true infection. Irritation may also be due to manipulation either by the girl herself or by another child. Children are curious; they examine themselves and each other. They love to play doctor and nurse. Older girls may impose on the meekness of the younger child and cause some irritation by the introduction of foreign objects. There is no serious physical harm in this, and there need be no dangerous psychological effect unless the adult interprets it for the child in terms of "dirty," "nasty," or "bad" and instills in her a feeling of guilt and shame. The management of these conditions should be mainly preventive, by teaching the child proper hygiene and by supervising her play with other children.

Gerda, age seven, had the most serious condition of the three—a thick, creamy, vaginal discharge. She was not made particularly uncomfortable by it, but it had persisted for several days and seemed to the frightened mother to be getting worse. In Gerda's case, which was carefully investigated, the mother's suspicion was confirmed—it was a specific vaginal infection. Infection, as a gynecological problem of childhood, is almost always limited to the vagina. The symptoms of such a condition are redness and swelling of the outer genitalia and a purulent discharge from the vaginal opening. Vaginitis may be due to any number of infecting organisms such as the streptococcus or colon bacillus, as well as the gonococcus, the bacteria that produce gonorrhea in the adult.

The course of the disease or infection caused by the gonococcus is quite different in adult women and immature girls. In women, the vagina is not susceptible, but the bacteria quickly make their way into deeper structures such as the urethra, Bartholin glands, the cervix, and finally the tubes. Thus in adults, it becomes a disease of the internal genital organs, which often causes an acute illness accompanied by pain and fever, and results in sterility. In immature girls, however, it is only the vagina that is vulnerable. The true internal organs are not involved, and therefore permanent injury does not occur. The seriousness of gonorrheal vaginitis in children is twofold; first, it is highly contagious and very easily transmitted from one child to another, second, the infection may be transplanted to other parts of the body, particularly the eyes, with dangerous consequences.

The most important aspect of handling gonorrheal vaginitis of childhood is that of prevention. First, little girls should be taught the safe use of public toilet facilities. While it is improbable that an adult ever acquires gonorrhea by toilet contamination, it is one of the most common means of transmission to the child. It is therefore of greatest importance that when an adult has the infection, care should be taken to prevent contamination of anything such as towels, bath cloths, toilet seats, and bath tubs, with which the little girl may come in contact. If the child does contract gonorrhea, she should be isolated from other children to the extent that she does not contaminate articles with which the others may come in contact.

When a little girl has a noticeable persistent vaginal discharge, the condition should be carefully investigated by physical examination, and vaginal smears and cultures should be taken. Treatment must be withheld until an accurate diagnosis is made. It is important to know the identity of the offending organism for several reasons. Such information affords the only means of selecting the most effective medication, since different organisms require different drugs for quick and adequate control. Repeated cultures afford the only accurate means of evaluating the response to treatment and assuring that treatment will be continued unremittingly not only until the symptoms subside but until a complete cure is effected. And only by knowing the identity of the organism can we know what measures are necessary to protect the child herself as well as to protect others.

Treatment nowadays is much simpler and vastly superior to that available only a few years ago. The antibiotics such as penicillin and tetracycline are quite effective; they work well, and they work fast. Equally important, they can be taken by mouth, which eliminates local treatments so arduous for all concerned. Furthermore, to the little girl's way of thinking, when local treatments can be avoided, her problem is on the same level as any other illness she may have. She is thus spared the feeling that she is somehow different from other children, and she does not become too greatly aware of or concerned about that part of her body.

One of the great bugaboos of childhood, in the minds of many mothers, is masturbation. She has been told that it is abnormal behavior, which may have all sorts of direful effects on both the mind and body of the child. None of this is true. Masturbation comes about in a normal way and causes no harm to the child. The handling of the genitals by a baby is part of the cruise of investigation that the baby makes of her body and by which she becomes acquainted with herself and her surroundings. She first follows objects with her eyes, but soon she uses her hands. The hands find the mouth, the feet, and finally the genital organs, no one of which has more significance to her than the other.

As the child grows older, she may seek relief from irritation due to tight clothing or uncleanliness by rubbing herself. During childhood, the act itself may elicit a pleasurable sensation, but it is only as the girl approaches puberty that it takes on a sexual significance. It does not result in any harm to the physical well-being or the mental capacity of the child and is usually outgrown by the time of puberty. When it persists after puberty, however, it becomes a problem that should have competent medical care. It portends trouble because it threatens, not the girl's physical health, but her emotional well-being. It represents a preoccupation with self that may make it impossible for her to make a satisfactory adjustment to the opposite sex later in life.

The only gynecological problem of children due to the disturbance of endocrine glands is that of precocious puberty, which has already been discussed. There remains, therefore, only one other of her peculiarly feminine problems to consider—that of sex itself.

THE SEEDS OF MATURITY

While infancy and childhood are periods of physical sex dormancy, they are probably the most important periods in life from the standpoint of the attainment of a full, happy, sexual adjustment in adult life. A girl's premarital training rightly begins when she is a baby and continues unabated throughout childhood and adolescence. The sex impulse or drive will awaken in the girl, and her fertility will mature when nature is ready. But the ability to procreate will not make her a sexually mature, well-adjusted woman. The ability to love must have matured also.

The first lesson is to love and be loved, to give and to receive. As the child grows and matures, the modes of giving and receiving change, but the fundamental character remains the same. A child is not spoiled by too much love, only by indulgence. The meanings of the two words have little in common. Parents may be afraid of spoiling the child by being too demonstrative of their love or seek to compensate for the little time they give by lavishing gifts and providing advantages of play and education. In both instances, they are failing in their objective. Love and affection, which the parents demonstrate to the child and allow the child to reciprocate, are the surest foundation for mature love. It gives her a sense of security because she belongs, of self-respect because she is important to someone else. She learns the meaning of rights, privileges, and responsibilities. She comes to know her own rights and to respect the rights of others. She learns to assume the responsibilities that are inherent in every privilege.

The second lesson is to teach the child to accept the biological functions of her body as natural and nothing to be ashamed of. She must be taught to feel that her body is one of the most wonderful and beautiful creations on earth and that her use of it is a privilege, and her care of it a duty. She may be taught all the facts of body function, including those of sex, but these will not suffice in her training toward sexual maturity unless such facts serve to strengthen and broaden this concept of the innate purity of her body.

There is no justification for the current teaching that a girl inherently feels herself to be inferior to the male because of her body structure. She may envy the male child his greater freedom in play and in rough-housing and resent being told that she must be a little lady. But she does not envy him his body, although she may be curious as to why boys and girls are made differently. If in later life she resents the fact that she is a woman, it is because of faulty training and unfortunate experience, and not because she was born to have a feeling of inferiority.

Children are curious about sex just as they are curious about everything else around them. Their most frequent utterances are "What is that?" and "Why?" Children will accept the facts of sex as natural if they are presented in a natural way. Answers do not have to be detailed or even completely explanatory, but they should always be truthful and given without evasion or embarrassment.

Sex education begins in the home, and the responsibility for it falls squarely on the shoulders of the parents. They cannot meet it by a "serious talk on the facts of life" as the child approaches puberty. Neither can they delegate it to others, such as the church or school or even the family doctor. But this does not mean that parents must know a vast array of facts of physiology or even psychology. This knowledge is of comparatively recent date, even to college professors and the authors of books. There have always been good parents who were successful in rearing their children to happy and full maturity. This is because sex is part of life, and true sex education is not the acquisition of facts and the perfection of technique, but training to live happily both with one's self and with others.

Parents lay the groundwork for sex education long before the child is ready for the acquisition of facts. This they do by loving the child and expressing that love in a meaningful way. Such love is not only affectionate care letting the child know that she is wanted. It recognizes the child as an individual with rights and privileges to which she is entitled. Such love gives guidance and teaches discipline. Every adult needs someone to turn to for guidance and respects the person who will help her to see the truth about herself. Why then should anyone think that a child must not be told what is right and what is wrong? She must learn to live in a world of people who also have rights and privileges. We have a culture, which children must learn to understand and to accept—and the learning is easier and will save many a hard knock if it is mastered or at least started in childhood.

Parents provide the fundamentals of sex education for their children by the way they themselves live together and meet the problems of life together. This includes their own attitude toward sex. If they themselves accept sex as a normal, natural, and wonderful part of life, they will impart this healthy attitude to their children, and the teaching of actual facts will be easy. If, on the other hand, sex is to them an unacknowledged part of life, concealed and distorted by fear, shame, and the taboos the experiences of their own childhood placed on it, their children will be handicapped in their progress to maturity.

Parents today recognize the danger of trying to ignore sex, and in their zeal may go to the opposite extreme, giving too many facts too soon for the child to assimilate them properly. They may fail to teach modesty and restraint for fear of inhibiting the child. The physical aspects of sex thus become isolated and exalted at the expense of the other components equally vital to the ideal of sex education. They are abetted in this error by our present-day concepts, which have been changing in this respect. It is just as bad—if not actually worse—to overemphasize sex as it is to try to ignore it.

Fortunately, facts are meaningful to children only when the children are ready for them. They will ignore what they do not understand if it has no bearing on what life means to them at that particular moment. This holds true for all of us. You may already have skipped some of the physiology in this book if you see no connection to yourself. You have never seen a pituitary gland or a hormone, and they therefore may not interest you at all. But when a real-life story is related, you can identify yourself or someone you know with it—and it has meaning and interest for you. So it is with children. If you try to explain the sex drive, passion, they would not know what you were talking about; or the sex act, they would only wonder why adults should do such things.

The facts of sex must be meaningful in terms of the child's experience and understandable according to her degree of maturity. The sort of sex education that provides this will teach sex in terms of love, oriented and integrated in family living. Sex thus becomes a personal, private, and precious gift that must be used with care and discretion as an essential ingredient to a happy healthy maturity. Thus the foundation for true sexual maturity is laid in early childhood, and the edifice rises with each passing year, which adds experience, knowledge, and understanding.

It should be pointed out that all that has been said of sex education for little girls applies equally to little boys. They too should be taught that sex is a precious gift not to be squandered and a responsibility not to be ignored. We should always remember (and so seldom do) that an older girl becomes a sex delinquent, her pregnancy illegitimate, because there was a male somewhere in the background who also was delinquent.

THE AGE OF YOUTH

XX

ᶠEMININITY UNFOLDS

ᴵᴰ ʏᴏᴜ ᴇᴠᴇʀ ᴡᴀᴛᴄʜ the heterogeneous assemblage of girls that pour out
f a high school door at the end of a day? Were you impressed by the
ariations in girlhood represented—the tall ones, the short ones; the skinny,
he fat; the quiet, the bumptious; the dowdy, the fastidious—in all grada-
ons and combinations?

I once spent a year teaching in a girls' finishing school and although
ore than a third of a century has passed since then, I still see clearly
he picture those girls made as they were being taught how to enter or
ave a room, how to go up the stairs and how to come down—all with
race and charm.

They had arrived at the opening of the school in all their finery of
r coats, silk hose, high-heeled shoes, and some with lipstick and rouge.
ome of them at least appeared to be quite grown-up. But when they
ut on the school uniform, a green peter-pan cotton dress, black cotton
ockings, and flat-heeled shoes, and their faces were scrubbed clean, they
ere reduced to a common denominator—girls growing up, ages twelve to
ighteen. The uniformity of dress served to emphasize the differences
hat existed among them in the degree of maturity in body and personality.

There were those who were still flat-chested and narrow-hipped, and
hose who popped their buttons in the blouse front and stretched the seams
f the tight little skirts in the rear. There were those who still had the
oft clear skin of childhood, and those who were agonized by the pimples
f adolescent acne. There were those who were shy and timid, homesick
t being away from the security of home and mother for the first time,
nd those who were joyous at being with girls of their own age with whom
hey could exchange confidences.

These girls, from a physical standpoint, were no different from the girls of their grandmothers' time or from girls of today. As a group they represented all variations in feminine form that characterize the transition from childhood to maturity—the Age of Youth. It is in the meaning each generation attributes to this age that we find a difference. In the 1920's they would have been "flappers" doing the Charleston; today they are "bobby-soxers" and "teen-agers," enthralled by "rock and roll."

Youth to the girls in the finishing school meant just a short period in which they attained maturity of physical form and some of the social grace to enhance the charm of their feminine maturity. This was the only preparation then considered necessary for the one future that lay ahead for most of them—early marriage and the security it provided in their own home.

It has been an accepted fact, from time immemorial, that there comes a time in the life of every feminine individual when she must cease to be a child and become not just an adult, but a woman. Her body must undergo changes that fit her for the role in life to which nature has assigned her. And she must learn to assume the responsibilities of her maturity. It is only the concept of what constitutes maturity and the preparations necessary for it that have varied with different times and cultures.

"Coming of age" for the youth of primitive peoples has always been an important part of their lives. It consists of a period of preparation at the end of which the youths must demonstrate by trials and tests their proficiency in the necessary skills of maturity. If successful, initiation ceremonies vested them with the mysteries, privileges, and responsibilities of maturity. Customs pertaining to the "coming of age," whereby a boy demonstrates his attainment of manhood by his courage, fortitude, strength, and skill as a warrior or huntsman vary with different tribes.

"Coming of age" for girls among primitive peoples, on the other hand, means just one thing, the attainment of reproductive maturity. As the physical signs of approaching maturity appear, or more often at a specific age, girls are segregated to await the event which would announce or confirm their maturity, the first menstruation. Such taboos as are placed on menstruating women usually also apply to her first menstruation. She is considered unclean, dangerous to man, beast, and crops. Therefore, she must remain apart until purification ceremonies render her again harmless and acceptable. Occasionally, the first menstruation has been given just the opposite meaning, that of beneficence, the dawn of fertility endowing the girl with supernatural powers to give strength and health to others. Then she is treated with great respect and reverence.

The test for maturity successfully passed, the initiation ceremonies follow. In some few instances they are brutal. The girl is subjected to circumcision by crude and exceedingly painful methods to which she must submit stoically. To allow fear or pain to mark her actions or even show in the expression on her face means disgrace. In most tribes the initiation ceremonies are no more than the tatooing of her body or the stripping from her of her childish apparel and ceremoniously placing on her the headdress and mantle of maturity. Varied as these rites are, they all serve the one purpose of announcing that the girl is now ready for marriage.

We should have to stretch our imaginations to find any semblance to " coming of age " in our modern American culture. We should find only the confirmation ceremonies of certain churches and coming-out parties among the socially minded. Modern society has produced instead a new age, the Age of Youth.

The Age of Youth is the result of the long lag between reproductive maturity, which may occur as early as twelve years, and the other aspects of maturity to be attained at some distant and indefinite time. There are no rigid standards for preparation and no tests by which a person acquires the status of an adult. Modern society has not yet crystallized its concept of the Age of Youth. On the one hand, youth is viewed as a turbulent period highlighted by the problem of juvenile delinquency. We hear a great deal about the troublemakers who constitute a small minority of youth today, but little about the large majority who go through the age without much difficulty to themselves or to others. From the discussions about youth one would never believe that there are girls and boys who go through the period placidly and happily. On the other hand, youth from the purely physical aspect is glorified as the ideal for womanhood. From sixteen to sixty, woman must always strive to appear " youthful."

As modern as we think we are, we, too, have taboos for the age, which are just as senseless and may be even more harmful than any primitive practices to the girl in her development to maturity. There has been and still is a taboo on sex education. We deny or fail to recognize that sex is a dominant force, which requires not only intelligent understanding but also respect and a sense of dedication if it is to be successfully integrated into a healthy, happy personality and a purposeful life. Rather sex is interpreted in terms of its purely physical aspects and as such is set apart and ignored as far as possible. The taboo cannot be lifted by giving youth the facts of physical structure and function. True sex education is instruction and guidance in a way of life whereby the child becomes a mature, responsible woman or man.

There is also the reluctance, which amounts to a taboo, to place responsibility on youth. Instead, parents and teachers have been taught to believe that youth must be furnished with all the necessities and pleasures of life without any effort on its part to earn them. Young people must be given education in the subjects of their own choosing rather than an introduction to all the rich fields of knowledge and practice in the disciplines necessary for acquisition of true understanding and for kindling the desire to search for truth. This taboo denies the necessity of guidance, discipline, the ability to conform, and punishment for wrong-doing.

We have been "modern" long enough to understand something of the meaning of the new Age of Youth, that it is a transition period whereby the child should achieve maturity on the physical, sexual, emotional, and intellectual levels. We have accumulated facts as to how this transition takes place, but we have not achieved any degree of skill in directing it. Modern woman is granted the freedom to develop on all these levels of maturity along with men. But it is up to her to do it on her own. She has few standards and no tests to guide her.

A girl entering the Age of Youth is really pioneering in a new realm. Her journey from childhood to maturity is longer than that of a few generations ago, and it is much more difficult. The route is not clearly marked, it is beset by many pitfalls, and there are false pathways that lead to dead-ends and sometimes to danger and disaster. Furthermore she is deprived of the guidance and protection afforded girls of yesteryear, which they may not have always enjoyed but which benefited them nevertheless. Finally, her destination is not a single, clearly defined goal, but one of several or even a combination of goals.

For the young girl of today, marriage is still the most important goal, but with two important differences. She is free to plan and train also for any other career she may choose. It is her privilege to pursue this career of work instead of marriage or to try to combine the two. As a matter of fact, however, there is really not so much choice because most girls may have to work at least a while before marriage and a large percentage will continue to work long after marriage. The second difference is that marriage itself as a goal has changed. It is no longer an indissoluble state, and too often it is looked upon as an adventure entered lightheartedly with the idea that if it proves to be too difficult or unpleasant it can easily be abandoned. Grandmother married for keeps. To her, failure in marriage was something to keep to herself, and she would live with it rather than run the risk of the censure of society by resorting to divorce.

PATTERNS OF FEMININE MATURATION

The Age of Youth starts with one thing and ends with something completely different. The little girl is changed into a mature woman. This transformation includes changes in the structure and function of her body and changes in her mode of life from dependence to independence, irresponsibility to responsibility, and asexuality to feminine sexuality. Like all periods of change, it is marked by instability, fluidity, vacillation. The girl must undergo the physical aspects of change in her body and learn to cope with them, which is not always easy. Growth and maturation processes are not necessarily smooth and gradual but are more likely to come in spurts of astounding abruptness. These changes she must not only accept as they come, but she must also learn to understand their meaning to her as a feminine personality. This is a difficult job, which at times may seem to be beyond her ability. Her physical appearance may be gangling and awkward, and her actions may have the outward appearance of being contradictory and perverse. It is a period when she is groping to find her way, sometimes advancing, sometimes retreating. One day she is a little girl who doesn't want to grow up, and another she may be trying very hard to be a woman.

Youth is the age when sexuality becomes a vital part of the young girl's personality. Its onset is imperceptible—something stirs, and her feminine sexuality begins to unfold. When the maturing factors controlled by her endocrine glands begin to function, the girl's body begins to change. The breasts swell, the hips broaden and become rounded, and she has her first menstruation. With these physical changes she becomes acutely conscious of her sex. Her feminine sexuality becomes the dominant factor of her life. On the one hand she is trying to understand it herself, and on the other she yearns for its recognition and appreciation by others and especially by the opposite sex of her own age.

This maturation process, which is the Age of Youth, does not mean a break with the past or the addition of anything new or mysterious. Youth is merely the unfolding of traits that have always been present. The kind of child she was, to a large extent, determines the kind of woman she will become.

There is only one milestone in the Age of Youth. That is the "menarche," or the first menstruation. Its occurrence is concrete evidence that she is on her way to physical sexual maturity but not that she has arrived. The facts that the beginning and end of the Age of Youth are vague and the menarche is the only milestone are brought out by the different names that are commonly used, but not always clearly understood, to identify the stages of maturation. Puberty means the attainment of a certain amount of sexual maturity, which in girls is the onset of menstruation. Thus, for her, menarche and puberty are the same. Prepuberty, or pubescence, is the period preceding menarche. Adolescence is the period following menarche, which ends at some vague time when full maturity has been attained.

Breaking of the Age of Youth into two phases, prepubescence and adolescence, is misleading. The onset of menstruation is only a single incident in one long continuous process whereby the girl attains maturity on the physical, sexual, and psychological levels. From one aspect the division is valid. Prepubescence is the period in which physical growth and maturation is most prominent, while adolescence is characterized by emotional and intellectual development. In other words, in the first stage the girl acquires the physical characteristics of her feminine sexuality, and in the second she has to learn to live with it.

The menarche does not occur at any fixed age. Rather there is a wide variation within the normal for the year at which girls experience their first menstruation. In this country, the average age at menarche is thirteen years, and the majority of girls are between twelve and fourteen years. But there are some who start earlier, even at nine or ten years, and some who are as late as sixteen years. Failure of menstruation to occur by eighteen years means that something is definitely wrong.

The time of the menarche is an inherited character, which may be modified by environmental factors. In some families an early menarche is the rule, in others it is late. Girls are apt to start menstruating at about the same age their mothers did. Identical twins frequently experience the menarche in the same month, while fraternal twins may be several months apart, just like any other sisters. Climate is usually considered to be a modifying factor, but this is not necessarily so. Girls of the United States have an earlier menarchal age than those of any other country including those of much hotter and much colder climates. And here only 25 per cent of girls start to menstruate during the summer months. Many of the girls who start to menstruate during the winter months will fail to have a period for the three or four months of summer and will then start again in the fall. They often repeat this pattern of summer amenorrhea (perhaps to their great delight, if mother doesn't become too alarmed) for several years. Eventually, they settle down to a full-time yearly schedule, and no harm is done by their brief years of summer vacation. The more important environmental factors that tend to delay the menarche are poor general health and poor nutrition. In girls who have severe illnesses in late childhood, all the processes of maturation are delayed, including menstruation. In the same way, anemia of a marked degree or undernourishment may cause delay.

Two other physical characteristics of youth, growth in body size and development of the secondary sex characters, are not so clearly defined in time of occurrence as the menarche, but they are equally important. All three are integrated to form the pattern of maturation. Each contributes to the process as a whole, and each is in turn affected by the contributions of the others.

Youth is the age in which nature must accomplish the tremendous feat of changing the size of the body from that of a child to that of an adult and of transforming childhood to womanhood. At only one other time does she have so much to do in such a short period of time. We have already witnessed this in the Age of the Unborn when the fertilized ovum, a single cell, infinitely small, grows to a weight of seven pounds and is transformed into a human infant. After birth, growth is still rapid but is slowing down, and by the first year it has reached the steady stride that continues unchanged until the years of childhood draw to a close. Then growth again slows down as if nature were catching her breath, preparing for the intense effort that must be made in the Age of Youth.

The Age of Youth is ushered in by a period of very rapid increase in size, particularly height, and the appearance of the secondary sex characters. This phase may last one to three years and ends with the occurrence of menstruation. Thereafter, the rate of growth slows down and ceases almost completely within one to two years after the menarche. All girls normally follow this general pattern. Some appear to differ because the timing within the pattern is different as to the age of onset, the rapidity of growth, and the length of time required to complete each of the phases.

Girls vary considerably in the age at which this speeding up in growth and the onset of sexual maturation, one to several years later, occurs. Rapid growth may start as early as the age of eight or be as late as fourteen years and still be normal for a particular girl. The girl who enters the period of accelerated growth early grows very rapidly for a short time, her body fills out to feminine contours, and she has her first menstruation long before other girls. Then growth slows down, and she soon attains her mature height and size. At the other extreme is the girl who matures late sexually. She continues to grow at a slow rate for several years. When her growth rate is accelerated, it is only moderately rapid, and her first menstruation occurs at a much later age. Thus there is a fixed relationship between acceleration in rate of growth and the onset of menstruation.

THE ENDOCRINE GLANDS AND FEMININE MATURATION

It is a tremendous feat, the transformation of a child into a woman, and it requires a complicated, efficient, and well-attuned mechanism for its accomplishment. Nature therefore uses all the beneficent forces available, not only the pituitary gland and the ovaries, but the adrenals and the thyroid as well.

We have already seen in "The Age of Infancy and Childhood" that growth is under the specific guidance of the growth hormone of the pituitary gland and that failure of growth may be due not only to pituitary deficiency but also to thyroid, adrenal, and gonadal dysfunctions or hypo-functions. During that age, in the normal, the pituitary has been func-tioning at a fairly fixed level, producing the growth hormone at a steady rate. Then suddenly, when the time comes for growth to be speeded up and sexual maturation to appear, the pituitary bestirs itself. It pours out more growth hormone, and it also pours out more of its specific tropic hormones, which stimulate the adrenals, the thyroid, and particularly the gonads.

The adrenals play a significant part in the growth and maturation process. Their cortical hormones are responsible for the increased de-velopment and strength of the musculature. This is, of course, more prominent in the male, but it is important in the female. There is also increased production of androgen, which is responsible for the appearance of the sexual hair. The changes in the glands of the skin, which often is apparent in the acne of adolescence, is also associated with excessive androgen.

What calls a halt to the growth process? Why doesn't it go on and on? What is the timing mechanism of the pituitary whereby the hormones are produced at different rates in different ages? What causes the pituitary to withhold the gonadotropic and growth hormones in the early years and then to speed them up suddenly in the Age of Youth? The answer to the first question, what stops growth, is not to be found in still another hormone, but rather in the action and interplay of the hormones already at work. Estrogen is truly a versatile and powerful director of growth and maturation, and it exerts a profound influence on the whole body and personality of the girl. One particular function is of interest—the effect estrogen has on the growth of bones. Estrogen calls a halt to growth. As the ovaries become more proficient, they produce more and more estrogen, and with this increase in estrogen, growth is progressively retarded and eventually ceases. We have seen that growth of the long bones takes place at the epiphyseal line, and as long as this area is made of cartilage, growth can continue. When the cartilage is transformed into bone, further growth (increase in length) is impossible.

Estrogen stimulates the deposition of calcium, that is, it directs the cells of the bone to speed up the process of taking calcium from the blood stream and depositing it in the areas needed to make the whole bone solid and rigid. This speeding up results rather quickly in the complete ossification of the bone and closure of the epiphyses. When this is accomplished, further increase in the size of bones is impossible. To slow the process of growth in the rest of the body at the same time, estrogen issues another command. It depresses pituitary function, which means that it orders the pituitary to stop producing so much growth hormone, as well as other types of hormones.

To meet the needs of accelerated growth and maturation, the thyroid also is called upon to speed up in order to maintain a normal rate of metabolism. That this is sometimes a strain is demonstrated by the fact that obvious swelling of the thyroid (adolescent goiter) is a common occurrence that subsides when maturation is achieved.

Maturity of ovarian function means two things: the production of the female hormones in adequate quantities, and the production of fertile germ cells. They are not always achieved simultaneously. The ovaries, which have been dormant in early childhood, probably start functioning some time before the speeding up of the pituitary, in some girls as early as eight or nine years of age because even then there is some production of the gonadotropic hormones. With the speeding up of the pituitary and increased production of the gonadotropic hormones, the ovaries wake up and begin to function.

Estrogen is really a special kind of directive hormone of female sexuality. By its orders, sometimes gentle coaxing, sometimes peremptory command, the child becomes a woman. It is estrogen that causes the breasts to grow, the voice to become lower and softer, the skin to take on the glow and the hair its lustrous sheen of youth. It is estrogen that causes the reproductive organs to grow, and when they have achieved adequate maturity, menstruation occurs.

The onset of menstruation means that cyclic changes have begun to take place in the lining of the uterus, changes that are initiated and controlled by hormones elaborated by the ovaries. This in turn indicates that the ovaries have matured to the point where they respond to stimulation by the pituitary gland, which they were not able to do during childhood.

The uterus-ovary-pituitary relationship is a very delicately balanced mechanism when it is functioning in regular recurring cycles in the adult. It is not surprising therefore that it sometimes takes quite a while for it to achieve perfect balance during adolescence. While acquiring the rhythm, there are apt to be many irregularities. A girl may menstruate once and then not again for three to six months, and thereafter at intervals of one to three months, or fairly regularly for a few months, only to skip. This means that the ovaries are not yet wide awake and responsive. On the other hand some girls will start by menstruating every two or three weeks and may have very long periods of flow, which means that the ovaries have not yet learned to go through a complete cycle. Irregularities are not considered abnormal for the first two years of menstrual life. By that time her type of cycle will be established. That is, what will be normal for her.

The occurrence of menstruation, even fairly regularly, does not necessarily mean that the ovary has achieved full maturity of function and is discharging each month fertile germ cells. There is considerable evidence that many of the first cycles are anovulatory. Specific data derived from hormone assays, temperature charts, and endometrial biopsy have demonstrated this to be true in individual cases. There are also clinical observations to the same effect. Among certain primitive people, sex play between young girls and boys is a common practice, but the girls rarely conceive. The reason suggested is that the girl has not yet started to ovulate, although her ovaries are producing sufficient hormones to cause menstruation and to play their role in the sexual urge.

Another bit of evidence that the first menstrual cycles have occurred without ovulation are that they are painless. By various means it has been demonstrated in adult women, who had no disease of their pelvic organs to account for pain, that only those cycles in which ovulation had occurred were painful. A girl is frequently brought to the doctor for examination because one or two years after the menarche her periods have suddenly become painful. The doctor can assure her that there is nothing wrong but that actually the ovaries are now functioning more efficiently (if not as pleasantly) than previously.

The timing mechanism of pituitary function, which causes not only the speeding up of the production of growth hormone but also the addition of new hormones, the gonadotropins, to arouse the ovaries, is our last aspect of this mechanism. The answer is not to be found in another endocrine gland or any hormone function. Rather it represents a phase in the pattern of growth and maturation inherent in the gland itself. That is, the time it takes the pituitary to attain its full maturity of function is an inherited character. We grow according to the pattern of our inheritance, and the form we attain at maturity—the height, the body build, and all individual physical characteristics—are pre-ordained by our inheritance. This explains why Mercedes and Kitty, whom we met as problems of childhood, were not problems of faulty endocrine function.

Mercedes, the short girl who wanted to grow taller, was of Spanish descent. Her mother and father were short. She first menstruated at the age of eleven and had attained full height by the age of fourteen. She had not been self-conscious about her height among her friends at home, who also were not tall. But when she came to boarding school in this country, she found the girls much taller than she and was unhappy about it.

Kitty, the tall girl of twelve, was the daughter of a tall mother and tall father. Her older brothers and sisters were tall. In neither Mercedes nor Kitty was there anything wrong with their endocrine glands, nor was there anything to be done about their heights. The timing and degree of the growth processes were inherited characteristics.

We may add the case of Catherine, who at 14 was quite small as compared to other girls of her age and had not started to menstruate. Catherine was very unhappy, bcause if there is one ideal for teen-agers it is to be just like all the other teen-agers. To be different is a terrific burden. So her mother brought her for examination to see if anything could or should be done. X-rays of her bones disclosed the fact that her bone age was less than her actual age by several years, and her epiphyseal lines were far from closed. She had not attained all the growth possible for her. As Catherine had no brothers or sisters, we could not say offhand that Catherine's pattern for growth was slow, but this seemed to be the case. This supposition was strengthened by the fact that we could find no evidence of glandular imbalance and that the first signs of maturation were appearing. The only thing to do was wait, not always an easy thing to do, but in this case it proved correct. Catherine did grow and mature to normal womanhood.

If I may be allowed to introduce a mere male into the picture I would like to mention Johnny, whom I saw in my early years of medical experience. His case is the counterpart of Catherine's. He was twelve and the runt of his class. In my youthful enthusiasm and eagerness I gave him all the hormones and vitamins I thought might help him grow. The fact that he became a handsome six-footer, a pilot in the Air Force during the war, was not because of my futile efforts. I might as well have given him sugar water, and the results would have been the same. Hormone preparations such as the growth factor that we had then were completely ineffectual and fortunately harmless as well.

Johnny's case points up this important fact. First, it is useless and wrong to put a youngster to the expense and trouble of treatment for delayed growth without complete understanding of what kind of pattern of growth the youth has inherited and is following. It is a wise plan in the problem of growth as in all phases of medical practice to give nature a chance. Help her if possible, but above all do nothing that will interfere with or impede her progress.

We have now seen how menarche fits into the pattern of growth of the body and the mechanism of endocrine function by which this is accomplished. But we have only mentioned or made casual reference to the maturation of the body in terms of appearance of the secondary sex characters.

Secondary sex characters—this is a very cold, impersonal way to refer to something that becomes of such vital importance to the girl in her Age of Youth and will remain so to a certain extent for the rest of her life. These include the roundness of her breasts, the texture of her skin, the contour of her body, the softness of her voice, the strength of her muscles, the structure of her bones, and indeed every feminine characteristic of her body (except the sex organs themselves, which are called primary sex characters). They are her badges of femininity, the basis of her physical attractiveness, and she yearns for their perfection. Her inability to achieve her ideal of perfection in these is the source of most of her problems during this age.

XXI

YOUTH NOT SO CAREFREE

AH YOUTH. Those were the happy days. How wonderful it would be if we could only turn back the clock, discard the cares of maturity and be sweet sixteen again, even just for a day. Or so we think. Cherished memories have created a vision of the past that has little resemblance to the reality. We recall the pleasant things—the first party dress, the boy next door, the first kiss—and forget the intensity of our feelings at that time, how much we wanted to be pretty, to be liked, even just to be recognized as no longer a child, and to what extremes we would go to try to achieve these. We forget how much even little things could hurt. No, they were not always happy days. One day of return would be more than enough to convince us that youth too has its problems.

MOTHERS AND DAUGHTERS

Mothers, of course, recognize that their daughters have problems, but too frequently they see them from the adult's point of view and seek to meet them in what has been the accustomed way—that of mother taking care of the needs of her child. Sometimes the problem arises from the fact that, in her overanxiety for her daughter to develop normally, the mother becomes disturbed by the slightest symptom she considers abnormal and takes the unwilling daughter to the doctor for examination. She forgets the painful modesty of youth that makes girls resentful of the intrusion of anyone, mother or doctor, on the privacy of her physical being. Sometimes it is the daughter who is anxious, and the mother belittles the problem, taking the problem of youth for granted as something that will be outgrown. At times the problem arises from the mother's desire for her daughter to attain the attributes of feminine maturity, which she considers desirable, and here again mother and daughter do not always see eye to eye. The daughter has her own ideals of perfection, which require her to conform not to adult standards but to those of other girls her own age. Finally, the mother expects the doctor to tell her what, if anything, is wrong and what she should do about it. She ignores the daughter's need to be independent and to do for herself.

Many of the problems of youth (and maturity, too) would never occur if the mother had a better understanding of the physical needs of youth and a mature attitude, which includes knowledge of her own femininity. Such a mother would have given her daughter information as she was ready to understand it and would have encouraged her to assume her individual responsibilities as early as she was able. More important she would also have been teaching her daughter, by precept and example, that it is a privilege and a responsibility to be a woman.

It is because mothers vary so in the part they play and girls are so different in their response to the changes within themselves that no two problems of youth are ever alike, although the physical symptoms may be similar. This is vividly illustrated in the stories of what the menarche meant to two girls, Elaine and Rose.

Elaine's story came to me from her mother, for Elaine was only eleven years old and had no reason to be a patient. It consisted of only one short incident, Elaine's reaction to a movie, but it revealed much. As a prelude the mother said that she had always tried to answer Elaine's questions factually and that a year ago she had tried to explain to her about menstruation. At that time Elaine was far more interested in baseball than she was in how she would become a woman. Recently however, the signs were beginning to indicate that Elaine would soon be faced with the fact of her femininity, and her mother was anxious that it should not come as a shock to her, but rather would be a source of satisfaction in being normal. The mother therefore was quite pleased when a film on "how life begins" was to be shown for mothers and daughters at her church. She said to me: "Elaine sat through it completely engrossed every minute. I wasn't sure how much she understood or whether I should have brought her. But all my doubts were quickly dispelled when we were home again. She came to me completely starry-eyed, put her arms around me, and said, 'Oh, mother, do you know what I really want most of anything? I want to menstruate.'"

Elaine, of course, will have many different thoughts about menstruation as the years go by, but this approach to the event as yet unexperienced banished fear and shame and laid the groundwork for a mature attitude, which would see her through the inconveniences and discomforts that it might later bring.

Rose, the second case, was twenty-two when she came for a premarital examination and gave as her reason for coming, "I can't talk to Mother about anything pertaining to sex. The few times I have tried she evades the question or cuts me off. I shall never forgive her for not telling me about menstruation. I have several older sisters, and as a little girl I had heard them speak of being unwell and knew that it had something to do with bleeding each month. Sometimes they went to bed with cramps, and Mother had her sick headache when she spent the day in a darkened room, and everyone had to be very quiet. In my innocence and ignorance I thought they meant what they said. If they were unwell naturally they were sick, and they must be sick because they didn't pay proper attention to their health. So I determined that I wasn't ever going to be sick or unwell if I could possibly help myself. I went to bed when I was supposed to, ate my spinach and took cod liver oil. I didn't know what else to do, and I couldn't ask, for obviously no one in my family really knew any better; but I hoped it would be enough. You can imagine how I felt when I realized that I had failed because I too was bleeding. I tried to keep the horrible secret to myself. It didn't help the situation when Mother found out and scolded me for being so silly. She said that all girls get unwell, it was woman's curse, and I might as well make up my mind to accept it, stop being a rowdy tom-boy, and try to act like a lady."

Most girls of today do not approach menarche with either of these extremes of bliss or ignorance. They know about menstruation long before they experience it and approach it with mixed emotions. Too frequently, the knowledge has come to them in such a way and so distorted by misin-formation or untruth that they are unable to achieve a healthy emotional acceptance of it. Menstruation becomes a burden of resentment, em-

barrassment, sometimes shame, and occasionally of severe physical discomfort.

ACQUIRING THE BADGES OF FEMININITY

The gynecological problems of youth may seem quite simple, and
medically speaking they usually are. Girls are rarely acutely or dangerously
ill because of them. But even the simplest physical problem has overtones
and complications that make it complex and not to be judged by the
standards of any other age. The new role of feminine sexuality leads to
problems each of which has three components. First there is the physical
aspect of the problem. The maturation process may not occur on schedule,
or it may be abnormal in some respect. Sometimes it is the result of the
physical strain incident to growing up, but more often it is due to ignoring
the girl's physical needs of adequate rest and nutrition (which are great)
and allowing her to become involved in too many activities. Second there
is the girl's emotional reaction to the business of growing up. And third
is the mother's handling of her own role. These problems are made easier
or more difficult to handle depending on the mother's interest, understanding, and assistance.

Menstruation

The menstrual abnormalities of the Age of Youth run the gamut from
too much and too soon through too little and too late. The extremes of
these we have already discussed. Precocious puberty, which represents
the too soon, we met in "The Age of Infancy and Childhood." Amenorrhea, the complete absence of the menstrual function, we found in "The
Age of Maturity" might be physiologically normal as in the case of Amy,
who was pregnant, or might represent profound glandular deficiency as in
the case of Claire. These are rarities.

The usual menstrual problems of adolescence are those of irregularity.
The irregularity may have to do with rhythmicity of the period or the
duration and amount of flow. In general these irregularities may be con-

sidered in two groups: the girls who have infrequent periods, and those who have too frequent periods that are prolonged and profuse. These appear to be quite different when only the symptoms are considered, but the basic physiology is similar for the two. Both represent a failure of the ovaries to complete a normal cycle of function within the normal time limits.

The abnormalities of menstruation in adolescence are mostly functional in origin. This means there is no disease such as tumors, cysts, or infection that causes the difficulty, but that the glandular mechanism, the uterus-ovary-pituitary relationship, is not functioning properly. This may be due to lack of maturity of the glandular mechanism, but more often it is due to some interfering external factor, such as poor nutrition, anemia, overwork, lack of rest, low thyroid function, or obesity. Furthermore, there are no physical problems of the age of maturation that do not have a large emotional component. When girls have menstrual problems, they worry about them. They don't like to be different from other girls. This unease may be intensified by an overanxious mother. To approach any menstrual problem in terms of the physical alone and ignore the girl's home environment and her daily routine and to fail to try to understand how she evaluates her problem is inadequate. The doctor must not only understand the whole problem but must try to help both the girl and her mother to recognize broad aspects of it and to understand each other. For this reason we will present each problem as a case history and then give some generalities.

Mrs. Waldrop and Hetty were finding it very difficult to play the roles of mother and daughter satisfactorily. To see them together, it was not hard to understand the reason. Mrs. Waldrop was petite, quite youthful, well-groomed, vivacious. Hetty, her daughter, was just her opposite, tall, overweight, and slouching in posture. Her oily black hair hung in strings about a face marred by a bad complexion. Mrs. Waldrop did all the talking while Hetty sat nervously twisting her fingers, eyes downcast, sullen, resentful, distrusting.

"I have two daughters and you would never know that they are sisters. Hetty here is my problem. Gwen, my older daughter, is so sweet and dainty, so bright and cheerful. We have wonderful times together, and she never gives me a moment's worry. But Hetty I just can't understand.

She doesn't like to go out with us or even other girls, and she hates boys. All that she really likes to do is eat. I keep after her all the time, but it just doesn't do any good.

"That is not what we came about," she continued. "I guess that is just difference in temperament. What I am worried about is Hetty's physical condition. Her periods have become so irregular and she is getting so fat that I know something must be wrong. She is sixteen now, and her periods started when she was twelve. They were all right for several years, but last year she menstruated only two or three times. At least, I think so. She is so very secretive about herself and is resentful when I ask her. Now Gwen is just the opposite, so confiding."

The mother rambled on at great speed, enjoying the picture she intended to portray of herself, an earnest, devoted, and sympathetic mother with one responsive daughter and an ugly duckling. Hetty's discomfiture was so great that I hastened to put an end to the interview by saying that probably Hetty did have some physical reasons to account for her difficulties and that we would try to find them.

Hetty's problem proved to be a complex one, the menstrual irregularity being only one symptom in a chain of circumstances. Hetty had started growing rapidly at the age of eleven and at the same time had begun to put on excessive weight. Now she was five feet, eight inches tall and weighed 170 pounds. This alone was sufficient to account for some of her difficulties. She just didn't have the physical energy to do all that was expected of her. The situation was made more serious by a low metabolic rate, indicating a deficiency of thyroid function, and anemia. Another factor, probably just as important, was the fact that Hetty was profoundly unhappy at home.

"Mother and I don't get along," she confided. "She is so disappointed in me because I'm so big and awkward. I wish that I could be little and pretty like Gwen, but I'm not, so what's the use?" She continued that she was not smart in school; the only subject she liked or did well in was home economics. She was not interested in going to college, nor was she looking forward to getting a job. Her one ambition was some day to get married and have a family like her Aunt Kate. She was rather hopeless about ever attaining this because she considered herself so unattractive.

Hetty's treatment consisted of a rigid diet to lose weight, thyroid extract for her low metabolism, and iron and vitamins for her anemia and lowered vitality. But most important of all, she was given big doses of encouragement through the months that followed, praise for the effort that she was so earnestly making to improve herself. She responded unbelievably well. She lost weight and began to carry herself with pride. Her menstrual periods became normal. Finally she emerged a nice looking, if not beautiful, girl, and a much happier one.

Years later she came again to see me, this time alone. She was then a very self-possessed, assured, well-poised, becomingly dressed, and carefully groomed young matron. She was even a little cocky. Her manner was understandable and forgivable in view of the struggle she had made to achieve this change. One could only admire her for the enthusiasm, devotion, and satisfaction with which she was giving herself so completely to her chosen career—that of marriage, with a home and a growing family.

Janice, a lovely girl of fourteen, graceful, and pretty, and her mother seemed to have an ideal mother-daughter relationship, but theirs too was heading for trouble. This, however, was far from the mother's realization when she sought medical advice. Janice was having excessive menstruation. Her periods were too frequent, profuse, and prolonged.

Janice accepted, for the present at least, her mother's devotion to her, and the mother's pride in having such a lovely daughter could be accepted as natural and her ambitions for Janice's success understandable. But already this ambition was getting out of hand. Janice started to take dancing lessons when she was quite young. She showed considerable talent and was encouraged to spend more and more time and energy perfecting herself in ballet. At present she attended dancing classes three times a week and practiced from two to four hours a day. This was in addition to her regular high school work and social activities.

A careful examination revealed no physical reasons for the fact that Janice was having menstrual bleeding every two weeks lasting from seven to ten days. The true reason was that Janice was carrying a schedule of physical exertion far greater than her body could stand, and the delicate mechanism of menstruation had broken under it. Dancing was discontinued for a while, and measures were instituted to rebuild her general health, which included an adequate well-balanced diet, more rest and sleep, some out-of-doors exercise. The anemia was corrected by appropriate medication, and the bleeding was treated just as we have described previously for the adult. Perhaps most important of all she was relieved of the emotional stress of trying to achieve perfection in her dancing and fulfilling her mother's ambition for her.

Janice responded well to this regime. Her periods became regular as her general health improved. After a time she was allowed to resume her dancing but in a more moderate way. But all was not yet clear sailing. As Janice and her mother, who always accompanied her, visited me from time to time, it became apparent that the mother was trying desperately hard to be on "we girls" terms with Janice. In her family, and there were other children, she was partial to Janice and sought to monopolize her attention and affection. Such an attitude of a mother toward her daughter could lead only to heartache in the future for one or the other. Happily Janice was able to break these ties by which her mother was endeavoring to bind her and found friendship and love outside her home.

It was the mother who was hurt. She came back to see me several years later, nervous, depressed, and upset. Eventually, she told me why. Janice, now eighteen, had obtained a place in a summer theatrical group for which her dancing had equipped her. She had made friends and went out frequently with other young people whom her mother did not know, and she had a steady boy friend. Mother felt that she had been rejected and was miserable in the situation for which she alone was responsible.

Not all girls are as fortunate as Janice in achieving independence when they have to struggle with the problem of a selfish, immature mother or a domineering one. Too frequently we see examples of women whose lives have been blighted by such mothers. Some do not marry, some have their marriages made more difficult. All lose the wonderful relationship that can exist between two mature individuals as mother and daughter.

Her Breasts

The breasts are woman's emblem of femininity. There is no other part of her body that has greater psychological significance to her. They become important to her as they begin to develop when she is a young girl and continue to be so for the rest of her life. What her attitude is toward them varies with the dictates of fashion, but she can never ignore them. In the flapper age of the 1920's when it was the style to be flat-chested and long-waisted, she bound herself unmercifully to deny their presence. Now in the age of the sweater girl she helps nature out with falsies. Their more serious significance is made clear to her in later years when disease threatens them. The removal of a breast is a psychological shock to a woman from which she sometimes has great difficulty recovering.

It was concern over the development of her breasts that first brought Cynthia to me as a patient. Cynthia and her mother represent one of the loveliest pictures of mother-daughter relationship that I have encountered professionally in all the years that I have dealt with the problems of girls and women.

Cynthia was just twelve years old the first time she and her mother came to my office. I asked what brought them. The mother replied, "Cynthia has a problem which we have discussed and because she was worried about it we decided to consult a doctor. Cynthia will tell you." From that day until Cynthia came for premarital examination and advice years later it was always so. She was encouraged to work out her own problems. Just as important, perhaps more so, the mother recognized that things that might seem trivial to an adult were real problems to a young girl and sought with sympathetic understanding to guide her in the solution of them.

Cynthia's home life was happy. She was loved and returned the love in full measure. She was encouraged to make friends and enjoy activities outside the home, but home and family were always waiting for her in time of difficulty. She was a beautiful, unspoiled girl. She was allowed normal social activities, but her mother did not push her to make a great social success of her. Her education in sex was adequate. From the time she was a little girl her questions were answered truthfully, carefully, and as fully as she could comprehend for her years. She knew about menstruation before her first period, and was prepared to accept it as a normal function. She respected and appreciated the femininity of her body as shown by her careful dress and the problem that had brought her for medical care.

Cynthia thought her breasts were too large and was quite self-conscious about them and fearful that they might continue to grow. She had been menstruating regularly for about a year and only recently her periods had become painful. Physical examination showed her to be a normal girl, a little on the chubby side. Her breasts, well developed, were perhaps larger than usually found in girls of her age, but not abnormally so. It was explained to her that the hormones from her ovaries caused the breasts to grow, starting years before her first menstruation. The fact that she was menstruating regularly indicated that her ovaries had settled down to a normal balance and probably would not cause further growth of the breast tissue. However, there was one way that she could do something. The whole breast consists of a large amount of fat. If she allowed herself to put on more weight, there would be more fat deposited in the breasts, and they would become larger. Therefore, she must watch her weight.

For every Cynthia, there are dozens of girls and women who are concerned about the smallness of their breasts. Some feel shamed or cheated and are convinced that they are somehow less women because they have not attained what is to them the most precious badge of femininity. The importance women attach to the size of the breasts is attested to by the number and diversity of means offered for their development. These means include mechanical gadgets, exercises, lotions, and creams, all of which are ineffectual. There have been various forms of plastic surgery to lift the breasts, to add an extra padding of fat from another part of the body, or to increase the size by implanting an artificial padding of paraffin or one of the new plastic materials. All are failures and may be dangerous.

Most women with small breasts do the sensible thing, albeit sometimes reluctantly, and accept the size of their breasts for what it is; an individual characteristic that is the result of heritage of body size and body form and of the degree of perfection of growth and maturation.

In childhood the breasts appear to be no more than little pinkish rosebuds to which the little girl pays scant attention. They are small, inconspicuous, and no different from what little boys have. But when her sexuality begins to unfold, it is the change in the breasts that she notices first and about which she becomes a little alarmed and perhaps ashamed. Something is happening to her body that others can see, and she doesn't like it. So she refuses to wear sweaters or tight blouses that reveal the new form of her breasts (ignoring the curves that are developing elsewhere and that are just as tell-tale). But this phase soon passes, and she wants to wear a bra whether she has any need for it or not.

Breasts have a way of developing that gives them peculiar contours at different phases. It is an interesting story that has its beginning in the Age of the Unborn.

Before birth, in the very early months of development, nature does a peculiar thing. She lays the pattern not for just two breasts, but for many pairs of breasts arranged in rows along the front of the body like buttons of a double-breasted suit. She doesn't follow through with this plan but selects just the upper pair, and the rest fade away. At birth there are only the two little pinkish nipples. Sometimes, however, the erasure of the others is not complete, and one or more of these little nipples remain and in youth increase a little in size and become deeply pigmented. Many women have these little "accessory nipples" and, not knowing what they really are, accept them for what they look like, brown moles.

At birth and all through childhood, the glandular element (which will comprise the largest part of the breasts in the adult) is only a tight little bud of tissue just under the skin and nipple, but it is capable of growth and development when the girl's endocrine glands furnish the necessary stimulation. The important fact is that the amount they are capable of growing has already been fixed in this little bud at birth or perhaps long before. This accounts for the fact that some women have small breasts, which hormone creams, hormone injections, massage, and the many devices advertised to develop their womanly bosoms will not change. None of these devices can increase in size something that is not there to grow in the first place. The buds had the potentiality to produce just so much glandular tissue—and no more.

The maturation of the breasts in youth consists of increase in size due to the development of the glandular tissue, which is padded with a varying amount of fat, and the growth of the nipple with its surrounding brown areolar. The appearance or contour of the breast goes through several phases, which is most apparent in profile. The first change from the almost complete flatness of childhood is the elevation of the nipple and areolar into a cone shape. As the bud of glandular tissue grows and sends out the finger-like processes, the breast mound begins to form with the little conical nipple above. Sometimes this increase in glandular tissue and fat is so rapid that the skin cannot accommodate it. The connective tissue fibers break under the stretching and red lines or striae appear. These later turn white but never disappear entirely. Finally, the mound of glandular tissue becomes rounded, the cone sinks down so that the areolar is flat and only the papilla projects above the domed or hemispherical breast.

Nature frequently does not accomplish perfect results, and in maturity the breasts are still small or cone-shaped like those of early youth. Occasionally, she overdoes it and the breasts are of excessive size.

Her Figure

The change in contour of the body is another manifestation of feminine maturation. Some of this is due to feminine directional change in bone structure, particularly the widening of the pelvic girdle. But most of the feminine curves are due to the change in the amount and distribution of subcutaneous fat. The girl loses some of the soft layer of fat on her chest and back and gains additional padding on the hips and thighs and within the breasts. The problems arising from this are not usually qualitative (where fat is) but quantitative (how much fat is distributed within the body as a whole).

Overweight is one of the most common problems of adolescent girls, and it can become one of the most serious if it is not properly handled. Many girls enter the Age of Youth considerably overweight. Mothers, even doctors, are prone to say that this is baby fat and that it will disappear when the girl starts to menstruate. This is only partly true. With the onset of maturation there is a change in the distribution of fat, but this does not necessarily mean that the excessive fat will be lost. When a girl does not lose this weight, she should have help, and she should have it early, for overweight can be a great trial to the girl growing into womanhood and may affect her whole life. Dr. Jane is a case in point.

Women and the careers they choose raise many interesting questions. Why are some content to lead leisurely existences while others exert themselves so long and so hard to perfect and establish themselves in a chosen career? There is a different answer for every woman. I asked Dr. Jane, a woman of middle age, why she had chosen the career of a research scientist. She hesitated a moment, smiled and replied, "I suppose because I was such a fat little girl." Seeing the surprised and questioning look on my face, she explained.

Dr. Jane was the youngest of three children in a family of two girls and a boy. Her sister, ten years older than she, was an attractive young lady having a gay social life when the future scientist was a chubby young girl entering the difficult period of adolescence. The sister represented an ideal that Jane thought she could never attain. The brother, a few years older and mother's pride and joy, teased Jane unmercifully, particularly about her weight, calling her "fatsy." Jane became self-conscious and unsure of herself, shy, refusing to participate with others in the normal activities of her age group. Instead, she sought some field in which she could excel and found it in her school work. She was never satisfied unless she made the highest marks in her studies. Meantime, no one ever thought to help her with her weight problem. By the time she had reached college, her pattern of work and academic achievement was established, and her interests led to science as a career. Along the way she had learned for herself what to do about her weight, and when I knew her she was streamlined.

Not many youngsters who are overweight are fortunate enough to be able to compensate in other ways, as was Dr. Jane, and few are able to control their weight without some help. Some are unhappy and find solace in eating and so get even fatter. Some try and with the tempestuousness of youth go on a starvation diet for a few days, only to break it, overeat ravenously, and gain back all and more than they have lost.

When a young girl is very much overweight, she has a serious problem, and it should be treated as such. But it is folly to force the issue. Little can be accomplished until the girl herself wants to lose weight and is ready and willing to assume some responsibility and to deny herself the pleasure of eating. The desire to be attractive and to look like other girls is characteristic of youth and will provide adequate incentive for a girl if she is encouraged rather then teased and scolded for her efforts. But she needs more than this. She needs guidance.

The mother can be of great help by providing a diet that is not only correct, but also satisfying, and by keeping the tempting but restricted foods out of sight. Her understanding and encouragement will also be helpful. Usually, however, this is not enough, and better results are obtained when the girl is placed under the care of a doctor who appreciates the importance of the problem and is willing to take the necessary time and trouble to correct it.

Such a doctor will give the girl a specific well-balanced diet, check her regularly not only to see that she is losing weight but to be sure that she continues to be well nourished. There will be times when the girl will falter or make mistakes. A little encouragement and sympathetic understanding of her problem will restore her perspective and determination. Thus good medical care for overweight is not just the restriction of food for a limited period of time. It is the teaching of new and better habits of eating that will serve the girl well the rest of her life.

Very often a mother takes her daughter to the doctor because she thinks the problem of overweight is a glandular one that can be cured by medication. This is never completely true. Obesity is rarely caused by glandular dysfunction alone and never can be corrected by medication alone. Occasionally, there is some glandular deficiency that appropriate medication will help. And the doctor may give the girl tablets to curb her appetite. But the fundamental and essential element of management of all cases of obesity is diet. Both the doctor and the girl can rejoice as they see their efforts transform an unhappy misfit into a well-poised, attractive young woman.

There is one other point concerning weight that should be emphasized—what constitutes normal weight and ideal weight. Girls have their own ideals about what they should weigh, which are quite often wrong. They want to reduce below what is good for their health. Sometimes this ideal is based on measurements of beauty queens and fashion models. The beauty queen's weight may be normal for her because she has a small frame, whereas the girl in question may have heavy bone structure and for her to reduce that extra ten pounds or so would jeopardize her health. Also those girls whose figures are their fortune maintain a figure that will photograph well. As we know, the camera makes us look larger than we are and is merciless in recording the little bulges here and there. So to be photogenic, these glamour girls are considerably underweight.

The ideal weight, therefore, must be determined for each girl. It may approximate that of charts and tables, but it must have as its final criterion the weight at which the girl not only looks better but feels better and is in the best of health. As a matter of fact, a few extra pounds are an advantage in youth in helping her maintain normal vigor and resistance to disease during the period the body is being subjected to the extra stress of rapid growth and maturation.

Her Complexion

The skin is a badge of femininity; it proclaims woman's sexuality. It is also one of the prime ingredients of her feminine beauty. As such, it may be a source of pride in its perfection, or a disfigurement that is a stumbling block in her progress to maturity.

The "bloom of youth" conjures up a picture of fair soft skin delicately colored, glowing with health, and free from wrinkles and blemishes. One might suppose it to be the rightful heritage of youth. It is certainly widely proclaimed as the criterion of perfection for woman in all her ages. This, however, is contradicted by the fact that adolescent acne is also accepted as commonplace to youth, a phase of growing up, another part of the awkwardness that is normal for the age.

The skin of a young girl can be beautiful, but frequently it is not. Blemishes of the skin are the source of much unhappiness. They not only mar her appearance, but they may affect her ability to enjoy her girlhood. Equally important, they may leave scars not only on her face but on her personality in the years that follow. One must not look on these pimples on the brow, the face, or the back as purely local blemishes that can be covered up or left alone in the hope that they will disappear. Rather, one must view them as a disturbance in the function of an important organ in the process of maturation.

As an organ and badge of femininity, the skin responds to the call to maturation by the endocrine glands and undergoes not only rapid growth in all its structural elements but also changes that render it typically feminine. Estrogen and the thyroid hormone exert a beneficent effect on the whole skin, causing it to maintain a smooth soft texture. The most apparent changes are the rapid increase in the size and activity of the sebaceous glands and the appearance of the sexual hair. These are due to the increased production by the adrenals of other sex steroids—androgens and possibly progesterone. Disturbances in these result in the two skin problems most typical of the age, hirsutism and acne.

Adolescent acne is so familiar that a case history is unnecessary. Acne has its beginnings in the abnormal function of the sebaceous glands. These are tiny coiled structures that pour their oily secretions into the base of the hair follicles. Only the oil glands of certain areas of the body are susceptible—the face, chest, back, and shoulders. In acne there is a plugging of the gland at its opening due to overgrowth and increased thickness of the skin and an accumulation of the fat secretion in the gland, producing at first large pores, blackheads, and whiteheads, which may lead to redness, swelling, and tenderness around each follicle, causing the pimple. When infection is added, pus accumulates and the pimple takes on the appearance of a miniature boil. When the process is severe, damage is done to the follicle, which leads to pitting and scarring after the acute stage subsides. This is a serious problem that involves one or many follicles at a time and moves on to others or recurs.

Thus acne is not one single reaction but the result of several—increased activity in the follicle, inflammation, infection, and local susceptibility at a particular age. To this may be added the genetic factor—some types of skin appear to be more susceptible than others. The fact that acne occurs at the time the sex glands become functional and pour their hormones into the blood stream is certain evidence that they are in some way responsible, but the question is—which hormones and why?

The sebaceous glands increase in size and pour out more oil as a part of the sexual maturation process reaching a peak sometime after puberty (menarche). It is during this period of growth that acne occurs, and after growth ceases, acne disappears. The male hormone, androgen, would seem to play the major role in the production of acne, as evidenced by many known facts. It provides a powerful stimulus to the sebaceous glands and will produce acne in either a normal male or female when administered in large doses. This would account for acne in the adolescent male whose gonads are accelerating the production of androgen. But the mechanism in the female is less apparent. It has been assumed in the case of the female that androgen is also the active factor and is produced by the adrenals. But there is other evidence that progesterone has a similar stimulating effect on the sebaceous glands, and that its excess or unbalanced action is the mechanism of the production of acne in the female.

Estrogen, on the other hand, produces no growth stimulus to the sebaceous glands but inhibits excessive keratinization or thickening. It therefore works to prevent rather than to cause acne. Thyroid hormone has a similar action—to keep the skin in normal texture and vitality.

There are other factors that contribute to the production of acne, such as diet. Fats and especially carbohydrates increase the production of oil. Vitamin A is important in the process of keratinization, deficiency of this vitamin leading to thickness. Acne flares with certain foods, especially those that contain iodine and chocolate, and with certain drugs. It is usually self-limited, burning itself out by the age of 20 or 25, but this is small comfort to the young girl who suffers the blemishes of youth and may reach maturity with a permanently scarred face. Therefore, correct treatment should be started early before damage is done to the girl's personality as well as to her complexion. Treatment is directed toward removing the plug that closed the gland, decreasing the activity of the gland that overfills it with oil, and eliminating the factors that cause irritation, flare-ups, and recurrences.

There are some things that a girl must do for herself. Perhaps the most important is recognizing acne for what it is and rejecting the many false ideas associated with it. There is no evidence that acne is due to bad blood, too much acid, allergy, constipation, or the result of improper sex practices.

Acne is helped by scrupulous cleanliness, and a young girl will certainly be tempted to use some of the medicated soaps, creams, and lotions so enticingly advertised with the promise of a beautiful skin. But self-medication is dangerous for many reasons. In the first place all blemishes are not acne but may be other disorders, which may require a different approach. Secondly, there is no one specific cure for acne. All skins do not respond to the same treatment in the same way. When acne is mild, the simple measures of cleanliness, good hygiene, and diet may be sufficient. In the really troublesome cases these will not be enough, and acne then should be considered a skin disease that requires the care of a specialist.

Ier Hair

Woman's hair is her crowning glory. Whether she wears it short or ong, curled or straight, it is always an important part of her feminine ppearance. On the other hand, hair on other parts of her body, which s especially apparent when a woman is wearing a bathing suit, is con-idered unfeminine and something that should be concealed or removed. Actually the hair on her body is a feminine characteristic that first appears s she begins to mature and usually follows a definite pattern.

The first sign that maturation is beginning is the appearance of a ew hairs in the pubic region, the mons and the outer lips. This increases n amount, spreading out to cover the outer labia and upward to cover he mons and forming a straight line across the lower border of the bdomen. In the male the pubic hair extends upward on the abdomen orming a triangle with the peak at the umbilicus. Occasionally girls vill have a little line of hair or even a small triangle on the abdomen and n later years a few hairs on the chest between the breasts and a few long airs around the nipple. None of these are indicative of abnormality. The ubic hair is usually well developed before any becomes apparent in the xillary region and both are quite apparent before menarche.

Complete absence of this sexual distribution of hair occurs only in the are cases of complete failure of maturation. Excessive or masculine distri-ution of hair in girls and women is fairly common. In most cases it has ittle or no significance from the standpoint of essential femininity and ertility. Only in rare cases does it indicate a serious endocrine problem. 'rom a psychological standpoint, however, whatever may be the cause, xcessive hair (hirsutism) may be a handicap of considerable importance o a girl. She considers it unfeminine, a masculine attribute. Many girls arry this problem to their doctor. Maria was such a case.

Maria and her mother came in together. Before anyone spoke, Maria ooked at me so searchingly and beseechingly that I wondered what could ave happened to one so young and lovely to induce such tragic appeal n her eyes. She told her story in a high sweet voice with a hint of a oreign accent.

Maria was 18 years old and had come to this country from southern Europe only two years previously. The cause of her present distress was

the appearance of hair along her chin line and a little fuzz over her lips.
She was in terror that she would develop a mustache and beard.

As she told her story, I looked at her mother and saw the probable
answer. Both were brunettes, and there was a strong resemblance between
the two. The mother had a heavy head of hair with the hair line low
on her forehead and dipping down in front of her ears. She too had hair
on her face, more than Maria. Perhaps, I thought, she has gone through
this same heartache as a girl and is hoping that something can be done
to spare her daughter the experience.

To understand how the problem of excessive hair is studied and what
can be done about it, we must first know more about the normal. We
are all part male, part female. During the Age of the Unborn, as we
have seen, there is a time when the primary organs of both sexes are
present. The body never loses completely this bi-sexuality or male-female-
ness. Thus every woman has potentially the same hair adornment as the
male. Furthermore, her glands produce not only estrogen as the dominant
sex hormone, but also an appreciable amount of the male sex hormone,
androgen. Whether she can keep these factors in feminine balance or
have the scales tipped in the direction of masculinity or hirsutism depends
on two factors.

The first factor in the production of hirsutism is the relative sensitivity
of the dormant hair follicles, which girls have in the same distribution
as boys. The hair follicles will always respond and grow when large
amounts of androgen are present or administered, but they are more
sensitive and responsive to small amounts of androgen in some women than
in others. The second factor is the actual amounts of estrogen and androgen that the glands produce. Thus a slight excess of androgen applied
to sensitive dormant hair follicles will cause the hair to grow and become
apparent. This balance is a hereditary character, that is, we inherit glands
that function a certain way and skin of a certain structure and sensitivity
just as we do the color of hair and eyes or the shape of the nose. Hirsutism
of this type is normal, and there is nothing we can do to prevent or
cure it. It can only be removed.

However, there are rare cases where hirsutism is a part of masculinization
of the body that results from congenital defects or abnormal function of
the endocrine glands. The abnormal function may be the result either

of tumor growth in the ovary, pituitary, or adrenal glands or of overactivity of the adrenal gland. The differentiation of normal hirsutism from masculinization may be a very difficult problem in some cases requiring a thorough study including physical examination, X-rays, and special tests to determine the relative amounts of estrogen and androgen being produced.

Maria's physical findings were normal. She had no other masculine features, such as heavy musculature, deep voice, or enlargement of the clitoris. On the contrary, she was quite feminine, with well-developed breasts, high-pitched voice, and normally developed internal reproductive organs. X-ray studies produced no evidence of a tumor of the glands. These examinations were not sufficient to rule out the possibility that the adrenals were producing excessive androgen.

Maria was instructed to keep a basal temperature record, and a premenstrual endometrial biopsy specimen was obtained. These are the same tests that we use in fertility studies to determine the character of ovarian function. Both indicated that Maria was having normal ovarian cycles with ovulation. This would not have been the case if there had been hormonal imbalance, for excessive androgen suppresses normal pituitary-ovarian function. That she was not producing excessive androgen was further indicated when no excessive amount of 17-keto steroids (the form in which the male hormone is excreted) was found in the urine.

When all the studies were complete, what could we tell Maria? Not very much that would make her happier, for her problem was one of heredity, and she would have to learn to live with it. But there was the consolation that there was no tumor, which would require surgery, and no serious endocrine imbalance. Furthermore, since she had reached sexual maturity with normal ovarian function, it would seem probable that there would be no further increase in amount of hair, as she feared. We could reassure her that she was in every way a very feminine person and should enjoy woman's normal life of marriage and children.

Maria accepted these explanations but was still concerned with the immediate problem of getting rid of the hair. Would hormone creams or pills or injections help? What about electrolysis? She had read that hormone creams, meaning estrogen, will make the excessive hair drop out. This is not true. Estrogen by whatever means administered—as creams, by mouth, or by injections—will in no way reduce the existing hirsutism and may have undesirable side-effects of temporary disturbance of the normal ovarian cycle.

The natural inclination is to shave or pluck the offensive hairs on the face. This is usually not advisable, for it carries the possibility of irritating the skin and hair follicle, and as the hair grows back, as it will, the blemish is still more obvious. Repeated bleaching, on the other hand, may be very helpful. It not only makes the hair less obvious but may in the long run suppress the growth by making the hair brittle so that it breaks off and reduces the follicle's ability to grow new hair. Electrolysis is the surest way to destroy the hair follicle, and when performed by a qualified person, it is a safe procedure. It has the disadvantages of being a slow, tedious, sometimes uncomfortable, and always expensive procedure. X-ray treatment should never be used for hirsutism. The results are apt to disfigure more than that for which it was used.

ADVANCING TOWARD MATURITY

The patterns of physical growth and maturation, at times beset with difficulties, are matched by equally defined patterns of change in two other aspects of a girl's personality, the psychological and the sexual. To achieve a successful transition from childhood to womanhood in all these aspects of her personality, the young girl needs understanding, training, and guidance. The importance of these needs becomes most apparent in cases where they have not been met, for the failure to achieve the physical badges of femininity may impede her progress toward maturity on other levels. Failure to advance toward maturity on the psychological and sexual levels has a similar effect and may contribute to delinquency in youth and serious problems of maladjustment in adult life.

Toward Emotional Maturity

We accept the fact that adolescence is an awkward age physically. It is apparent that the girl is growing rapidly and that she is having difficulty in learning to handle her new body proportions gracefully. At times she seems all arms and legs. She slouches, she stumbles. We make allowances for her clumsiness. But when we come to her emotional reactions, we may forget that here too it is an awkward age.

Mr. and Mrs. Brown were very unhappy and bewildered parents as they told about their fourteen-year-old daughter. Their's had been a late marriage, and it was several years before their only child, Jo Ellen, was born. Her childhood had been a source of great joy and satisfaction to them. She had been a sweet, quiet, obedient child. But lately she had changed to a complete stranger to them. She did not want to have any part in home affairs and resented being asked to help her mother with household tasks. She was critical of her parents; nothing they said or did pleased her. She had suddenly grown to a tall gangling girl, careless of her dress. She was secretive about herself and her activities away from home. Recently she had developed a crush on another girl whom her parents did not approve of and she sulked when denied permission to associate with her after it was learned that the two were secretly meeting boys they knew little about. The Browns were sure Jo Ellen was headed for disaster unless something was done.

In seeking a solution, they wondered whether there was something physically wrong with her glands or whether they should take her to see a psychiatrist. They had no insight into what was happening to Jo Ellen —that she was trying to launch out from home port and take her place as an adult in an adult world. She was not making a very satisfactory job of it. The failure was partly a result of her own inadequacies but more because she had had no preparation through childhood and was without sympathetic understanding and guidance from her parents at this difficult period in her life.

The way a girl will react in this transition period will vary greatly, depending on the temperament of the girl, her family background and training, and the type of social contacts she has at the time. But at best it may be a period of great emotional instability. It is a period of weaning away from home and family. She feels the need to make new social contacts and receive emotional satisfaction from people outside the home. She must give up her protected place as a child in the home and stand on her own. Often this first emotional contact outside the home is intense and takes the form of crushes on other girls or teachers—and later love affairs. This transference of emotional interest is not always easy. She i torn between being a protected child and an independent, responsibl adult. Childhood impulses and memories are all mixed up with glimpse of adult independence. Because she is unsure of herself, she is very sensi tive. Failure, teasing, ridicule are unbearable at times. She is on th defensive, and because of this she may give the impression of being self assertive.

Her problems pertaining to self are greatly exaggerated. The factors o the orbit of her life—her personal self, her clothes, her house, her parents– and whether they measure up to what she thinks they should be are al important. She has not as yet acquired a philosophy of life. She has no learned to take the good with the bad, success and failure. Failure i crushing, and success is just as hard for her to take gracefully—she struts For most, full emotional maturity is finally attained after many readjust ments, with acquisition of skills in co-ordinating, organizing, evaluating and accepting the experiences of life. But many never attain it.

Toward Sexual Maturity

There is an Age of Youth because our complex culture dictates tha there must be an interval between the physical acquisition of fertilit and the assumption of that responsibility in marriage and parenthood Failure on the girl's part to understand and to conform may lead to tragi situations, the most obvious being illegitimate pregnancy.

The story of Amy (a case of amenorrhea cited in "The Age of Matur ity") is an example. She frequently went to the house of neighbors ir the evening to "baby-sit." At first she was alone and then her boy frienc started meeting her there, a fact unknown to her parents and the coupl for whom she was baby-sitting. One evening study gave way to pettin; and petting to experimentation, and Amy became pregnant.

This case is typical of most teen-age illegitimate pregnancies. The scen or opportunity may be different, but they have the same causes. The are the result of lack of training and discipline in the sexual aspects o life, which include not only the physiological facts of sex and the potentia results of sex activity but also the meaning of sex on the psychologica level. The far more important failure, tragic as such a pregnancy is, doe

ot stem from the mere premature exercise of a biological function. Rather
is the failure to achieve understanding and acceptance of the meaning
f sex, which is the common experience of far too many young girls.

The awakening of sex, the consciousness of her femininity, is the domi-
ant characteristic of the Age of Youth. Sex impulses begin to emerge
when the girl begins to feel the need to broaden her horizons. She is no
onger satisfied to be loved only because she is a member of the small
ircle of family. She seeks to be an independent person in the whole
world of people. But she is not sure of herself. At first she is attracted
o girls of her own age. This is the age of crushes, exchange of confidences,
nterminable telephone conversations, and withdrawal from the family.
Attraction to the opposite sex is idealistic and impersonal, but girls may
lmost deify older males, giving them adulation and expecting nothing in
return. Boys of her own age are of less importance, partly because they
ag a year or so behind her in entering the period of maturation. But the
period of homosexual attraction passes, and the stage is entered where
he girl must seek her sexual satisfaction from the opposite sex.

The awareness of her sex takes the form of awareness of the femininity
f her body as a whole, and she gains satisfaction in the recognition of her
ttractiveness to the opposite sex. The sex impulse in the girl toward
ctual mating is not strong. Even sex experience is indulged in more out
f curiosity and desire to please the male than for personal physical satis-
action. In juvenile sex delinquents it has been found that girls enter sex
lay not to relieve an inner sex tension, as does the male, but to please
he male. Unfortunately, this interpretation of the meaning of sex to
woman is halted at the juvenile level as the ultimate goal of feminine
exuality.

Nature announces to the girl that she is on the way to maturity at about
he age of twelve. She sees her body growing rapidly to adult size and
aking on the form and characteristics of an adult woman. And she begins
o experience nature's urge for fulfillment of her sexuality. She suddenly
ecognizes that males are interesting creatures and becomes intensely
lesirous that the male should find her interesting also. So she begins
er quest for a mate. But it is not to be as easy as that. Society says she
must wait. The fact that she will not be legally of age until she is
wenty-one, although some privileges will be accorded her at eighteen,

does not bother her at all. She is little concerned with legality except when it obtrudes itself on her quest for a mate by saying that she is too young to be married or that her intended mate must serve his time in military service.

To satisfy this need for recognition of their sexuality by the opposite sex, youth has taken into her, and his, own hands—too early and too strenuously—the selection of activities they consider appropriate. As the result we have the spectacle of formal parties for the two' sexes at ages as young as 12 and 14, of dating and "going steady" at twelve or even earlier and of "being engaged to be engaged" in the early teens, of "fan clubs" devoted to the worship of some crooning or hip-swaying male entertainer—the epitome of maleness, and of the mass hysteria invoked by the cacophony of sounds considered music, which arouses the most primitive of instincts and emotions. All of these lead to early sexual experimentation, beginning with the casual kiss and embrace, and advanced by necking and petting. Add to this the ingredients of alcohol and drugs too easily available, and the stage is set—not for fulfillment, but for catastrophe.

Meanwhile, her elders stand on the sidelines—sometimes apprehensive, sometimes ignoring the situation, but too frequently failing to give her the guidance so desperately needed. They allow to pass unchallenged the propaganda continuously aimed at her that the acquisition of sexual allure is all that she needs to be a success, and fail to impress on her that being an adult in the complex, highly technical world of today is a serious business and that success is attained by self-restraint through a long period of training and education. Sexuality is a powerful force that she must learn to control and use wisely.

Sex Education

While boys and girls may intuitively know how to gratify the sex urge and can perform the sex act, the biologic significance is not intuitive. They must be taught. Primitive people did not understand the relationship that existed between intercourse and a baby that arrived nine months later. For her own protection a girl should be taught early. Adequate sex education teaches the difference between the meaning of sex and the meaning of love and that the two are not synonymous. Sex is a physical drive for self-satisfaction. Love is giving for the happiness and welfare of another.

The actual facts of reproduction should be given when a girl is ready, in answers to questions as they arise. It should be given by the mother, because a good mother knows her daughter, understands her needs, her moods, and has her confidence. She is the one best suited to instruct her daughter and to establish sex as a part of the high ideals of marriage. She can teach that final sex gratification should be an act of giving supremely to the one most loved for their mutual happiness and not just for what she can get out of it for herself. Thus premarital training has as its aim a way of life for which a person gradually matures. Full attainment of such maturity is made easier if careful guidance has always been a part of the girl's life.

Parents ask what is the best way to give their daughter sex education. The answer is that, in the broader sense, they have been doing it ever since she was a baby and will continue to do so until she leaves home. A child is born into a world differentiated as to sex—mother and father, brothers and sisters, aunts and uncles. What she accepts as her adult place in life as wife and mother is determined by what she sees in marriage every day—love, courtesy, mutual respect, co-operation, and sharing of responsibility. Parents may be consciously giving or withholding the actual facts of reproduction during these years, but they are establishing attitudes toward sex by precept and example for good or bad. A healthy attitude toward sex is the parents' responsibility. To establish such an attitude, the parents must have such an attitude themselves. They must be informed as to general facts and must be able to impart these facts with clarity and dignity and with no feeling of embarrassment, guilt, or shame.

Parents may be reluctant to talk about the physical facts of sex, but that doesn't mean the girl will not learn them. It is literally thrown at her in magazines, novels, the songs she hears, the shows she sees. But the tragic fact is that the physical act of sex is masqueraded under the name of love. A great deal is now being said about the necessity of sex education in the schools, which apparently means giving children the "facts of life," with the reasoning that if they know the intricate biologic facts of the reproductive function, meaning primarily sex desires and sexual intercourse, they will avoid sexual problems and unwanted pregnancies.

There is nothing wrong with giving girls all the information they want and are able to understand about the facts of reproduction. It is a wonderful story, and the truth will dispel doubts and fears. Some will want a lot of information; some will be disinterested. The truth about sex is never harmful if it is the simple truth, in which sex is integrated with other aspects and ideals of life, not magnified or distorted, and if it is given at a time when the individual is able to accept and understand it. The actual teaching of sex should be a part of revealing the wonders of nature—the science of life, which encompasses the world of living things as well as that of the children's own bodies. This can and should be started in the first grade and added to each year.

The atomic age, which came on us so suddenly and has advanced with such breath-taking speed, has accentuated the need for the teaching of science in the early years. This has been directed largely to the fields of mathematics, chemistry, and physics, which deal with the physical world, the laws that govern it, and the uses that man has learned to make of his knowledge of those sciences. In teaching science, more stress should be placed on revealing to young people the wonders of the living things that are so easily available to everyone but so rarely seen. Not the least of these is the marvel of reproduction. A great deal of ridicule has been directed at the teaching of sex in terms of "the birds and the bees," ridicule that may be deserved when this is taken out of context and used as an illustration for sex to be taught in one single lesson. In the complete story (which really is endless) of the world of nature, one learns the true meaning of sex, as well as the physical facts of reproduction.

There is an added bonus to this teaching of nature that will pay dividends for the rest of life. The atomic age has changed man's environment and broadened his horizons, but it has not changed human nature and the age-old problems of individual peace of mind and of people living together in harmony. Rather it has presented the individual with greater difficulties in satisfying his need for achievement, independence, responsibility, belonging, and in finding the meaning of life. An understanding and appreciation of nature is a source of peace and inspiration. We may see on every hand examples of man's desire to identify himself with the world of nature—in the trek to the suburbs, outdoor sports, gardening, hiking, bird study, travel to nature's beauty spots, and the effort of some to increase their knowledge of the out-of-doors, and of the conservation associations to preserve our heritage of nature's gifts.

Toward Intellectual Maturity

There is a wide difference in the ease with which youth today may achieve maturity in the various aspects of personality. On the physical level there is a positive approach with the accent on health based on sound knowledge of how best to achieve good health and how to correct the abnormalities that may arise. On the sexual level there is a recognition of the importance of sex, but there is also a lack of sound knowledge and understanding and a great deal of misinformation. But there is no lack of discussion. One sometimes gets the impression that some "moderns" consider the greatest discovery of the atomic age to be sex.

When it comes to the intellectual phase of a girl's development, there is a great void. Often she is not told why she needs to continue her formal education; she is not told what kind of education will be meaningful; she is not even told that she needs education. This may stem in part from the present-day concept of education. There is great pressure for conformity, social adjustment, equal and free education for all. At the same time, intellectual attainment finds little favor. For the most part the content of education is aimed at security for the individual and, recently, at the advancement of science for our national security. The needs of maturity would best be met by the kind of education that seeks out each individual's intellectual potentialities and emphasizes her responsibility to develop and utilize to the fullest these capabilities.

There is no general agreement on the amount of education that is desirable for a girl. While it is true that a large proportion of girls go through high school and many go to college, only a small percentage of those who have the mental capabilities for advanced education are receiving it. In recent years there has been an increase in early marriages, which usually means that the girl drops out of school and frequently takes some small job to help her husband through school. Others stop to take a business course that will enable them to earn a small salary until they are married.

It is not difficult to point out the error in this and to give valid reasons why a girl should have as much education as she is capable of assimilating The hard fact is that many women are now working whether from choice or not. One fourth of the labor force today is made up of women and mostly married women. The number decreases in the specialized fields in proportion to the amount of training required.

In our present complex world education has become essential in order to earn a living, to get ahead, and to acquire status. More training is needed to fill the jobs that science has created. But that very fact carries the danger of overspecialization and loss of individuality. Most jobs will include repetitive function in a very limited area, which yields little in the sense of accomplishment. An equally important product of the modern age is an increase in the amount of leisure produced by the shorter work day and week, longer vacations, and, particularly earlier retirement. If woman is going to work, she should have training that will not just equip her to earn but will aid her in selecting the work that will bring her not just a pay check, but satisfaction in her job, and that will open avenues for real enjoyment and personal growth in her leisure time.

These same general facts hold true if the girl chooses marriage and homemaking as her main career, for these require many talents and broad training for true success. This is also a short-term career. It becomes part time when all the children are in school and she is advanced to a consultative capacity as they leave home for college and careers of their own. Thus her retirement comes early, at forty-five to fifty years of age, and she still has twenty-five to thirty more years ahead. How will she fill this leisure time unless she has acquired and nurtured other interests, of which education is the richest source? Whether work or marriage, or a combination of the two, is to be her career, a woman should make the most of educational opportunities available to her.

When we come to the question of what kind of education a woman should have, there is no simple answer. We have not yet achieved "ideal education" and have not formulated opinions as to what constitutes ideal education for woman. Modern education has made two concessions to woman in the opportunities afforded her. First it has allowed her to pursue any field that she may choose although she has not yet received equal recognition or recompense for her achievements. It also has added a special technical course for her in home economics, the skills women have usually seemed able to acquire on their own at home.

Education for a woman, even if she goes on to advanced study, is not directed toward self-discipline, the search for truth, and the recognition of her individual responsibility to be a contributing member of a democratic society from the feminine standpoint. Rather it is the same education offered the male, which for the most part has evolved into merely training for a way to earn a living. She may pursue it and enter into competition with the male, trying to fulfill herself at the expense of her feminine function, or she may try to do both. More often the only attraction such education affords is a chance to conform to what others are doing and to kill time with the added attraction of a greater opportunity of finding a husband.

Recently there has been some change. We have been scared into realizing that education should be directed toward the individual's development to use his or her ability for the national good—especially for scientific advancement. We should pause for a moment and realize that we also need mature individuals with the capabilities of applying and integrating these advances for human welfare on levels other than national security, as expressed in the arms race, or even than other sciences, including health.

Merely pointing out some of the needs for educational attainments as they pertain to woman's maturity as an individual does not offer any solution for the problem—nor is a solution at present in sight. It may be best that marriage is early and the lines of responsibilities of the sexes not drawn so rigidly, but if this is so, there must be other changes made to compensate. Perhaps education should be speeded up so that an adequate amount could be obtained at an earlier age. This could be done if some of the frills were omitted and more concentrated effort required on the part of the students.

The content of education might be changed from accumulation of facts to the pursuit and appreciation of truth and orientation in our rich heritage of knowledge, and the emphasis shifted from "life adjustment" to the responsibilities of maturity. Perhaps students should be divided according to individual abilities and aptitudes. Perhaps woman's education should be along the lines in which she excels, which includes the humanities, and not merely toward earning money as the male's competitor. The world is certainly in dire need of trained people in this area.

Whatever time may prove to be the ideal education for woman, there can be no doubt that the young girl of today should take advantage of the education now available to her. She will need it in the Age of Maturity and the Age of Marriage and Motherhood. But the true significance of her education may have its greatest impact as she experiences another period of transition, for she will require the use of all her potentialities if she is to have and enjoy an Age of Serenity.

THE MENOPAUSE

XXII

THE SECOND PERIOD OF TRANSITION

THIS SIXTH AGE OF WOMAN has no appropriate name, that is, one which is truly descriptive of its nature and meaning. The reason is simple: it is different for every woman. There is no fixed pattern, no chain of events that must transpire. The onset is imperceptible, the end unpredictable, the duration indefinite, and the experience different for every woman as she passes through it. It is a transition period in which a woman passes from fertility to infertility, and the one and only experience common to all women is the cessation of menstruation. "Menopause," meaning cessation of menstruation, fails to convey the true significance of the age.

You may think that it should not be called an age, and that would be correct except for two reasons. It is a period of readjustment that involves every aspect of feminine personality—woman's moods and emotions, her mind and body. Usually, this readjustment is accomplished smoothly and without obvious symptoms, but for some women it may be a period of many and varied discomforts and occasionally of acute illness. Most important, woman herself considers it an age, which she approaches with reluctance and sometimes with fear because of the many misconceptions, myths, and superstitions that are passed on to her.

WHAT'S IN A NAME?

The false concepts about the menopause are revealed in names that are given to the age, such as "the change of life," "the changing years," "the climax," "the climacteric," "the critical years." All these carry the implication of impending doom, that a life of happiness and fulfillment is possible for a limited time only and then the hour strikes, and woman's life is over. There remains for her a barren and futile future. No wonder woman dreads such a change. But a few moments of consideration of each of these names will reveal their falsity, and a little knowledge of the basic physiology of this age of woman will dispel the doubts and fears.

"The change of life" is the most commonly used misnomer and carries the most dire implications. It signifies that when a woman reaches a certain age, there will be a change or transformation from which she emerges as something entirely different. She, it seems to say, will lose the cherished characteristics of her femininity and be less a woman. She will suffer not only loss of fertility but also her feminine sexuality and will become the "neuter sex." She can no longer be attractive to her mate or even present a satisfactory physical appearance, for she may very likely become fat and take on masculine characteristics. She may even grow a mustache! The name implies further that the menopause is the only change a woman experiences. Nothing could be more untrue or more absurd than these implications.

The truth is that woman has been changing all her life. Each age, as we have seen, is one of continuous change. We need recall only some of the highlights of a few of the ages to see that this is true. The Age of the Unborn witnessed the change from one single cell to the complex being that is the newborn baby. There follows in orderly procession the change from a helpless baby through the many phases of childhood to the emergence of femininity in the years of youth. All of these changes are building up to the Age of Maturity, which itself has an ever-changing meaning as marriage and motherhood are experienced. Menopause is merely a transition to another aspect or level of her maturity, another age with its own peculiar significance to her as a person. Life means change and when these vital changes cease, life itself ceases. Why then should we imply that there is only one period of change in a woman's life?

The "critical years" of a woman's life, a term often applied to the Age of the Menopause, is another misnomer that should be recognized as such and discarded. This carries the implication of danger—that woman is on the brink of disaster, that her health, her happiness, and her very life is in jeopardy. It further implies that this is not merely a time of crisis that can be met forthwith and dissolved, but rather years when she must feel her way along a narrow ledge of safety, at any moment of which by one false step she might fall into the abyss of a mental breakdown or serious physical illness. This is, of course, absurd. The Age of the Menopause does not carry a greater threat to her health and happiness than any other age. It can be uncomfortable, but it is not necessarily dangerous. The danger is determined by the degree of maturity with which she approaches the age, and how well she has attended to attaining and preserving good health.

The fact that child-bearing days are over should not mean that she can no longer continue to grow intellectually and enjoy the fruits of her knowledge, or that her emotional life will dry up. Neither will she lose her mind, have a nervous breakdown, or sink into melancholia because the menstrual function ceases. Furthermore, this transition period in the mechanism of her body function does in no way make her more susceptible to any disease, especially those that she has been lead to fear, such as cancer and heart disease. She may have symptoms suggestive of many, but they can be prevented or controlled, and most will disappear spontaneously after a time. She can, of course, have any of the illnesses to which flesh is heir at the time of the menopause, but not because she is in the Age of the Menopause.

The " climacteric," still another way of designating the age, is not particularly apt, for it is derived from the Greek word meaning " rung in the ladder," which could be applied to any age, for all life consists of one step after another. Women themselves do not often use or even know this term. It is a medical term that doctors use to include all the physiological characteristics of this period. To doctors, this age of woman includes more than just the cessation of menstruation. It begins when the ovaries begin to slow down and become less efficient, and it ends when the body has achieved a new equilibrium in glandular function. Thus the age consists of three phases—the premenopausal, menopausal, and postmenopausal.

In most instances, nature accomplishes this transition smoothly and successfully. But occasionally she falters, and the doctor must give her a helping hand. The symptoms of these phases are different. Those of the premenopause are due to failing ovarian function with menstrual irregularities and nervous and emotional disturbances. Those of the postmeno-pause are primarily associated with the period of pituitary hyperactivity—vasomotor and metabolic disturbances—as the body seeks to achieve a new endocrine balance. It is important for women to recognize this broader concept of the menopause, which should be a coming of age to a new level of maturity in the Age of Serenity.

We might add one other title to the long list of names for this age and call it the Age of Questions. The woman asks not only what is happening to her but how and why. She starts early to wonder when it will begin, and she is eager to know when it will end.

THE QUESTIONS

The questions at this time arise because the woman notices a change in the way she feels physically, in her moods and emotions, in the way she meets her everyday problems, and even in her outlook on life. As a rule these changes are only moderate lapses or deviations from her usual feeling of well-being. They may be subtle, indefinable, and fleeting, or occasionally cataclysmic.

How the woman will find the answer to her questions will depend largely on a question's significance to her. She may keep the question to herself, confiding in no one because she thinks that it is unimportant, that she knows the answer, or that if ignored the changes will cease to exist. Or she lives with her questions in silence, because she fears to know the truth.

But if woman is wise, she will face the fact that she has passed another milestone, that she is entering another age. She will cast aside her re-luctance to leave one age and will press on with eager anticipation for what another will add to the meaning of her life. She will seek the answers to her questions from the only person who can give her facts, her doctor, who will reassure and guide her in the solution of her problem.

What are these changes that a woman may notice? What are the questions that she will want to ask her doctor? The following are actual questions and are a fair sampling of the many reasons that women give for seeking medical care.

"Why Do Women Have To Go through the Menopause?"

This is a question one often hears, as if menopause were another curse of Eve placed on woman, another trial that she must bear because she is a woman. Nature has decreed that woman's fertility, her reproductive capacity, shall terminate at the time in life that is most advantageous for all concerned. It comes earlier (but not always as much earlier as you might think) than in the male, for woman's reproductive responsibility is far greater than his. Therefore, she should be called on to bear it only during her most vigorous years and be relieved of it when she still has many years of health and strength to care for her offspring during their years of immaturity and dependency.

For several reasons, woman today comes nearer to fulfilling this destiny than at any time in history. More women are living to experience this age. Only a few decades ago the few women who escaped the dangers that threatened her life in the earlier ages arrived at this age with her health impaired by the burdens of everyday living—strenuous physical work, poor nutrition, and repeated pregnancies. Today, she arrives at the age physically young and vigorous with the prospect of many active years of life ahead. Moreover, it is only in the past few decades that we have come to understand the physiology of the menopause. Now we know that the unpleasant symptoms of the menopause have a definite physiological basis, that they are not the product of a woman's imagination or the manifestations of a neurosis. Furthermore, hormones are now available that can control the menopausal symptoms without any danger to her. Finally, new opportunities for fulfillment have been provided by the change in the concept of woman's place in society. She has passed from the state of dependency, in which the sexual aspect of her personality was her only function, to independence, where she may achieve, and continue to enjoy even more after the menopause, the fruits of maturity in all the facets of her being.

"What Is Happening to Me?"

Eve said: "I don't know exactly what is the matter with me. I'm not really sick. There is no one thing that bothers me, no particular ache or pain, but I just don't feel like I used to. I don't enjoy living with myself, and I'm sure my husband and children are finding me difficult to live with. I'm nervous and irritable. Little things that in the past would never have bothered me may throw me into a tantrum, or I'm ashamed to say, a crying jag. What is worse, I seem to have lost my zest for living. I don't get the pleasure out of the little everyday family things that I used to. All these symptoms sound like I'm getting cantankerous, reneging on my job as a wife and mother, but I'm really not. I'm quite concerned about myself.

"I have tried to find the reason. I've watched to see if there was some one thing that pointed to a physical disability, but there was none. I thought of the menopause, but it can't be that. That is over, because I finally had my last menstrual period six months ago. There have been lots of little things that annoy me, all probably completely unrelated, but I've jotted them down, and here they are: I'm troubled by insomnia; sometimes I find it difficult to go to sleep and other times I wake up frequently and always earlier than necessary. I never sleep the eight hours that I need to feel well. The back of my neck gets tense and aches. I have pain in my arms and legs, especially at night; sometimes they go to sleep, at other times they are numb and tingle. Sometimes I have a peculiar choking feeling, especially when I'm tired or upset."

This is quite a long "chief complaint," as doctors would call it. However, it is a fair example of how many women describe their problem.

Other chief complaints are very brief. Each woman has one symptom she fears indicates some specific serious physical condition, so she names it and asks one question, such as:

"Am I Going Insane?"

Anne said: "I have been crying for five weeks. I can't eat, I can't sleep, I can't work. There is no reason for it, but all the world has gone black. Do you think I am losing my mind?"

"Am I Pregnant?"

Elizabeth stated: "I am two weeks late with my period and that has never happened to me before except years ago when I was having my babies. But I can't face having another baby after all these years."

"Do I Have Cancer?"

Carol reported: "My regular period came the first of the month and was normal, and just two weeks later I started to bleed again, and it has continued for ten days. You read so much about bleeding as a symptom of cancer." Dotty said: "My breasts have been hurting. They feel swollen. They used to do something like this before each menstrual period, but I haven't menstruated in over a year. I can't actually feel a lump, but I am afraid that something might be starting, that I may be getting cancer."

"Do You Think I Have a Brain Tumor?"

Ethel complained: "These headaches are driving me mad. I've had headaches before, but I could usually account for them, either because I was tired or worried or had a digestive upset and could find relief with a couple of aspirins. But these are different. They hit me for no reason at all and knock me out completely. I'm nauseated, thoroughly miserable, nothing helps. I have to go to bed and just let it pound."

"Did I Have a Heart Attack?"

Frances reported: "I was awakened last night with my heart pounding. It was beating so hard and so fast that I thought it would surely stop at any moment. I couldn't get my breath. This didn't last very long, but it left me exhausted and afraid to go back to sleep."

"Do I Have Arthritis?"

Gladys complained: "Look at the knuckles of my hands, they are getting so large. They don't hurt too much, but sometimes my hands get numb and tingly. My knees creak. But the worst thing is the pain in my legs. At night they ache like a toothache, and I can't find any comfortable position to put them in, so I toss and turn and get up and walk the floor."

"Do I Have High Blood Pressure?"

Helen said: "I have been having these attacks sometimes during the day but more often at night when suddenly I get hot all over. My heart pounds so that I can hardly get my breath. I might think they were hot flashes and that I was having the menopause except that it is impossible because that was over long ago when I had a hysterectomy."

There is one other group, who know what is the matter with them and ask for help, as Hilda did: "I guess Father Time—or Mother Nature—has caught up with me and I might as well admit it. I'm tired of trying to be strong-minded. I've tried mind over matter, but it doesn't work. These hot flashes are really getting me down. Oh, I feel O. K. but what a spectacle I must be, with my red hair and ruddy complexion. When the hot flashes hit me, I feel that my whole face is redder than my hair and the sweat just pours. I work in an office with other people, and it is embarrassing, besides being darned uncomfortable. Now they are getting so frequent that they interfere with my work. I can't even play bridge. At the most interesting moment when everyone else is completely cool and absorbed in the game—suddenly all I want to do is rush away from the table and open all the windows. I did it once, to my great embarrassment, but now I just sit and mop my brow and pretend nothing is happening, hoping that no one notices."

These problems, as each woman has related hers, may seem on first consideration to represent the whole gamut of human ailments and to be totally unrelated. Actually, they all have several important things in common. They were all related by women, and all these women were in the same age group 45-55 years. In each story, the underlying theme was anxiety over the loss of a feeling of well-being. Their symptoms were different, and each interpreted her symptoms in terms of some physical disability. But the fact is they were all menopausal problems, which adequate and appropriate therapy promptly relieved.

No one case history, or even a dozen, can reveal the complete picture of the menopause, for no two cases are ever exactly alike. There are many changes or symptoms that occur at this time, none of which are peculiar to the menopause (except hot flashes). No one woman has all of them. Rather, the symptoms occur not only in an endless variety of combinations but also with a tremendous variability in intensity. Each case is further individualized by the woman's reaction to her symptoms and how she interprets them. What is important to one, another will ignore. What is incapacitating to one, another will take in her stride.

THE ENDOCRINE GLANDS IN THE MENOPAUSE

The basic physiologic reason for the menopause is simple. The ovaries go to sleep. They stop producing their hormones in the cyclic manner characteristic of the Age of Maturity.

The ovaries have a life cycle that is different from that of any other organ of the body, a limited number of years in which they are called upon to contribute to woman's body function and personality. Other organs start functioning before birth, achieve maturity at a steady pace, and continue to function (with varying degrees of efficiency, to be sure) for the rest of her life. But not so with ovaries. They do not begin to wake up or mature until she is nine or ten years old and then they require years more to acquire proficiency of function. They function as mature organs for a limited span of thirty to forty years and then go to sleep. All in all, with woman's life expectancy of seventy to eighty years, they are major contributors to her total body physiology during only about half of her lifetime.

The ovaries during maturity play an enormous part in the total body economy. Their hormones become a vital part of the endocrine symphony. Their removal requires considerable readjustment on the part of other glands. To understand their adjustment, let us review briefly the physiologic status of maturity.

As we have seen, in maturity the control of the body is effected on three levels—the central nervous system, the autonomic nervous system, and the endocrine glandular system. All work efficiently together in a delicate, intricate balance, each dependent on the others, each contributing to the efficiency of the others. When anything happens to upset or change the balance in one system, this imbalance is reflected in the efficiency and mode of action of the other two systems.

Also, as we have seen, the endocrine system is made up of several glands

.nat are mutually dependent. That is, either overactivity or underactivity of any one gland will affect the way the other glands function. This is especially true or marked in those glands involved in the female functions —the ovaries, pituitary, thyroid, and adrenals.

The ovaries during maturity are dependent on adequate pituitary function to stimulate them through the regular cycle of follicular growth, ovulation, and corpus luteum formation. During this cycle, the ovaries produce their two hormones, estrogen and progesterone. These ovarian hormones in turn act on the pituitary gland to regulate the cyclic production of the gonadotropic hormones. Each monthly cycle consists of an increasing production of estrogen by the ovary, which causes a decrease of the pituitary gonadotropic hormone. The estrogen level attains its maximum and falls abruptly, releasing the pituitary to activity again, and another cycle is started. A similar mechanism is effected between progesterone and its pituitary gonadotropic hormone.

This see-saw arrangement or changing balance between ovarian and pituitary function works with a remarkable degree of regularity, uniformity, and efficiency during the years of maturity. It maintains not only the woman's menstrual regularity and her fertility, but it contributes to her whole body economy, her physical health and well-being, her feminine personality.

When the ovaries begin to slow down, there is an alteration in ovarian-pituitary balance. The loss first of the progesterone-pituitary gonadotropic hormone function affects primarily the woman's fertility while the loss of the estrogen-pituitary gonadotropic hormone balance affects not only her fertility but her whole physical mechanism on all the levels of control. The loss of the progesterone phase of the cycle can pass almost unnoticed. It corresponds to the period of adolescence before fertility is attained. The ovaries go through anovulatory cycles with a fair degree of regularity, and because there is adequate estrogen produced each month, the ovarian-pituitary balance is maintained. It is only when the ovaries are no longer able to produce an adequate amount of estrogen that the balance is upset, and repercussions are felt in all the levels of control. For estrogen deficiency results for a time in pituitary overactivity. To put it another way, as the ovaries begin to slow down in their work, the pituitary puts on more steam and exerts a greater effort than usual to urge the ovaries to do better. But the ovaries have reached the end of their ability to respond, and eventually the pituitary gives up and settles down again to a normal level of activity.

In simplest terms, then, the endocrine basis of menopause and all its symptoms is estrogen deficiency and pituitary overactivity. Doctors are not quite agreed as to which causes the characteristic symptoms of the menopause, such as hot flashes and other vasomotor phenomena. As for the other symptoms, some are the result of lack of estrogen and some of excessive pituitary function. If we recall all the functions of estrogen, the change it induces in adolescence and maturity, we can understand what its abrupt loss to the total body economy will mean and that any number of symptoms may be produced. The important thing is that both states of imbalance are relieved by the administration of the estrogenic hormone.

Nature has provided for this. She does not expect the woman to have to continue what could be a third of her life span without the sex hormones so essential to her well-being. So she has provided a source other than the tiring ovary, which she now calls into action. It happens this way.

We have noted previously that the adrenals produce the sex hormones, not only the female hormones estrogen and progesterone, but also the male hormone androgen. When the ovaries begin to falter, the pituitary becomes overactive, not only in urging the ovaries to another last effort, but also in calling on the thyroid (by its thyreotropic hormone) and the adrenals (by ACTH) to speed up. The adrenals respond by producing more of the sex hormones. As the estrogen from the ovary depresses the pituitary, the adrenal sex hormones also slow the pituitary down. But there is an important difference. There is no cyclic adrenal function so that a steady equilibrium is achieved. The ovaries do not cease completely in their function at the menopause. They continue to produce estrogen for years thereafter and are therefore quite important.

The physiologic basis of the menopause is the transition from one type of glandular equilibrium to another, from the glandular balance that we have examined in great detail in " The Age of Maturity " to the glandular balance that we shall inquire into later in " The Age of Serenity." The most significant change that occurs at this time is the loss of the cyclic production of estrogen.

THE VARIED SYMPTOMS

The symptoms of the menopause are real. They are not imaginary or indications of a neurosis. They arise from specific physiologic changes. The woman whose menopause is mild or without symptoms should not congratulate herself for her strong-mindedness, but be thankful for her good fortune. Nor should the woman with severe symptoms be condemned as neurotic and denied the help that she needs. The symptoms that any one woman will experience at the menopause will depend on three factors: the smoothness with which the change in her glandular balance takes place; the state of her health when she enters the menopause; and the emotional maturity and stability with which she faces this period of change.

Why are the symptoms of the menopause so varied? Why do some women have only mild inconsequential symptoms while others are completely incapacitated for a time? Why do women have any symptoms at all if menopause is just a normal transition period?

The descent from high ovarian function to low ovarian function may be like a meandering path down a hillside, gradual and unexciting with the level of the valley below reached without effort or even awareness that a descent was being made. Or it might be like a roller-coaster, a series of abrupt rises and falls. The shock of the first fall takes your breath away, then the tension eases as you slow down on the next climb, only to have the calmness shattered by another abrupt fall. Eventually, this too comes to an end, and you reach solid ground, shaken but still all in one piece. So, too, in the menopause, if the descent (loss of ovarian function) is gradual, the body is able to adjust and no symptoms occur. But the withdrawal may be erratic, with marked rises and falls to which the body cannot adjust, and symptoms result.

It is most important to realize and to understand that the symptoms of the menopause arise because the body is trying to adjust to a changing level in the production of estrogen by the ovaries. Just as the body functioned well during the period when the high and cyclic level of estrogen obtained, it will function well again at a low level of ovarian function.

The symptoms of the menopause are modified by the degree of general good health that the woman is enjoying as she enters this age. A woman who is healthy and strong is better able to make a smooth adjustment than a woman in poor health or one who has neglected the aspects of healthy living. We have seen how nutrition, rest, and exercise affect the normal function in maturity and all the other ages. They are equally important in the menopause.

This does not refer to specific diseases particularly. If the woman is ill with some specific disease such as heart trouble, the menopause may pass unnoticed. If the menopause is particularly stressful, the symptoms and seriousness of the illness may be increased. Such diseases are no more likely to occur at this age than in any other age. But they may be discovered because the woman is moved to seek medical help by the discomforts of the menopause.

In general, it is the physical stamina that woman has built up through the years that will contribute to a smooth transition. The symptoms will be modified by the degree of emotional maturity the woman has attained. Maturity is never a complete and static or absolute state. Woman is better able to cope with the problems of the menopause if she has absorbing interests and is busy, happy, and willing to face up to her problems.

Menopause may be a stressful period physically, as we have seen. It may also be a stressful period emotionally. The stress comes from two sources: the problems a woman must meet in everyday living—family affairs, finances, or job—and her attitude toward the meaning of menopause to her as a person. There are some women with disturbing symptoms who are reluctant to seek help for fear of being called neurotic. They think and have been told that menopause is a natural period in which there are no symptoms. There are others who cling to the ideal of youth, fear to grow old, and will not admit that menopause is the cause of their symptoms. There are a few who are overwhelmed by the symptoms of the menopause and do not realize what is happening to them. They lose their perspective and only know they are miserable. And there are some women who make menopause the scapegoat. They blame everything on it and enjoy talking about their symptoms. As with every fish story oft repeated, the fish gets bigger with every telling. Some use it as an excuse for their failures, for their instability and irresponsibility.

We have been speaking of symptoms of the menopause in a general way—what causes them, what makes them vary so from woman to woman.

But "symptoms" do not tell us specifically what the woman feels, how she is made uncomfortable, what makes her uncomfortable. Let us try to answer the question: What are the symptoms of the menopause?

We can appreciate what the loss of estrogen means and how symptoms are produced if we recall the multitude of functions of this hormone. First, estrogen is the growth hormone of the reproductive system. When it is decreased in amount, growth ceases and regression sets in. The first symptom of this is the waning and eventual cessation of menstruation. Retrogression of other of the reproductive organs does not become apparent until some years later when aging decreases the auxiliary supply. Second, estrogen as part of the total glandular mechanism has played an important part in the maintenance of stability within the three levels of control of the entire body. When estrogen is removed, there may be repercussions in any or all of these, with symptoms referable to disturbance in function of mind and emotions, the automatic functions, particularly the circulatory system, and practically every phase of body metabolism.

Changes in Menstruation

The cessation of menstruation may occur in any number of ways, all of which are normal. In general, there are four basic patterns that lead to the final disappearance of the menstrual function: sudden cessation of menstruation; regular cycles with gradual diminution of flow; loss of regularity with periods occurring further and further apart with a fairly normal amount of flow; and shorter cycles with profuse flow.

A woman may be menstruating regularly and suddenly stop and never menstruate again. Or, she may remain amenorrheic for a few months, six months or a year, and then have another period of flow. There is no fixed time after her last period when a woman may say: "This is it—I won't ever menstruate again." She may or she may not. There are instances in medical reports of women who have had recurrences of bleeding years after their last menstruations, which a curettage revealed to be normal fertile cycles. This probably accounts for "change-of-life babies." In such cases, the woman has a few months of amenorrhea and, assuming that her age of fertility has passed, abandons the means of contraception that she has previously used and becomes pregnant.

In the second type of change, the menstrual cycle maintains its regularity, but the actual flow gradually becomes less and less. This decrease may be a shortening of the length of flow—that is, a woman who has normally menstruated six to seven days finds that her periods are lasting only two to four days, then one day. Or the length of the flow may remain the same, but the actual amount diminishes to the point where there are only recurrent periods of spotting. Occasionally, the periods of scanty flow or spotting will last longer than her normal periods. The important thing is that the period of bleeding remains cyclic, that is, it occurs at regular intervals, lasts a few days, and stops. It is not an off-and-on affair. Irregular spotting, even during the menopause, should never be passed over as menstrual irregularity. It must be investigated.

In the third pattern, the menstrual periods maintain a similarity to previous periods as to amount and duration of flow but become further and further apart. The delay at first may be a matter of days, then whole months go by between periods, and eventually there is no recurrence.

In the fourth type, the woman goes through a phase that corresponds to functional bleeding as we have seen it in maturity. The cycle may remain fairly regular with the flow longer and profuse. Or the cycle changes, and bleeding occurs at two-to three-week intervals or as long as seven or eight weeks apart. All similarity to regularity may be lost, and bleeding may occur at varying intervals for a variable period of time.

These four basic patterns are not rigidly followed. They may occur in any number of combinations—short cycles followed by long cycles, scanty flow by profuse. Hence it is apparent that no two women will have the same experience during the months or years that her menstrual function is changing.

There is one important fact that needs to be repeated and stressed: Not all vaginal bleeding is menstruation. A woman should keep an accurate calendar record not only of the regularity of the cycle but also of the character of the flow. During the menopause years she should have periodic physical examinations and present this record to her doctor. More important she should present herself for examination at any time when there is the appearance of spotting. Spotting before the period, after the period, or irregularly between the periods and spotting or slight flow after a period of amenorrhea is important to note. Most of the time this spotting is not significant, but that is something that her doctor must evaluate. She can be as strong-minded as she likes about hot flashes, depression, and the other symptoms of menopause, although she will be foolish to put up with them and inflict her moods on others. No great physical harm will come of it. But she must never assume the responsibility of interpreting the meaning of bleeding. She must be alert and informed in order to recognize bleeding that might be of serious import. The most significant type from a health standpoint is spotting, which is painless, inconspicuous, and easy to ignore. We are speaking, of course, of spotting as a symptom of cancer of the uterus.

While the cessation of menstruation is the only sign that all women have, the only objective signal that ovarian function has reached a low level, there are subjective symptoms that women experience, and these may appear long before there is any great change in the menstrual pattern and continue for some time after it has ceased. The hot flashes are the most typical subjective symptom, but they are not necessarily always present. There are a multitude of other symptoms, involving every aspect of body physiology, that are the result of estrogen deficiency. These symptoms may appear before or after the cessation of menstruation as well as during the more clearly defined menopausal phase. Their significance is more easily appreciated when hot flashes are present, but they may occur in the absence of hot flashes.

Nervousness

When a woman states that nervousness is making her ill, unhappy, ineffective, and inefficient, she may be referring to one or a combination of several possible sensations that may detract from her sense of well-being, self-control, self-confidence. They lessen her ability to live comfortably with herself as well as make her a person who is hard to get along with.

"Nervousness" thus may mean that she feels tense, keyed up all the time, and unable to relax. She experiences an inward drive that keeps her on the move, going from one thing to another, never finishing anything, never satisfied with anything. With this tension there may be loss of appetite or compulsive eating, headache, inability to sleep or to concentrate, apprehension of something unknown, or depression.

"Nervousness" may mean excitability, that she responds excessively to any and all stimuli. Good news lifts her into a dream world of unreality, while bad news sinks her to the depths of despair. The demands of usual routine excite her to excessive activity or loom so ominous that she gives up without trying. Common everyday occurrences cause a flurry of excitement.

"Nervousness" may also mean irritability or sensitivity to little things, such as noises or slight mishaps in everyday living, that one ordinarily accepts without much ado. The threshold for annoyance is extremely low or varied. Anger, even rage, is easily aroused. She says things or does things for which she is instantly sorry. In turn she is sensitive, her feelings are easily hurt, and she feels herself imposed upon. Sometimes she may lack insight as to what is happening to her and projects her own short-comings onto others. All the world is wrong or against her. Sometimes she recognizes that the fault is within herself but feels helpless to do anything about it. She is always tired, easily exhausted, and loses the physical ability to carry on her usual activities efficiently.

Insomnia

Disturbance in the normal pattern of sleep is a common, even a char-acteristic, symptom of the menopause, and it is debilitating. A woman may no longer enjoy the experience of a good full day of work and play, which should be followed by a night of deep restful sleep. Rather, she may reach the end of the day so exhausted that she goes to bed earlier than usual or even drops off to sleep in a chair but awakens in an hour or so and further sleep is impossible. She may retire at the usual time, but sleeps lightly and fitfully, waking at the slightest noise, or she may have her rest disturbed by dreams. She may toss and turn until daybreak, when she drops off to sleep and thus is still unrested when she has to arouse herself for the day's activities a few hours later. With any of these disturbances in the pattern of sleep, she gets up more tired than when she went to bed, and the continued loss of sleep results in increasing nervous-ness and exhaustion, both mental and physical.

Headaches

Headaches occur with declining ovarian function and may be just as typical of it as the hot flash. There are usually two kinds, the sick head ache and the tension headache. The sick headache is a feeling of fullnes or severe pounding that involves the whole head, a feeling of a tight banc above the eyes, and a heavy pressure on the top of the head. A woman in describing this kind of headache says her head feels like something foreign, useless, and uncomfortable that she would like to lift off and throw away. When the pain becomes severe it is followed by nausea and vomiting. These headaches are associated with the menstrual cycle even years before there is any change in menstruation and may occur before, during, or after the flow. They may become exaggerated at the menopause, and they may persist after the menstrual cycle ceases, but they have a cyclic nature occuring at fairly regular intervals. They may be quiescent for a while and be reactivated by periods of stress. They disappear when the transition to stability is completed.

The tension headache is located in the back of the head and upper part of the neck and is a feeling of rigidity and dull ache or pain that extends over the back of the head and down the shoulders. It has no cyclic time of occurrence, may come and go, or develop as the day progresses. It may be a more or less permanent dull nagging sensation and is exhausting.

Migraine is a third kind of headache that may occur at the menopause, but it is not specifically menopausal in origin. However, migraine head-aches that a woman may have suffered for years can be counted on to disappear when the transition period is completed. The term " migraine " is frequently applied erroneously to any and all kinds of headaches. A typical migraine headache involves only one side of the head (not neces-sarily the same side each time), is preceded by an aura—symptoms that warn of the approach—and often leads to nausea and vomiting. The pain, which is severe, may last a short time or several days, and when it finally subsides, it leaves the scalp and eyeball on the side affected sore and tender.

There are other discomforts in the head that are not actually head-aches but are due to involvement of specific nerves of the head or the blood supply. These include neuralgias, dizziness, ringing in the ears, loss of sense of balance, spots before the eyes.

Mental efficiency may suffer transitory lapses—periods when the woman complains that she cannot concentrate, think clearly, or follow a problem to a successful conclusion. She reads and finds that she is not comprehending, or she may find it no longer a pleasure to read. She finds herself forgetting things, usually recent events such as where she put things or what she started to do.

Depression

Of all the nervous changes, the emotional are the hardest to bear—the moodiness, the sense of impending disaster, tears that are always close to the surface and spill over at the slightest provocation or for no reason at all. The most disturbing of all is the depression.

I do not believe that anyone who has not experienced depression, the feeling of being lost in a dark cloud, can fully appreciate what it means. I am not referring to the depression that comes as the result of some sorrow, disappointment, failure, or worry—a mental state that is the result of events in life taking the wrong turn. That depression is real and unpleasant but understandable, for it comes from without the person. It has a cause, and one can expect or hope for a solution or learn to accept it and move on. But the depression of menopause is something different. It is as if you have lost your way—the lights have gone out and you are engulfed in a fog. In your own private world nothing seems very important, nothing very meaningful. This is oppressive gloom and with this a loss of drive, hope, and meaning to everyday living. You become nervous, irritable, and more vulnerable to all the little stresses of everyday living. You lose your perspective. You can't account for it, you can't explain it, and you can't rise above it. It engulfs you.

To dispel this cloud, to bring back the sunshine of purposeful living, the joy of accomplishment, and the thankfulness for just being alive by changing the body chemistry is the wonderful accomplishment of the estrogenic hormones.

Circulatory Symptoms

There are many symptoms referable to disturbances in the circulatory system in any or all parts of the body. They are the result of irritability and instability of the autonomic nervous system, which is charged with the responsibility of keeping this system functioning smoothly, efficiently, and effectively.

The hot flash, or flush as it is sometimes called, is such a symptom and is perhaps the most typical of all menopausal symptoms. Flashes are sometimes considered as the characteristic symptom, and when they are absent, other symptoms that are present, even though incapacitating, are not recognized as menopausal in origin. The hot flashes are also the most variable as to character and intensity as well as in frequency of occurrence. Some women do not have them at all, but experience other equally disturbing discomforts.

A hot flash may be nothing more than a feeling of warmth, which comes on suddenly and gradually subsides. A typical flash is a sudden sensation of heat, which seems to start in the neck and quickly spreads upward to the face and head, and the woman is conscious of the fact that her face is flushed. There is usually some increase in perspiration, which varies in intensity. Flashes may be unpleasant and embarrassing during the day, but they also occur at night to disturb sleep. A woman may be aroused enough by the heat to fling the covers off only to be awakened later shivering with cold. In winter, if she is an open-window addict, the cold blast that hits her when she is uncovered and her clothing is damp makes her the victim of frequent colds and aches in the muscles and joints similar to neuralgia, bursitis, or arthritis.

A woman quickly recognizes a hot flash for what it is, but other circulatory symptoms she rarely identifies as menopausal in origin. Sudden palpitation of the heart, when first experienced, is almost always interpreted as evidence of heart trouble. A woman may wake suddenly from a sound sleep with her heart beating rapidly, and she becomes apprehensive and short of breath. The spell may last only a few moments or what seems to be hours. Spells also occur during the day. The fact that she tires easily and finds herself short of breath on moderate exertion, with palpitation, also suggests heart trouble to her. A feeling of pressure on the chest is another disturbing symptom. It may be in the midline or to one side or the other, a feeling of constriction of the chest. There may also be fleeting pains, which are difficult to localize.

There are also disturbances in circulation in the extremities, which give rise to numbness and tingling of the hands and feet. She is also bothered with cold hands and feet. Her rest may be disturbed by pains in her feet and legs, twitching, and jerking of the muscles, making it difficult for her to find a comfortable position.

A mild hypertension is frequently found on examination, an expression of her state of tension rather than of vascular disease. On the other hand, hypotension, poor cerebral circulation, is the cause of dizziness and black-outs, especially when a woman arises from the recumbent position or after she has been stooping over.

All of these disturbances are purely functional in origin. They do not herald the onset of disease of the circulatory system. They subside and disappear as stability after menopause is achieved, and they respond quite readily to appropriate treatment. There is a further reassuring fact for women at this age in life when they hear of so many dying suddenly of heart attacks. Women seem to have some kind of built-in protection against heart attacks for coronary occlusion is only one fourth as common in women as in men.

Changes in Metabolism

There are many signs of metabolic imbalance due to over- or under-activity of one or more of the glands of internal secretion that may appear at menopause. This is understandable in light of the fact that estrogen plays an important part in the regulatory mechanism of the glands involved —the pituitary, adrenals, and thyroid, and in turn in the efficiency of their function.

The most frequent finding is a change in thyroid function, which may go either way, hyper or hypo, depending on the condition of the thyroid before the onset of menopause. If the thyroid has been potentially hyper-active, it may be thrown into full blown hyperthyroidism by the stress of menopause, which includes not only the glandular stress of readjustment, but the mental and emotional stress as well. If, on the other hand, the thyroid has been sluggish before, it may be unable to meet the increased needs of menopause, and a frank hypothyroidism develops. In most instances the thyroid is normal at the onset and is able to ride the tide of menopause and maintain its equilibrium.

In some women there is a disturbance in carbohydrate metabolism resulting in an elevation of the blood sugar and a spilling over of sugar in the urine. This may return to normal with proper menopausal therapy and relief of stress, especially with proper diet and control of weight. Occasionally, a latent diabetes develops and must be treated as such.

Most of the other metabolic changes that are the result of loss of ovarian function and the aging process are slow in developing, such as a disturbance in calcium metabolism, which leads to deficient deposition of calcium in the bones. Osteoporosis is an example. These will be discussed later. There are, however, two that are apparent and bothersome at the menopause—arthralgia and obesity.

Arthralgia and pain in the joints are quite frequent. The joints of the fingers are perhaps the most often affected. This may be only pain and stiffness, but there may also be some thickening of the knuckles leading to a knobbiness. This is not evidence of a progressive arthritis, and the greatest injury is to the appearance of the hands, and the woman's pride, for the pain and stiffness go, but the enlargement of the joints remains.

Obesity can be a serious problem at the menopause when women tend to put on weight. It is true that this may sometimes be attributed to a decrease in activity or increased intake due to nervous eating, but that is not the whole story. We do not know all of the facts of fat metabolism and the storage of fat and what leads to a general excessive storage and obesity, but there is certainly an endocrine factor not only in the amount of fat stored, but also in where it is stored. For instance, a young girl achieves her curves at adolescence not only by growth of the gland tissue of the breasts and the sexual characteristics of maturation of her bone structure but also by the increased deposition of fat in the breasts and specific locations on her body. She does not suddenly lose these at menopause, but there is a gradual decrease during the postmenopausal years. When a young woman is surgically deprived of her ovaries, castrated, early in the age of maturity, a peculiar type of obesity develops. Large pads of fat appear on the upper parts of her thighs, at the level of her hip joints, while she loses the fat in the breasts and around the shoulders. At the time of menopause, the deposition of fat is more apt to be around the waist line and to increase in amount in the lower abdominal pad. This, with the increased abdominal distention due to poorer intestinal function, makes the abdomen quite large proportionally.

The listing and description of all these symptoms might suggest a depressing picture of the menopause, which is not true to life. These symptoms have been listed in detail for a definite purpose—not to frighten, but to reassure. First, however unpleasant a woman may find her particular menopausal symptoms to be, they do not last forever, and they do not threaten her life, her health, her happiness, or her longevity if they are recognized for what they are and are properly handled both by the woman and by her doctor. While they mimic serious illnesses, they are functional and not symptomatic or precursors of organic diseases. No woman ever has all of these symptoms. Most women experience only a few. In the vast majority the symptoms are mild and not greatly disturbing.

It is true that menopause is a natural period, but few women pass through it without some symptoms. If we tried to state this in terms of statistics (which have little significance for the individual), we might estimate that 50 to 60 per cent of women go through menopause with symptoms so mild that they pay little attention to them and 20 to 30 per cent have symptoms that are disagreeable but easily controlled with proper treatment. About 10 per cent of women have a difficult time.

" Am I starting the menopause? " " How long will it last? " These are questions that occur to a woman regardless of what her age may be when she first experiences some irregularity of her menstrual cycle.

If she is asking whether or not she is going to stop menstruating, we can say: " Yes, some day." If she is asking when she will stop menstruating, we can only say: " Time will tell."

This is not being facetious or evading the question. There is no clear-cut answer that we can give her, for the simple reason that the Age of the Menopause is not clear-cut as to its beginning or its end. The occurrence of the last menstrual period is the decisive symptom of declining ovarian function. It may come abruptly or be preceded by a period of slowly declining ovarian function.

A mild degree of ovarian deficiency may start years before the actual loss

of menstruation with many of the symptoms of tension, headaches, occasional flashes, and scanty and irregular periods, but that does not mean
that menstruation will cease for one, two, five, or ten years. No one can
predict how rapid the decline in ovarian function will be.

While we cannot predict the time element of the menopause for any
particular woman, there are some general facts that are of interest. Most
women, statistics show, complete the menopause between the ages of
forty-five and forty-eight. Of the remainder, about one half will be forty-
to forty-five and the other half forty-eight to fifty-two. This leaves a few
scattered cases before forty and between fifty-two and fifty-five. Percentages
for each of these groups have been reported by different investigators, but
they do not agree on the actual figures. Practically, the percentages mean
little. What is significant is the range of normal, that these general facts
give us.

It is my impression that more women today are older chronologically
but younger physiologically when they experience the menopause than
they were even one of two decades ago. This is only another way of saying
that women today are healthier and younger for their age than the women
of earlier times.

The occurrence of the menopause before forty is unfortunate, as it indicates an underlying endocrine imbalance or deficiency. The failure of
menopause to be completed by fifty-two—that is, continuation of bleeding—
should always be suspect. A delayed menopause after fifty-two may be on
a natural basis. There have been a few cases reported of women in whom
menstruation continued into the sixties and seventies with a rare pregnancy,
but these are medical curiosities. Any continuation of bleeding after fifty-
two should be investigated. It may be due to prolonged ovarian vitality, but
it may also indicate some pathology, which should be corrected.

Where will a particular woman fall in this range of normal? There
are certain factors that influence the time element of the menopause that
we may apply in order to come up with a slightly more educated guess.

First, there is heredity. Just as young girls tend to have the same or
similar menarchal age as their mothers, so do daughters and mothers
and sisters have similar menopausal ages. Furthermore, those who had an
early menarche can expect to have not an early but a late menopause; those
who started to menstruate at about the usual age of twelve to fourteen

can expect to fall in the usual age group for the menopause, and those who were late starting may expect an early menopause. These, of course, are only generalities. There are always many exceptions, many who fail to conform, that prove the rule!

Second, there is the experience during the Age of Maturity. Women who have had children will have a later menopause than women who have not experienced pregnancy. And a woman who has had several children is likely to continue to menstruate later than a woman with only one child. Perhaps more significant today than the incidence of fertility, which may be a matter of choice, is the character of the menstrual function. Women who have had regular and lusty flow can expect to continue this function longer than those whose flow has been irregular and scanty.

Previous illnesses and operations also contribute to an earlier menopause. Pelvic operations that do not involve removal of both ovaries (which results in abrupt surgical menopause), such as suspensions, removal of the tubes or the uterus, which eliminate menstruation but do not precipitate the physiological menopause, are apt to cause an earlier cessation of ovarian function, probably because the blood supply of the ovaries has been disturbed. When does it end? Again only time will tell.

XXIII

TRANSITION MADE SMOOTH

WOMEN APPROACHING this age sometimes ask: "Can't you do something to prevent my having the menopause?" "Won't you do something to get this menopause business over with in a hurry?" "Isn't there some way to delay the menopause?"

The answer, of course, is "no" to all these requests, not because the doctor is unsympathetic, but because such requests arise from a false concept of the true meaning of the menopause. The menopause is an age in the life of a woman that she cannot skip, she cannot hurry, and which she should not try to delay.

Menopause is not a disease and therefore requires no treatment as such. On this basis, woman is sometimes denied the help she needs by doctors who are either disinterested, unimpressed, or labor under the false idea that woman should endure it. On the other hand, some women do endure it without treatment because they think they should be strong-minded or are ashamed or shy and reluctant to seek help. In such instances there is a failure to realize that menopause is a period of stress that involves all levels of control in the woman's physical make-up. The severity of the stress is variable, the ability to meet the stress is variable, and the stress may be greater on one level than another. There is much that can and should be done during this period, according to each woman's need, to prevent it from being disabling or even unpleasant and uncomfortable.

It might seem, in the light of our understanding of the cause of the symptoms of the menopause, that the treatment is simple and clearly indicated. The cause is lack of estrogen; the cure should be the administration of estrogen. It is not as simple as that. Woman must first realize that

494

self-help is fundamental and essential. Self-medication, however, may be dangerous. There are things only her doctor can and should do for her.

THE WOMAN'S PART

The severity of the symptoms of the menopause depends to a great extent on the woman herself, on what attributes of physical and mental health she possesses at this time and the manner in which she meets the problems of this age. It follows therefore that self-help will come through preparation for this transition before it starts as well as attention to the specific needs as they arise.

The first requirement for a tranquil menopause is that woman must accept her age gracefully. This means a true acceptance within her innermost self, her mind and heart, not just a "front" that she displays to the world while she smolders inside. A woman who rebels at the thought of the menopause, who asks why it has to happen to her, and who sees nothing left in life when youth is gone can expect trouble. She is in fact creating much of her difficulty. A rebellious woman is certain to be an unhappy woman not only because her rebellion is futile and doomed to failure, since she cannot stay the natural cycle of life. She is also unhappy because her rebellion arises from her own shortcomings—immaturity and ignorance. The menopause doesn't make her unhappy. She makes herself unhappy.

Maturity is not the end of the road, an empty useless period of life that must be forestalled as long as possible. Rather, it is the achievement of proficiency in living—loving, serving, broadening our knowledge and understanding of the world about us and of ourselves—with enthusiasm, and appreciation for the reality of today, and with hope and expectation for tomorrow. Maturity should be a woman's true quest in life. It is the goal that she must be forever striving to achieve, for it has a different meaning for each age. Menopause is merely a transition from one type of maturity to another.

A woman can greatly ease the tension of menopause if she enters the age with accurate information concerning the physical aspects of it. Just as a young girl approaching the Age of Youth should be forewarned of the physical changes she is about to experience, so should woman have an understanding of this second transition period. But the woman, unlike youth, must seek this information for herself. She must make an effort to know the truth and understand the basic facts of her body function at this age. By such knowledge she is not only forewarned as to what might happen, therefore lessening the impact, but more important she is reassured as to things that will not happen, thereby eliminating the source of fear and dread that ignorance brings. The mature informed woman can recognize and accept the importance of the physical aspects of herself as a personality and as a woman. This means that she will be able to steer a straight course between the dangers of trying to ignore the physical aspects on the one hand and of overemphasizing them on the other.

The physical needs of this age, which are the basis of good health and normal feminine function, are those that we have stressed as being important for normal menstruation and normal pregnancy. They are no less important for a normal menopause.

A woman may seem to have "gotten by" for years not helping nature, even doing much to hinder her by disregarding the rules for good health, but eventually she must pay for this abuse and neglect. Menopause is likely to be that time. On the other hand, if she has striven to maintain a high standard of good health, menopause is the time at which it will really begin to pay dividends. The basic physical needs of good health for all ages are good nutrition and the proper balance of rest and exercise, work and recreation. They may require some quantitative adjustments during the Age of the Menopause.

Good nutrition, as we have stressed, means the proper food to supply all the body needs and maintain normal weight. The menopause brings no change to this. A woman does not get fat just because of her age, but because she eats too much and exercises too little. If she has allowed the pounds to accumulate, then reduction by the realistic way we have described will bring rewards. It will relieve stress on the normal body functions, increase her life expectancy, and bolster her self-respect and self-confidence.

What physical exercise should a woman take during the Age of the Menopause? Some have become so fixed in the habits of sedentary existence that the very thought of exercise is abhorrent to them. Others say: "I get enough exercise with my house work," or "After standing on my feet all day at work I'm too exhausted to think of exercise." Others, seeing unwanted bulges of fat, subject themselves to physical contortions, pounding or rolling on the floor, or they seek the easier way and resort to the miraculous machines that do the exercise for them while they lie placidly on rollers or shakers. A few will undertake strenuous physical exercise to which they are not accustomed, and which may be dangerous.

There are so many ways to get the proper amount and kind of exercise that every woman should be able to choose one that meets her needs. Good and healthful exercise has certain basic requirements. It should involve the use of all the body, thereby stimulating all body functions; it should be pleasant, diverting recreation; and it may leave the woman tired and ready to rest and relax, but it should not exhaust her. It should be regular—a little every day, not just one big dose once a week or once a month.

"Get enough rest" is always included as one of the basic rules for good health, but this is rarely defined. Rest means two things—complete rest or sleep, and periods of some relief from tension during the waking hours, that is a change of pace, a diversion.

WHAT THE DOCTOR CAN DO

I never cease to marvel at what a few drops of a certain liquid in a syringe or even a few gayly colored tablets can mean to the well-being and happiness of a woman. I refer, of course, to hormones.

We are accustomed to think of medication as a means of saving life, curing an illness, and restoring health, and the advances that have been made in the past few decades through new drugs and new techniques and even new concepts have been spectacular. It seems almost unbelievable that so much could have been accomplished in such a relatively short time. But to me, the use of hormones in woman's problems, especially the menopause, is something different. We are not using them to treat a disease but to help woman maintain the stability of her personality and physical well-being. They too have become available within my medical lifetime, and they have revolutionized not only the treatment of the menopause but indeed our whole concept of the meaning of the menopause.

The hormone that relieves her symptoms is not one of the "wonder drugs." It is not a drug at all. It is a chemical substance that her body has been accustomed to having all her life. It is not just any hormone. It is the specific hormone estrogen.

Previously sedatives were the only available medication. They might have had some numbing effect on woman's nervous tension, but they changed the problem very little. Many doctors thought then—and some still do—that menopause symptoms are fabrications of woman's imagination. Some think she is just "enjoying poor health." There was at first great skepticism that estrogen had any basic physiologic power to relieve, other than the power of suggestion. The woman wanted help, it was believed, and she had confidence that her doctor could give it to her. Anything he might do, even giving a sugar pill, would help her.

On being given estrogen patients often say: "The relief is so wonderful. How did woman ever get along without hormones?" The answer is twofold. It is only in the last few generations that many women lived long enough to reach the age of menopause, and those who did just accepted it as another one of the "trials of being a woman." She was told that all women must go through it. She wasn't called "neurotic" if the ordeal was too much for her, for the term had not become so popular as it is today. Modern woman is impatient of such an attitude. She refuses to allow her sex to limit her activities, and she demands and can obtain relief from the unpleasant symptoms of the menopause. She is indeed fortunate.

We have come a long way since the female sex hormone was first discovered. Once its identity was known and its physiologic activities established, further research quite rapidly gave us potent forms to be used in many different ways, by injections, by mouth in liquid or tablet form, and in creams for application to the surface of the body. These estrogenic hormones are, for the most part, derived from natural sources and are chemically identical with those found in the woman's own body. There are synthetic hormones, such as stilbesterol, which are different chemically but have some (and only some) of the physiologic properties of the natural estrogens.

With this plethora of means of treatment, it follows that many methods have evolved. However estrogen is used, by tablet or by injection, there is only one guiding principle. Its purpose is to smooth the transition, not to delay or defer it, and certainly not to prolong it. Each method has advantages and disadvantages according to the doctor's evaluation, which does not always coincide with the woman's evaluation.

The advantages of injections over tablets are the accuracy of dosage, the regularity, and the smooth prolonged action. When a tablet is taken by mouth, the amount which gets into the blood stream to become effective is quite variable and is always only a fraction of the amount ingested—usually no more than a fifth. On the other hand, all that is injected is absorbed and made available for the body's use. Moreover, the amount the woman gets by oral medication is still more uncertain because it is so easy to forget to take the tablet. When estrogen is injected, it is in solution or suspension, which acts as a reservoir from which the hormone is liberated slowly over a period of time from three or four days to two weeks or a month depending on the nature of the hormone preparation. This assures a smooth and prolonged action.

The disadvantages of injection as the woman sees them are the possibility of discomfort, the trouble of having to go repeatedly to the doctor's office, and the expense. These are more than offset, if she has a doctor who sees his patient each time, talks with her, and helps her to make adjustments incident to the change, guiding her in the things she must do for herself and watching her general health. Treatment must be individualized to meet the needs of each case. There is no fixed routine or course of treatment, such as injections once or twice a week for so many weeks. Some will require more than others to get the symptoms under control and keep them so. And the doctor must be alert for untoward side effects or overdosage. There is sometimes a narrow margin between what is enough to control the symptoms of menopause and the amount that will bring about uterine bleeding.

When the doctor prescribes tablets, the control is out of his hands. True, the intelligent patient can be trusted to follow directions carefully and to report anything unusual. But it is amazing what a patient's reactions to taking pills can be. Some forget, especially when they begin to feel better, while others seem never to tire of taking them. I recall a patient who returned after a five-year interval between visits. The last notation on her chart was a prescription for twenty estrogenic tablets and the instruction to return after a month. When asked how she was she replied that she was just fine, that the tablets were wonderful. To my amazement, she had been taking the pills for five years! How she had persuaded the druggist to give them to her for that long is a question unanswered, for the laws prohibit the refilling of such prescriptions without the doctor's permission. In doing so she had defeated the purpose for which the estrogen was given—to ease the transition. She had maintained a high blood level of the hormone so that her body had never learned to adjust. No medication should be taken in this fashion for an indefinite period without medical supervision.

Since moodiness, depression, nervousness, and insomnia are the most trying symptoms of the menopause, the ones most likely to exert a disruptive influence on the woman's life, one may ask why should not the new tranquilizing drugs be used for their relief. The answer is that it would be just as sensible to rely on cough medication in the treatment of pneumonia and neglect to use such medication as the antibiotics, which can cure the infection. Both would simply be treating a symptom and ignoring the cause of the symptom. Mild sedation has long had an important place in the treatment of the menopause, and it will continue to be useful as an added means of helping a woman over the rough spots. This is especially true in the beginning of treatment before estrogen has had time to do its beneficent work.

Tranquilizers and other mood-changers may do a quicker and in some ways better job at the beginning of treatment when the nervous symptoms are severe. But they should be used only for a short time. Then they serve the useful purpose of lifting the woman from the depths of depression and allowing her to regain her perspective. Even here the tranquilizers must be used with caution. Sometimes the age of the menopause merely coincides with the occurrence of a severe nervous illness and is not the cause of the symptoms at all. The use of the tranquilizers will make it difficult to be sure what the situation really is, while the use of estrogen will make a positive diagnosis. For instance, when a woman is nervous and depressed she may blame it on the menopause. Estrogen alone will bring her relief in a matter of a few days or weeks from menopausal symptoms but will have little effect on a true nervous illness. Tranquilizers may relieve the moodiness of either, and she may go on blaming her troubles on the menopause, failing to face up to her problems or to seek the special kind of help that she needs for more deep-seated nervous illness.

The ideal of treatment of the menopause, as in all other conditions, is to give the woman a true insight into her own problem, to relieve the physical stress by all means possible and to encourage her in her efforts to solve her problems, or at least to make the best of her personal situation. Tranquilizers alone will do none of these things. They only mask the need for doing so. True they will usually relieve the anxiety and depression, but they do not restore a feeling of well-being. Instead, the mood evoked is one of disinterested detachment in which nothing matters too much, neither does anything bring very great satisfaction. To become a disinterested onlooker is no way to live a good life. One must care even when it hurts. One must continue to strive against odds, and one must hope. To fall into the habit of meeting life's problems, the stress and strain of everyday living, by taking a drug so that there no longer seems to be any problem is not living.

Estrogen, on the other hand, not only relieves the anxiety and depression of menopause but also restores a feeling of well-being. Woman's problems too are lessened, not because she can ignore them, but because she feels fit to meet them with courage and determination, which is more than half the battle. Furthermore, tranquilizers act on only one type of menopausal symptom, the mood, and can do nothing for the host of other discomforts such as hot flashes, arthralgias, and night sweats. But estrogen will relieve these also. So, we can dismiss the tranquilizers by saying that occasionally they may be used as palliative treatment for a short time, but for corrective therapy, which will lead to restoration of health, we must rely on estrogen.

ARE HORMONES DANGEROUS?

Some women are afraid to take estrogen and will at first reject the offer. The reasons they give are several. They have read or been told that hormones cause cancer, hormones will make hair grow on the face, hormones are dangerous, hormones do not relieve the menopause but delay or prolong it. Of course, no woman should be forced to take hormones or duped into taking them. Neither should hormone therapy be offered on a take-it-or-leave-it basis. Rather, we can give a woman the truth behind each of these statements, relieve her of false ideas and misconceptions, and let her make the decision as to whether she wants the relief that hormones will bring or will work it out the best that she can without them.

In treating the menopause, we do not use just any hormone. We use one specific group of hormones, the estrogens. "Hormone" is a general term that applies to all the active chemical agents poured into the blood stream by the endocrine glands. Estrogen is one kind of hormone, androgen is another, and cortisone is still another, to name only a few. It is the failure to understand the meaning of hormones that gives rise to fears. Hormones are many, varied, and powerful chemical forces within the body. Some do cause hair to grow, some may be dangerous when administered under certain conditions, and some hormones do have some relationship to the growth (not cause) of cancer. But these are instances of a specific kind of action, not general physiological properties of all hormones. To illustrate this, we may answer three of the questions most commonly asked about the use of hormones in the menopause.

Will hormones cause excessive growth of hair? Some hormones will cause hair to grow on a woman's body in the male distribution, but these hormones are the androgens such as testosterone, not estrogen. And androgens have been used in the treatment of menopausal symptoms. It came about in this way.

In the early days, when estrogen first became available for use in potent amounts, too much was used and unwanted side effects were produced, such as swollen and tender breasts and, most important, uterine bleeding. The occurrence of this bleeding—sometimes irregular spotting, days of slight flow, or profuse and long flow—after a period of several months to a year or so of amenorrhea was disconcerting. As we have stressed over and over—but never too much—any bleeding after menopause is suspect and must be investigated. Many women were subjected to a curettage, and the bleeding was found to be benign. The bleeding was due to excessive stimulation of the endometrium by the estrogen that had been administered. To obviate this, some doctors looked for another hormone that would relieve the symptoms but not cause bleeding. (Some merely rejected all hormone therapy without further question.) It was known that all the steroid hormones—estrogens, androgens, progesterones, and corticoids—are very much alike in their chemical structure and also have some biological similarities, that is, one can pinch-hit for another for some purposes. Testosterone, it was demonstrated, would control to a certain extent the hot flashes, although not as well as estrogen. It could, however, be relied on to reduce them in frequency and intensity. Thus, testosterone was hailed by a few enthusiastic clinicians as the treatment of choice because it would not cause uterine bleeding.

There is nothing unnatural about giving androgen to a woman. It is not foreign to her body or necessarily antagonistic to her basic femininity, because it has been a part of her normal body chemistry all her life and serves a useful purpose. But androgen also has its side effects— not bleeding, but others equally undesirable. Women who were given large doses to control the symptoms of menopause developed a fuzzy growth of hair on the face, an acne that was worse than they had experienced in adolescence, and their voices became husky. No wonder they were disturbed and wanted no part of this method of treatment and quickly spread the word about that hormones caused symptoms that were worse than hot flashes. Fortunately, these side effects, just as in the case of estrogens, do not occur with small doses (what is small varies with the woman's sensitivity to them, which is variable), and they are temporary. As soon as the hormone is discontinued these signs disappear.

Today, most doctors believe that there is no need to resort to androgens to replace estrogens, but rather that a more careful regulation of the dosage of estrogen is the answer. The side effects of bleeding can be averted by giving smaller doses, breaking the course of treatment, with intervals of no hormones so that excessive reactions do not develop. Some doctors use testosterone in combination with estrogen, both in small amounts, with good results, particularly in postmenopausal problems, as we shall see later. But androgens alone cannot replace estrogen in the treatment of menopausal symptoms.

Do hormones cause cancer? No one can say with certainty that hormones do or do not cause cancer for the reason that we do not know the cause of cancer, although the intensive research now going on is accumulating information that leads to the optimistic hope that this goal will someday, perhaps soon, be achieved. We shall go into the subject of cancer, what it is and what can be done about it, in "The Age of Serenity." The question that we are concerned with now is not hormones in general and any relationship they may have to cancer. It is the specific question: Does the administration of the estrogenic hormone cause cancer in women? How did the question come to be asked in the first place?

Estrogen has been accused of complicity in the crime on circumstantial evidence, which is far from sufficient to convict. Yet the stigma has persisted. The facts of the case are these:

In the early days of cancer research and hormone research (and they are largely contemporaneous), certain chemical substances administered in certain ways to certain laboratory animals resulted in cancerous growths in those laboratory animals. These chemicals were labeled "carcinogenic" and included many widely different substances. Among them were some substances that were also estrogenic. On this evidence was based the accusation that estrogens cause cancer. But what did these experiments really prove as far as women were concerned? Very little, if anything, for several reasons.

It is never wise to translate biological reactions from one specie of laboratory animal to another. The effect that a chemical, such as a drug or hormone, produces in a mouse is not necessarily the same in a cat, guinea pig, or monkey. This becomes even more pronounced when laboratory data supplied by experimental animals is applied to the human. There has never been a duplication of these results in humans. Furthermore, there has been not one authenticated case in all of medical literature of estrogen causing cancer in a woman.

There are still other facts in the laboratory experiments that make it doubtful that estrogen *caused* cancer in those laboratory animals and reduce further their potential significance to humans. These facts relate to what kind of laboratory animals were used, and how much estrogenic substance was administered to them. There are strains of laboratory animals, particularly white mice, that have a high incidence of "spontaneous cancer."

This means that if one hundred such animals were kept for their natural lifetime under optimum conditions and nothing done to them, no chemicals administered, a large percentage, fifty or more, would develop cancer. Certainly nothing is proved even if ninety to one hundred develop cancer after the administration of estrogen. It merely demonstrates that more cases occurred in already "cancer prone" mice suggesting a speeding up rather than an initiating, inciting, or causative action. Yet this is the laboratory data on which estrogen was indicted. These were a pure strain (inbred for hundreds of generations) of animals. We have no such situation among humans, and we have very little factual data as to human "cancer proneness."

There is still another factor that makes the results of these experiments inapplicable to women. That is in the matter of dosage—the proportionate amount given and the proportionate length of time administered. If a white mouse is given one gram of the chemical weekly for six months, that might not seem to be much until we consider that a mouse weighs only 50 grams and lives only two years. Actually, therefore, the mouse has been given what amounts to almost half of its body weight over a period of one fourth of its total life span. Translating this to woman is ludicrous. It would be impossible to administer a proportionate amount, and certainly no woman would submit to it for twenty years.

There is one reassuring fact about estrogen that should clear it of the guilt of being carcinogenic to women in the menopause. Estrogen is something that her body has possessed, and benefited from, all her life, even long before birth. There are two periods in which the estrogen level is extremely high, during the Age of the Unborn and during pregnancy. Here the placenta and its precursor pours estrogen into the mother's bloodstream in amounts as much as ten times that of the peak of a menstrual cycle, and this also passes into the unborn's blood. After birth, the baby's blood level of estrogen falls rapidly to a low level but does not disappear entirely. Rather it maintains a low constant level until her own ovaries start the production of estrogen in appreciable amounts at about the age of nine or ten.

The amount present in both the mother and the unborn during the communal existence of the two would be difficult to attain by artificial means. One dose as usually administered to women is 1 to 2 milligrams by injection or 1.5 to 2.5 by mouth. It would require up to or at least thirty times this amount every three days to simulate the state of pregnancy.

There is, however, one restraining fact in the administration of estrogen. Estrogen is a growth hormone in the restricted sense that it induces growth in tissues normally sensitive to it particularly the breasts and the uterus. In the abnormal, cancer cells derived from these tissues might be stimulated to grow faster. For this reason doctors are reluctant to give estrogen to women known to have had cancer of the breast or the uterus. In such cases, estrogen will not cause recurrence if all the cancer has been removed. It can only stimulate cancer cells that were not removed.

As we review this Age of the Menopause, we find that it is different from all other ages in several important ways. It is the least well-defined age as to the time of occurrence and duration, as well as to the quality and intensity of a woman's experience. It is the least understood by women themselves and also by many doctors. It is the age that women have approached with fear and dread, burdened by misinformation and superstition. Because menopause is so different, there are reassuring facts worthy of repetition.

The menopause is a real age in a woman's life, and the symptoms and discomforts she experiences are real, not imaginary. It is an age characterized by changing body physiology and body chemistry, which produces changes all women feel and recognize. The symptoms and discomforts may be mild, as they usually are, or occasionally severe. They are nothing to be ashamed of or to be feared and hence borne in patience and silence.

Menopause is not a dangerous age. There is no special threat to her mind, her emotions, her health, her beauty, her efficiency, or her capabilities if the menopause is properly understood and handled, mostly by the woman herself but with medical help when necessary. Control of all the symptoms of the menopause is both possible and safe. Hormones and other properly selected medications are effective and safe, and do not prolong the age.

Menopause is a transition period, not a climax. It signifies only one thing, a release from the responsibility of fertility. It is not the end of being a mature woman, with all the term signifies. It is not the beginning of old age or senility.

The fact that in this Age of Questions woman asks not only what is happening to her, but also why and what can be done about it, is reassuring, for it indicates that woman no longer accepts or even considers this to be the end of a useful, purposeful life. Rather she thinks of these years as a change to a somewhat different outlook on life.

We might call this the Second Coming of Age. The successful passage of its trials and achievements and readjustments opens the door to a new kind of maturity, long years in which a woman may fulfill herself as a person. Browning has expressed this approach to the Age of Serenity very well:

> "Grow old along with me!
> The best is yet to be,
> The last of life, for which the first was made."

THE AGE OF SERENITY

XXIV

THE CHALLENGE

SERENITY. What meaning has the word? What picture does it bring to mind? It might be a scene from the world of nature, a wide river moving quietly onward, unruffled by winds, unhurried, tranquilly yet with undeniable force and direction seeking its destiny in union with the sea. Whence comes this serenity? Perhaps from the strength and purposefulness acquired in its experiences as many smaller streams. Some have rushed from their mountain springs past rapids and falls; others have quietly meandered through peaceful meadows. All are now merged into one calm entity, moving silently but always moving onward.

What is the meaning of serenity as applied to a person? How may we visualize a " serene woman "? She is composed because she is at peace with herself and with the world about her. Her serenity does not result from inactivity or withdrawal from life but, in accordance with her ideals, from participation in and acceptance of the world in which she lives. She has not avoided or missed the vicissitudes of life, but she has met them with reason and judgment. She radiates her feeling of well-being and happiness, which comes from a life of activity, usefulness, and warm human relationships.

Dare we apply serenity as an attribute of that final age in life, an age that must include infirmities for some, decrepitude and senility for others, and, for all, death as its destiny? " Serenity " is a valid title for this age when it is interpreted to mean three things: (1) There is a second plateau of maturity in life on which woman must reorient herself in all the facets of her personality—physical, psychological, and social. (2) Aging is not a disease or disintegrative force, nor is senescence a state of pitiable decrepitude of mind and body to which we must all succumb—if we live long enough. Both aging and senescence are inherent parts of life that we must acknowledge, accept, and seek to understand and thereby enjoy. (3) It is a challenge to woman and the society in which she lives to recognize and exploit the potentialities of this final age to the end that it will be vital and productive for their mutual benefit.

At present there are many who are denied the experience of this age, and for many who do survive, it is not an age of serenity, but one of frustration, invalidism, aloneness, uselessness, or helpless dependency; and society is more apt to consider the age a burden than a blessing.

The fact that few achieve and maintain serenity into old age does not deny the possibility that many could. It is not a right, God-given or withheld. It is a privilege that must be earned. And it can be earned only through the combined efforts of the individual and society. Any real hope of such achievement must be based on understanding. We, as individuals, and society as a whole, must know what the full potentiality of the age is, how good it can be, how long it can last. We must recognize and accept the starting point. We must understand what the aging process is and what the threats to serenity are before we can formulate our plan of action whereby many individuals may enjoy, and society may be enriched by, this final Age of Serenity. The age is now a reality. The serenity is still a dream.

This is a new age for womankind because only a few generations ago a mere handful lived long enough to experience it. Now there are millions in this phase of life, and there will be proportionately more with each succeeding generation. And, because it is a new age, the pattern of woman's behavior has not crystallized. She may therefore make of it what she will if she realizes that serenity must be planned for and worked for with strength and enthusiasm. Her success will come in proportion to her early recognition and acceptance of this age and her preparation for it. It is not the beginning of the end, but the dawn of a new kind, a second age of maturity.

THE DURATION OF THE AGE

A long life has always been the cherished desire of mankind. In ancient days, the means for this accomplishment were sought in elixirs or potions, alchemy, witchcraft, and sorcery. Even today, those who celebrate their hundredth birthday are congratulated on their achievement and questioned as to their secret of long life. Singly, their answers are interesting, but collectively they are a mass of contradictions. Some counsel complete sobriety; others a daily resort to the little brown jug. Some have adhered to a restricted diet of one kind or another; others have eaten heartily every day of whatever was put before them. Some advise a life of work and earnest endeavor; others caution against taking life too seriously.

From the ancient past to the present, there has always been a quest not so much for long life as for the retaining of youth, or return to youth—rejuvenation. Ponce de León, as every schoolchild knows, sought the Fountain of Youth in Florida. From long before his time, we have pictures and stories depicting man's quest for youth: magical streams whose waters would restore the vigor and strength of those who passed through them; baths that crippled old ladies approached in carts or on crutches and left on dancing feet, youthful and eager to join their waiting swains. We have not lost this wistful longing for eternal youth, even today. There are cults whose aim is to teach their devotees how to look young, act young, and stay young. Novelists have entertained us with the stories of mysterious places where time stands still, youth is perennial, and no one grows old. There are also stories of mystic elixirs or magic formulas that restore the potency, strength, and beauty of youth. We are intrigued by these fantasies and, while denying the possibility that they could ever come true, deep down inside there is the thought that perhaps it would be nice. But would it, really?

The search for boundless youth has not been entirely within the realm of man's fertile imagination and daydreams, of mysticism and magic. Even in the early beginnings of medicine, centuries before it became a science, some who were impressed with the mystery of body function, of life and death, observed that the aged were cold and dry while youth was warm and fullblooded. They concluded that to alleviate the infirmities of age, if not to restore youth, these qualities should be restored. Old men (women have not often been in the picture) were advised to take unto themselves a young woman, to absorb her warmth; to search out warm springs or imbibe special elixirs to restore the body's turgesence. Even the early beginnings of endocrinology sprang from this concept. The heart of a strong young animal was eaten for the strength and virility it might impart. And always there has been the belief that aging and sex potentiality have a reciprocal relationship; when sex activity wanes, aging, begins. Therefore, if sexual vigor could be maintained, aging would not occur.

The dawn of scientific knowledge of endocrinology, particularly that pertaining to the sex glands, opened new vistas to be explored. Reputable doctors experimented and proclaimed that they had found scientific ways of prolonging youthful vitality, for the male at least. As far back as 1889, one doctor at the age of seventy-two injected himself with the extract of animal testes and enthusiastically reported to his colleagues in Paris that he had benefited gre~tly. They, however, were unimpressed. A reputable surgeon of Vienna postulated, in 1920, that the physiologic life of the male sex gland could be prolonged by closing off the ducts (vas deferens) leading from them. He was not lacking in patients who submitted to "vas ligation" for the prolongation of youth. One of his colleagues went one step further by implanting in humans new sex glands derived from animals, and "monkey gland operations" enjoyed a flurry of popularity. An enterprising American substituted goat glands for the operation. Both amassed a fortune!

Following a somewhat different line of reasoning, a Russian in the late 1930's arrived at the conclusion that aging was due to changes in the connective tissues of the body whereby cells were deprived of normal metabolic requirements. He prepared a serum by injecting extracts of certain human tissues into a horse, which was supposed to revitalize these supporting tissues. This serum is said to have been used with beneficial results on many individuals, including some European notables. Although the scientist received the Order of Lenin for his discovery, he died at the age of sixty-five without using it on himself.

Whether rejuvenation is possible or even desirable is still an unsolved problem. It does not seem very important in comparison to the real problems facing us today—those associated with longevity.

The probability that many would ever live out the possible life span has always been small. But since the beginning of this century man's potential life span has been increased more than during all the previous centuries of the Christian era. In the days of the Roman Empire, 2000 years ago, the average length of life was twenty-three years, and only a few years were added as each of the centuries rolled by. In 1776 in the United States the average life span was thirty-five years and in 1900 less than fifty years. But a girl baby born in 1950 can expect to live to the age of seventy-six, her less fortunate brother to sixty-six or the average to sixty-nine years. To put it another way, Alexander the Great died at the age of thirty-three and Napoleon at fifty-two; both were old men in the life experience of their times. But in 1950, 15 million Americans or 8 per cent of the population were over 65 years of age and at the present rate of increase, it is predicted there will be 22 million such oldsters or 15 per cent of the population in 1980.

The questions arise: What is the ultimate in human longevity? How much can science hope to delay senescence and death?

Biologists tell us, from their study of the life cycle of many different kinds of organisms, that under controlled and optimum conditions the total life span in any species is about six times as long as the period required for the attainment of biological maturity. (There are of course exceptions and individual variations.) If we consider that humans attain biological maturity at 20 to 25 years, the longest life span that could be envisioned is 120 to 150 years of age. This is in accordance with actual facts. The oldest authenticated recorded age is that of a Danish seaman born in 1626 who lived a checkered life, was married at 111, and died at the age of 146. Recently a Colombian Indian who visited this country was said to be 167 years old. The prediction is that sometime in the future the expected life span will be increased to 100 years. What are the factors that modify this biological fact and determine whether one individual might live to be 20 or 100 and the average would be 35 or 75 years?

In the life history of the individual, longevity is primarily hereditary, long life runs in families. Some fabric is just more durable than others. But fragile fabrics can be preserved by care and protection from harmful influences far beyond their expected durability, and even the strongest fabrics will give way when exposed to excessive strain. Environment is therefore the second general factor determining longevity. Not all members of a long-lived family live to a ripe old age; nor do all members of another family die young. In each individual there are qualities both for and against longevity. There is individual variation in the qualities of the total personality, of mind and body, which enables an individual to meet the stresses of life long and successfully.

Sex plays little part in longevity, although prevalent figures seem to give women the advantage in maturity. It is true that more women pass through that age successfully, but when they reach old age, the advantage is lost. To put it another way, more women attain old age than men, but they do not attain a greater age.

When we turn to the general question of why more individuals are reaching the old age group, we find that increased longevity has been the result largely of changes in the external environment. The injuries inflicted so frequently and with such devastation in early life, before and during the age of maturity, have been reduced or eliminated by the conquest of infectious diseases, the lowering of infant and maternal mortality, and the attainment of better living conditions, better nutrition, and better medical care for a larger number of people. On the other hand, the hazards of the seventh age, which we are seeking to understand and eliminate, are largely those of the internal environment of the individual. These are the chronic illnesses and probably have their beginnings long before the seventh age.

Since the beginning of recorded history there have always been individuals who have achieved old age—seventy, eighty, ninety years. Judging from these writings, however, it was never a particularly happy fate, since much is said of their infirmities and little of their rewards. The problem now is not only to lengthen life but to make longer life better, to remove illness and decrepitude of mind and body from these later years. The goal therefore is old age that promises not to be one in which life is a burden to the individual or she a burden to society, but one of continued health, purposeful participation, and serenity.

In the normal pattern of life, death comes as a result of the gradual diminution of the vital forces. It is a natural consequence of living even when disease does not enter the picture. The ultimate hope for the end of our life cycle might be to repeat the experience of the " One Hoss Shay," to enjoy a hundred years of purposeful living and then to have a quiet and sudden end. More realistically, we may hope that our life cycle will follow the pattern we enjoy in our daily living. At the end of our day's activities we lay aside our cares in the companionship of our family, relax in the feeling of accomplishment, and retire to a night of peaceful sleep. In the same way, at the end of life's day, may we again be at home and again lie down to peaceful sleep—in dignity and unafraid.

We may also hope that medical science will some day help more of us to achieve this aspiration. But it will not be done by finding ways to keep the heart beating longer when disease has drained our strength, reduced us to helplessness, and clouded our minds. Nor will it be accomplished by removing us from the comforting presence of our family and depriving us of dignity and privacy of mind and body. Rather it will be by prolonging the life of the individual as a total functioning personality.

THE BEGINNING OF THE AGE

When does the Age of Serenity start? What day marks its beginning? What event heralds the arrival at this last stage of the journey of life? There is, of course, no such marking. The ages that have gone before are defined as to time and meaning. There can be no question, for example, about what constitutes the Age of Maturity nor, from the standpoint of reproduction, that this age comes to a close with the menopause.

We have been reluctant to recognize that there is another age in life, and we have been vague and evasive in referring to it. Instead, we hang on to youth and speak of old age or senility as a state that happens to other people but will never happen to us. We seek refuge in middle age when we can no longer lay claim to youth. But middle age has meaning that varies with the age of the viewer. When we are very young anyone older than the teens is middle-aged or even old. As we add years, middle age moves further ahead to include those who are a few years older. Sooner or later, a chance remark of a youngster or our body crying out in remonstrance makes us reluctantly admit to middle age, and we cling to it until the infirmities of old age will no longer allow such subterfuge and self-delusion.

From the medical standpoint, also, the last age has been denied the recognition and respect that it deserves. Woman's physiology, her health, and her problems as they occur at the end of reproductive maturity have been classed as menopausal with sometimes a vague reference to post-menopausal to bridge the wide gulf between menopause and senility.

This is a real, vital age that leads eventually to senescence, not senility, and we must find a starting point. Let us say that the Age of Serenity is marked by the fiftieth birthday. There can be no rigid definition but rarely will a woman's fiftieth birthday pass without some implication to her personally. Whether she chooses to acknowledge it, ignore it, or deny it, the fact that half a century of living lies behind is startling, sobering, and thought-provoking.

At the fiftieth birthday, a woman may have completed the menopause, be in the middle of it, or still have it before her. Some women look and feel old at forty, some are still young at sixty or eighty in that they are active, interested, and enjoy life. Mentally, some have ceased to grow years before, while for others the world with its fascinating kaleidoscope of people and events and its storehouse of knowledge is still a challenge even after their eyes are dim and their ears have lost their acuity.

The fiftieth birthday too often brings the distressing thought to a woman that her active life is over, that she is no longer young, and therefore that she is getting old. The woman who has devoted herself to rearing a family and making a home finds herself without the many chores that filled her days and at times made life quite hectic. She may feel that she is no longer needed. The creed that a woman should never acknowledge her age fills her with fear that she is losing her attractiveness as a woman. She sees ahead only loneliness, boredom, and dependency. Her incentives are no longer valid, and she has no new ones to take their place. The woman who has been employed in work other than homemaking faces the fact that there are several generations of younger women behind her, and retirement is not so many years ahead. She may see their youth as a threat to her security and further achievement in her work and may try to compete with them on their level. Having no other interest, no close human relationships, she fears the loss of her job, and the specter of old age and loneliness looms ominous. Then there are some women who close their eyes to the fact of their age and try to hang on to youth, hugging the thought that these things associated with old age will not happen to them. For all such women, the last age will not be one of serenity but of stagnation.

A woman's fiftieth birthday can be one of her best. The fiftieth anniversary is called the golden anniversary for a good reason. Gold is a symbol of something precious, durable, and lasting. In the measure of years, the very number speaks for stability, achievement, and progress and marks the entrance to the golden era. In any venture, business or otherwise, this anniversary is recognized as the time to pause, to be congratulated on past accomplishments, and, on the basis of the stability and know-how established through experience, to look forward to richer, more fruitful years ahead. It is not the acme to be followed by decline, but the promise of more to be accomplished. This designation is also valid for the greatest venture of all, life itself.

A woman's fiftieth birthday should also be a golden anniversary, symbolizing not the passing of maturity and entrance to old age but rather the achievement of another level of maturity with assets for a long, healthy, and happy life still to come. By recognizing the potentialities of the age and her own responsibilities to invest for it wisely, she may look forward to years of rich returns even through old age, which still lies far ahead. But this anniversary is not merely a milestone from which she may glimpse new vistas ahead. It is also a time to pause and reflect on the realities of today.

Facing realities can be quite reassuring, even a relief to woman, if she recognizes this age as a second chance for achievement of a new kind of maturity. The biological responsibilities of being a woman are a thing of the past, and her sole responsibility is to exploit her potentialities as a mature individual. But the fiftieth birthday is also a warning that the time is now. As a younger individual she may have compromised the present for the ambitious plans for the future, neglecting or foregoing many of the pleasures of each day, or she may have been content to muddle through with the hope that tomorrow would be better. By her fiftieth birthday she should have come to know herself and to realize that what life has to offer may also be enjoyed today. The future may hold many tomorrows, but what they will be, even how many, depends on how well she attends to the needs of today. The reassuring fact is that not only are more women living to this seventh age and enjoying its rewards, but they are reaching it with a new kind of vigor and vitality.

Let us examine woman's assets as a feminine personality as she enters this second age of maturity, which only she can develop into an age of serenity. It can be a phase of vigorous well-being and stability in all components of her mature personality—the physical, sexual, and psychological.

QUALITIES OF SECOND MATURITY

The body achieves stability of structure as it grows to maturity, and stability of function, or homeostasis, is maintained by the various regulatory mechanisms, of which the endocrine glands are a dominant element. Once maturity is achieved, there is little change, either in the structure of organs or the way in which they function. For example, the heart reaches its maturity of function early, and there is no change in the way in which it functions throughout life. The changes that impair its function, even in old age, are not primarily physiologic aging but are the results of stresses or disease that impair its structure. Many an oldster who dies in a traffic accident or succumbs to pneumonia still is truly young in heart. The brain, the most highly specialized organ in the body, also has its life cycle. Its rate of maturing follows a definite pattern and is not slowed down so much by aging as it is by injury, abuse, misuse, and disuse. If some of the faculties of learning are slowed down, these are more than compensated for by the wisdom that can come with age and experience.

Glandular Stability

There is only one organ of woman's body the life cycle of which is different, and that is the ovary. Because of the part the ovaries play in the endocrine symphony, this difference is of paramount importance. The fact that there is an " Age of Serenity " is due to a change in balance of endocrine function that results from change in the quality of ovarian function.

In maturity the body is subjected to the cyclic ebb and flow of the ovarian hormones, which has its repercussions in all the other endocrine glands. Exquisite adjustments must be made if stability is to be maintained. This state of affairs is occasionally interrupted by the longer cycle of a different endocrine balance that is in effect during pregnancy, but the system swings back to the normal monthly rhythm of maturity. In this, the ovary experiences youth, maturity, and old age over and over again in the life cycle of its functional element, the follicle. It has just so many to spend in a lifetime, a few each month.

This refers to the life cycle of the ovary as the organ of fertility, the source of the germ cells and the hormones that support the changes necessary for fertility. In the normal course of events the loss of ability to produce ova occurs before the loss of hormone production, which may continue for years after the cessation of menstruation. The sex hormones, particularly estrogen, are always important to woman, and it is well for her that the ovaries continue to produce some estrogen for years after they have ceased to be organs of fertility. But even this is not the whole picture. The feminine body does not have to experience the effects of a gradual decline and eventual total disappearance of the sex hormones as the ovaries go to sleep. Rather there is a period of readjustment of the whole endocrine gland balance; and there is a second reserve source of the sex hormones that continues to produce after the ovary bows out.

The readjustment of endocrine balance begins as the ovaries slow down in their production of hormones, particularly estrogen. After the menopause, the cyclic production of estrogen is absent, and the pituitary continues to produce and in increasing amounts. A state of hyperfunction develops that involves not only the gonadotropic factors (which may be increased ten to twenty times in amount) but also the adrenotropic and thyreotropic factors with resultant increase in adrenal and thyroid activity. This happens rarely enough to cause unpleasant symptoms but actually may be quite beneficial. (Remember the role that the adrenal and thyroid hormones play in strength, energy, and efficiency of total body function.) Eventually the pituitary hyperfunction subsides, and a new endocrine balance is achieved.

This new endocrine balance is truly a basis for serenity, for it contributes to increased physical strength and stability. The cyclic nature of endocrine balance, which is more vulnerable to stress, is replaced by a stable continuing equilibrium. The ovaries probably continue some secretion of estrogen, but more important, the adrenals become a steady source of the sex hormones—estrogen, androgen, and progesterone—as well as of their own specific hormones. Each of these hormones contributes to woman's general well-being.

Physical Fitness

The degree of physical fitness woman will enjoy during the seventh age will depend to a large extent on how well she has achieved maturity on all levels of her personality during all the ages preceding. Health, as was first pointed out in the Age of Maturity, is attained through adequate physical exercise, proper nutrition, and psychological growth. It may, of course, be impeded, injured, or destroyed by the hazards of life, illness, and disease. Being a woman and bearing children need not cause impaired physical fitness. Rather, being female gives woman an advantage toward longer life and a degree of protection from certain obstacles.

In general, physical fitness, as measured by the amount and kind of exercise that a woman is able to perform at this age, is largely dependent on the habits and training of her earlier years. The character of her training is largely cultural in origin. In some countries, physical exercise is an important part of everyday life. Gymnastics are stressed in schools and colleges. Family outings that include hiking, mountain climbing, and bicycling are considered desirable recreation and fun as well. Individuals well past middle life can perform with a dexterity, stamina, and strength that compares quite well with even the youngsters.

In our culture, exercise is not so highly regarded; in fact, it is largely ignored. Even the physical exercise of everyday living is reduced almost to the vanishing point. Housework is no longer arduous, office work is largely sedentary, and we have almost ceased to think of our legs as a means of transportation even for one or two city blocks. Furthermore, in the mad rush of today's living, we do not think that we have the time or the opportunity for physical exercise. So, if a woman is to have adequate physical exercise, she must make an appropriate and effective effort to obtain it, and she will be amply repaid in increased physical well-being.

That an individual in our prevailing culture can succeed in attaining and keeping physically fit is demonstrated in the cases of women such as dancers, swimmers, and actresses, whose careers are dependent on it. Exercise is part of their business, and they continue it not only through the Age of Maturity but far into the Age of Serenity.

What is the effect of aging on the woman's ability to perform physical exercise? Very little, really. As a young woman of twenty to twenty-five she reached the peak of her ability in the kind of exercise that requires a quick burst of energy. She could run for the bus or play a strenuous game of tennis and not be winded. If she had continued training for this sort of activity, she would have maintained a good deal of the reserve needed for it. Even with only a modest amount of regular exercise she can expect to have a greater amount of endurance for a somewhat less strenuous type of exercise than she had in youth. And this, with only a little effort, she can maintain with its resultant physical fitness to the end of life.

All that has been said about physical exercise is contingent on normal nutrition. Malnutrition detracts from the ability to perform physically, and in turn exercise is helpful in maintaining normal nutrition by healthy appetite and optimum weight.

The basic requirements of nutrition at the Age of Serenity are the same as they were for maturity, and they will continue to be the same throughout healthy old age. Woman still needs protective foods and sufficient calories to maintain energy and normal weight. As the years go by, she may encounter some problems in maintaining normal nutrition. Teeth go, and dentures do not always make eating a pleasure. Members of the family are not always there to share meals, and eating alone is not conducive to a good appetite. If a woman has paid proper attention to nutrition in the earlier years, this is the time that it begins to pay dividends, and if she has ignored, either through carelessness or ignorance, the body needs for normal nutrition, now is the time that she begins to pay the price. Many of the chronic progressive diseases of old age, which make their appearance at this time, are associated with, if not actually caused by, faulty nutrition.

We do not know many of the answers as to the role that nutrition plays in body metabolism, mental health, physical illness, and aging. The search is going on, greatly accelerated in the past few years, and will some day remove some—perhaps many—of the obstacles to a healthy, happy old age. But these are the "why's" and "wherefore's" that are within the province of research. The fact remains that enough is known to enable an individual to maintain normal nutrition, and this information is understandable by anyone who makes an effort to learn.

Sexual Tranquility

It has been said that women and men in this seventh age become a "third sex, the neuter sex," and lead a vegetative existence. This implies that when they have passed the age of fertility, maleness and femaleness cease to be characteristics of their personalities. This is, of course, nonsense. Sexuality continues on all levels of personality. Sex-identification is the result of years of living, thinking, and acting as a man or woman, which is not destroyed by the loss of sex vigor. Men and women remain physiologically different with different life potential, life expectancy, and vulnerability to disease. Woman never loses her femininity even though she loses her fertility. All the aspects of her personality—intellectual, emotional, physical, and sexual—that characterized her as a mature woman continue to characterize her in the second maturity and old age.

The only basis for such a characterization of the age is the fact that the gonads bow out of the picture, taking with them the hormone balance that obtained during maturity. With this may go some of the physical aspects of sexuality, the physical drive for sexual activity. But this decrease in sex hormones is a slow process and in the healthy individual not only a late one but one for which the body is able to compensate for a long period of time. The body will eventually miss the functioning of the gonads, but not until it also feels the effect of decline in efficiency of all the other functions of the body. The real difference in this age as to sexuality in individuals, male as well as female, is the change in emphasis from a role of dominance to a supportive role. Thus the age should be one of sexual tranquility not asexuality.

This concept of sexuality is not often presented to woman as she seeks to understand what the later years hold in store for her, but not because there is any timidity in the discussion of sexuality. As a matter of fact, sexuality after the menopause is given more attention than any other aspect of woman's personality.

The usual admonition to woman in referring to the postmenopausal years is that she has nothing to fear—she need not lose her sex urge or her sex attractiveness, but can actually gain in proficiency and enjoyment. The reason given for this apparent rejuvenation is that menopause relieves her of the burden of reproduction and the fear of pregnancy, and she is free to indulge in sex for pure pleasure, unhampered by dread of consequences. The truth of the matter is that woman cannot expect any sudden blooming of her sexuality just because she no longer menstruates and can no longer conceive. The satisfaction of her marital relations is dependent on far more than the physical, which is only a part of the successful marriage that comes with the integration of the physical relationship with companionship and compatibility. Unless a man and woman have grown together through the years on these other levels of their personalities and relationship, there is little chance that a magic spark will be added by the removal of the possibility of pregnancy.

A woman will have sexual responsiveness on the basis of her maturity not as a result of the loss of her fertility. Any increase that may come as the result of the increased physical vigor and well-being of the age, enhanced by relief from other demands for her strength, such as care of children or work, is only another means of expression of a deep abiding love—the need to give, the ability to receive.

If a woman has a deep-seated neurosis that prevents her from accepting her sexuality and the achievement of a satisfactory sexual adjustment during maturity, she will not be suddenly blessed with it at this later date. This is not to say that a woman is neurotic if she does not have the same vigor of sex drive and reactions as her mate. It would seem that some of those who are urging woman to fulfill herself forget or choose to ignore the fact that fundamentally sex is different in the male and female. From the very nature of his physiology, the male is aggressive and his urge is active and recurrent and often indiscriminate, while the female's role is receptive and highly selective. And love is not a physical technique that must adhere to one pattern for all people. Many women have never experienced this " joy of being a vital wife " and are perfectly satisfied with their married life unless they perchance read somewhere of how much they are missing and are lead to believe that there is something wrong with them.

If a woman's lack of interest in sex during her mature years has been due to a lack of general physical vigor, then the release from the demands of her daily routine and the increased physical vigor of the postmenopausal period can allow the fires of sex to be rekindled. On the other hand, when a woman resorts to an increased attention to sex as an effort to hold on to her mate and exhibits too great a concern about losing her attractiveness, this is an indication of her immaturity. If, after all these years, she has to hold her husband by physical attraction alone, she has failed miserably to achieve all that marriage should mean to her. Furthermore, her actions may be more detrimental than helpful. The husband might not welcome the increased demand on what may be his waning powers. A man experiences a decline in his sexual potency that he cannot conceal and that can be far more devastating to his ego than a woman's decline is to her. There is no unanimity of opinion regarding whether there is such a thing as a male climacteric, but there can be no doubt that men experience change. For some it comes early, for some late. There are men who have fathered children in the seventh and eighth decades of life, but they are no more numerous than those who slow down° and lose their sexual potency in the third and fourth decades.

Equanimity

There is only one constancy of maturity through the ages, and that is change. The mature woman recognizes this and honestly means it when she says on her fiftieth birthday that she would not turn back the clock. Certainly, she will look back to her sixteenth birthday, her twentieth, and others, each with its special significance, but only as cherished memories. She also looks forward realistically to the years ahead, recognizing that change is inevitable. This is to be the age of fulfillment. There will be changes that she will like, and some that she will dislike. Some things she can continue to have, some she will have to forego. She must learn to make the most of what she will have and to compensate for the things that she will lose.

Perhaps the most important thing for her to realize is that there are changes that old age will bring. All the goals of maturity that she has striven for—self-respect, achievement, the respect of others, all the abilities she has sought to perfect, become no longer goals for future fulfillment but acute needs in old age. She will need to be loved, to be wanted, to have someone to love, to be interested not in self but in others and in things impersonal, and to be a functioning and contributing member of her world.

The dawn of this second age of maturity is her last chance to determine whether the last years of this age will be a second childhood of dependency, ineffectiveness, deterioration, and senility, or years of continued fulfillment in serenity. This is, of course, not a mere matter of choice and determination on the part of the woman. She must have physical health and an adequate supply of material needs—food, shelter, and clothing. And she must be allowed by the society in which she lives to pursue her aims and be accorded a respected place in that society. There will be obstacles that make full realization of these goals difficult, the most important being the lack of qualities of maturity within herself and the continuing desire to grow and to learn. The problems of life, illness, the loss of family, and the narrowing of her circle of old friends as the years go by will decrease her assets of physical health and security. Through no fault of her own she may have lost or been unable to establish the kind of material security that she needs.

These obstacles need not be insurmountable. We have only to look around us or to page back into history to see that there have always been some who achieved the fullness of serenity whatever their surroundings, and others who seemed to have everything but still failed miserably. For serenity comes from within. It is arrived at through a mind that continues to grow. There must be continuous and unrelenting cultivation of native intelligence, a continuation of learning and above all an achievement of understanding. The capacity to grow through the ages brings knowledge, experience, and wisdom. There must also be self-discipline, which leads to the acceptance of reality, whether pleasant or unpleasant, and not to expectations impossible of fulfillment.

GROWING OLD

As we examine these qualities of second maturity that woman may abundantly possess at the beginning of the age, the questions arise: What changes will the years bring? How and why do they occur? What is the point at which she too will become an "old woman"?

To find the answers, we may compare woman's personality as an old lady to that of the young woman she was on that day long ago when we first saw her at the seashore. The place where we will find her will be indicative of the differences. She will not be by the seaside, walking alone, scantily clad, dreaming of the future. Rather, let us hope, she will be by her own fireside, for she needs now the warmth of the fire and the warmth of the love of her family. We would have to search to find any resemblance to the fresh beauty of youth. Her hair is sparse and grey, her skin like thin parchment, her curves are gone. Instead she has her own beauty that experience has drawn in the wrinkles of laughter about her eyes, the creases of worry on her brow, and the light of understanding in her eyes.

She is not so tall, nor so erect. Her movements are slower and do not give the impression of boundless energy and strength. Her steps are not so firm and sure, and she does not pause in a leisurely stroll to look dreamily into the future. If she were on that same beach again, she would not see the far distances over the water, she would not hear the slight sound behind her, and she might not recognize the friendly face in the twilight.

The wonderful mechanism that is her body is still functioning in harmony but in a different gear, at a different speed, with a different degree of efficiency to serve, in some respects, different needs and purposes. We call her healthy, not only because she has no disease, but because she possesses the qualities of mind and body still to enjoy life and still to be doing. We call her old because she has experienced years of living that have wrought changes. The change in appearance of her body is obvious, but the more important changes from the standpoint of health are those within—in the wisdom of the body in its ability to regulate, to maintain a healthy balance of controls and functions, and to meet stress.

We think of her as frail and needing to be protected because we instinctively realize that age has robbed her of resiliency and powers of recuperation. We know that youth can heap abuses on the body that, for a time, the body can take. This the oldster cannot do. She is more vulnerable also because she has lost some of her resistance to infection and bears the scars of indulgences and the injuries of youth. She no longer has speed and skill in her body movements. She is quiet because when her body is at rest, subjected to no stress, its functions are adequate, but they cannot rise to the occasion of great stress, such as heat and cold and physical exertion.

When did these changes that we now see start? How did they progress? There is no one answer, for the onset is insidious, and the time of occurrence and rate of progress is variable for each facet of change in body structure and function and from one individual to another. In the healthy individual, senescence, or old age, is a normal physiologic state and has its own characteristics of bodily structure and function. Senescence is the result of the normal process of aging. It is not to be confused with senility with its qualities of decrepitude, which is the result of illness that has impaired the normal function of some part of the mind or body.

The Aging Process

Aging is a characteristic of all things, those of the world of nature and those made by man. The world satellite, so new and intriguing to us, is an example. Its life cycle depends on the way it is made, the forces built in, which send it into its orbit. Whether it achieves its goal and how long it will last depends on its driving force, the amount of wear and tear it encounters, and its ability to withstand the stresses both from within and without. But its life, long or short, is limited—there will be an end. The purpose behind its launching lies not just in how long it will last but in how fruitful its cycle will be. Aging is an integral part of the life process, beginning when life begins. It is not some vague destructive force that makes its appearance late in life and heralds the beginning of the end. The character of the aging process for each individual, whether it be the body as a whole or any of its parts, is dependent on the same three factors that contribute to longevity—those of heredity, external environment, and internal environment.

The cause of aging has not received the intense investigation that other aspects of the life processes have, perhaps because it represents the inevitable. Only recently has old age—how, why, and when it occurs—come under surveillance. Modern physiologic research has revealed the mechanisms and regulation of body control and function in regulatory systems with checks and balances. When the mechanisms and requirements for normalcy of function near the perfection of maturity are revealed, it becomes apparent that many factors are at work. Each of these has been sought out and examined as the key to the aging process.

The process of aging has been attributed to the loss of efficiency of the endocrine glands, and with some justification, because the endocrines contribute to so many of the regulatory processes of the body. The process of aging, from time immemorial, has been associated with sexual activity, and certainly the sex glands and their hormones play a part. Estrogen, for example, besides its role in the reproductive process, is part of the regulatory mechanism of bone structure, cholesterol metabolism, and fluid balance. Androgen contributes to protein metabolism and muscle strength. But administration of the sex hormones will not delay the process of aging. The thyroid might reasonably be suspect, due to its over-all control of the rate of metabolism. Slowing down of thyroid activity leads to decrease in efficiency of body functions, which is also a characteristic of aging. Administration of the thyroid hormone may be beneficial, but it will not prevent ultimate aging. The adrenals are certainly important in their contribution to the ability to perform work, to stand stress, and to adapt, as well as in their specific metabolic activities. The result of their deficiency has many similarities to the findings in old age. The same might be said for the pituitary gland.

The nervous system is responsible for the direction of the vegetative functions of the body and plays an important part in many endocrine mechanisms, including the ability to adapt and to stand stress.

The vascular system supplies nourishment and oxygen to tissues and the kidneys, which play an important role in maintaining the normalcy of blood constituency and are essential to health and vigor in maturity. When they function with less efficiency, tissues suffer.

The loss of efficiency of function in every one of these systems is present in old age in varying degrees. Yet we cannot rightly attribute aging to their decreased function, because they themselves have aged, they too have undergone changes in structure. We cannot differentiate cause and effect of aging in any one particular system. The answer must be sought not in the regulatory mechanisms but in the tissues themselves and in the basic unit of life in the body, the cell.

Tissues grow old when they lose their ability to grow, for cells to divide and produce succeeding generations of cells, which are normal, vital, and young in structure and function. Why do cells loose their ability to stay young? We do not know. The answer is being sought by study of the various structural elements of the cell (the mitachondria, the nucleus with its chromatin material, the genes), the chemical constituents.

The aging of cells has been demonstrated in tissue culture. Pieces of tissue such as embryonic connective tissue has been maintained for long periods of time by optimums of nutrition and environment and protection from contamination and infection. The tissue grows and the cells reproduce, with increases in total size, and must be divided. But such growth slows down with time and eventually ceases, and the cells die.

Another type of culture is that of animals whose total life processes are contained in one cell, the protozoa. The paramecium reproduces by simple cell division to form two new animals similar in size and structure. But vitality is lost, and this type of reproduction eventually fails. Renewal of vitality is obtained by the union of two cells with a pooling of their resources and then equal division to form two rejuvenated mature cells.

Signs of Aging

If we define aging as the natural decline in efficiency of function (which goes hand-in-hand with structural changes) from the peak of normal, we will find signs of aging early in life. We could detect early signs of aging through all the functions of the body and their underlying structure. Aging is revealed by X-ray quite accurately from early in the "Age of the Unborn" throughout all the seven ages in the characteristic changes in bone structure.

In practical, everyday living, however, we do not look for signs of aging in internal function of the body. Instead we relate aging to personal appearance. But even the physical signs seem less significant today because there are ways by which we may maintain efficiency of function in spite of age. Eyeglasses, for example, are no longer unattractive spectacles, the crutches of old age, but are acceptable accessories worn without hesitancy or embarrassment, sometimes even for adornment. Hearing aids, while still not quite so acceptable as glasses, can be worn with comfort and concealment (thanks to the miracle of the transistor) and have replaced the ineffective tube and trumpet of only a few decades ago. We lose our baby teeth to a new and stronger set, and although there is no hope of further natural replacement, such as some animals enjoy, modern dentistry has taught us how to preserve our teeth longer and to replace them with comfortable, attractive, and functional appliances.

Woman should not look only in the mirror for signs of aging, however. She should also watch her behavior and performance in thought, speech, and deed to see whether growth is slowing, and recession is taking over. One sign of old age is a tendency to reminisce. Memories of past events come back clear and precise, while those for recent events are fuzzy and indistinct, if they come in at all. There may also be a loss of zest for living and less satisfaction in, or even desire for, accomplishment. This lethargy may be intensified by a timidity to undertake new projects or even a resistance to new ideas and change. But these and other changes represent only the rust accumulated by time, which may be polished off. It is not corrosion, which is insidiously destroying.

In the physical changes that take place as woman becomes older, there are three elements that she watches for signs of aging—her skin, her figure, and her hair.

The process of aging is especially noticeable in the skin, where we can see and feel the changes. The skin in some measure reflects the health of the body as a whole in the characteristics of its texture, moisture, color, tone, pigmentations, and blemishes of one kind or another. In the same manner, it shows characteristic changes in each of the ages of youth and maturity and in old age.

The aging of the skin is the result of changes in structure, which are representative of the process in other organs of the body. In old age the skin is thin, wrinkled, and dry as the result of atrophy, dehydration, loss of elasticity, and change in the colloidal state. These result in decrease in size and amount of the functional elements, loss of some of the essential elements, and their replacement by fibrous tissue.

The thickness of the layers of cells comprising the skin is actually decreased, and the cells are replaced more slowly. The hard outer layer continues to be formed (keratinization), but desquamation is not as efficient. The glands of the skin—both the oil and sweat glands, do not function as efficiently, failing to supply the skin with moisture and lubrication. The blood supply and nerve supply may also be decreased. These changes lead to dryness, scaliness, and loss of elasticity. There is also a loss of subcutaneous fat, which normally cushions the skin and fills it out, and the skin is thus thrown into wrinkles and folds.

With these changes in structure, the skin is less able to function efficiently as an organ for the welfare of the body as a whole. And it is exceedingly more vulnerable. It is less able to stand the stress of heat and cold and external irritants, or to resist infections. When injured, it heals more slowly. It is also more vulnerable to internal stress, such as nutritional deficiences and metabolic imbalance.

The skin of old age is subject to blemishes that are typical for the age, most of which are only disfiguring, but a few are of a more serious nature. "Liver spots" is the common name for brown areas that appear most frequently on the exposed surfaces of the body, the hands and face, and like freckles are due to aggregations of pigments that cannot be bleached out. They have no relationship to the liver and are of no particular significance. "Warts" and other dry crusty areas should be seen by the doctor for diagnosis.

The signs of aging in the skin are usually late in making their appearance, but vary in time (as do all the other characteristics of aging) among individuals. They may occur prematurely. Accelerated aging of the skin can be caused by overexposure to the sun rays. In relatively young, healthy individuals who spend a great deal of time out of doors, such as farmers and boatmen, the exposed areas show the signs of aging. Excessive sunbathing over a period of years to attain the dark tan that some think so attractive may in reality destroy the youthful appearance of the skin.

The use of cosmetics has increased and they have become a necessity to the average woman. There is no reason why she should not, and every reason why she should, use them to improve her appearance and increase her self-assurance and sense of well-being. What she will use for beauty is a matter of personal choice, but what she can use for health with any expectation of success is a matter of fact.

With the rapidly increasing number of women in the older age group, we can expect that the cosmetic business, which now involves billions of dollars each year, will not fail to exploit this fertile field. Besides continuing their claims to methods of maintaining youthful loveliness, the next step will be rejuvenation, with proposed ways to turn back the ravages of time, by skin foods, skin tonics, wrinkle-removers, or nourishing creams. We already have some, such as the " miracle " ingredients of the queen bee or hormone creams. Cosmetics can serve very useful purposes in alleviating skin dryness, covering blemishes, and giving an attractive appearance to the skin. But their ability to reverse the aging process is questionable, to say the least.

The feminine figure will eventually show signs of aging by change in weight, body proportions, and typical curves. But contrary to popular concept, this is normally late in occurrence, and there is much that woman can do to stay the process. The middle-age spread and mature figure involve gain in weight with increased padding around the hips and abdomen, which is not an inevitable attribute of aging. Gain in weight in this age has the same origin as obesity in the other ages. In the aging process, the typical finding is loss of fat in all parts of the body. The change in contour is due to the loss of subcutaneous fat in the typical areas of feminine padding—the breasts, hips, and thighs. This is increased by the gradual atrophy of breast tissue. The abdomen may become more prominent due to loss of muscle tone of the abdominal wall and flatulence due to altered intestinal function.

Advanced old age may bring its own types of curves, the stooped shoulders and increased curvature of the spine. These are due to loss of muscle strength, which holds the body erect, and to changes in bone structure.

It is apparent, therefore, that woman can maintain her figure for many years by adherence to proper nutrition, which not only prevents the addition of excessive weight, but which will maintain normal body function and muscular strength. To this must be added adequate exercise with attention to postural habits.

Hair is one of woman's most typically feminine attributes, an emblem of her femininity. The hair of her head is a cherished adornment, which she uses to express her personality by her choice of arrangement. The color classifies her more than anything else, but this too she can change. The sexual distribution of hair that appears with puberty she accepts and copes with as she sees fit. But she abhors any obvious growth on the rest of her body, particularly that suggestive of masculine distribution. The aging process may bring changes in any or all of these—the color, the texture, the amount, and the distribution.

"Gray-haired" and "old lady" used to be synonymous, but this is not true any longer. If a woman keeps her youthful face and figure by attention to her health, gray hair may be an asset, not the sign of old age. This change in attitude is good and probably reflects the acceptance of a common occurrence, for few women reach fifty without a few gray hairs. Many have a noticeable amount in the mid-thirties and a few even in the twenties.

The age of onset and the rapidity of change of hair color is mostly hereditary just as the original color is. Usually the progress is slow with long intervals when there is no perceptible change. Sometimes the change starts early and is rapid. The fact that the white forelock is fashionable may be because it has no relationship to aging but is a congenital or hereditary character. Some persons are born with an area of hair completely white that remains so for life.

It has been said that graying is associated with a decline of ovarian function. Premature graying, when heredity is not a factor, may be the result of premature loss of ovarian function. Certain nutritional deficiencies and glandular disturbances contribute to the loss of luster, brittleness, dryness, and thinning, but not to the graying process.

Is there anything that woman can do to stay this natural aging process, to prevent the hair from turning gray or to restore its youthful color (other than by tints and dyes)? Some years ago there was a short flurry of excitement over the use of a vitamin, calcium pantothenate, to prevent graying and restore normal color. This was based on observations in certain laboratory animals. The fact that one hears little of it today is proof that it did not produce similar results in humans.

There is some change in the sexual distribution of hair. The axillary and pubic hair is gradually diminished. And there is occasionally some increase in the facial hair, but rarely to the point of being disfiguring.

Aging of the Reproductive System

Since the maturation and maintainance of function of the reproductive system is dependent on normal endocrine function, which centers about the ovaries, it is to be expected that with the cessation of ovarian function regressive changes in these organs will follow. This, however, is neither an abrupt nor necessarily a rapid progress. The rate of involution will depend on the available supply of estrogen, which may be supplied by the ovaries for years after the menopause and which is supplemented by the adrenal glands.

The uterus grows and attains maturity of function at the call of the ovarian hormone. It has this sensitivity at birth, and it never loses the ability to respond—and response is in proportion to the amount and kind of hormones supplied to it. Thus the uterus could be maintained in size and function, with recurrence of bleeding simulating menstruation, by the administration of the estrogenic hormones for years after the menopause. Even women in their seventies or eighties who have not experienced menstruation for many years, when given large doses of estrogen for other reasons, may have episodes of uterine bleeding.

In the normal course of events, with the gradual depletion of estrogen, the uterus decreases in size and becomes harder and more gristly as the musculature is replaced by fibrous tissue. This is the same process of atrophy that we have already seen in the skin. Fibroids (nonmalignant overgrowth of uterine tissue), which grow with estrogen stimulation, can be left if they are not causing trouble by bleeding, pain, or pressure, because they too will undergo regression or shrink when estrogen decreases after the menopause.

The vagina attains its maturity as a soft, elastic, moist pouch under the beneficence of the estrogenic hormone. When the hormone is withdrawn, it loses these properties. It shrinks in size and loses its elasticity and moisture; its lining instead of being soft and moist, becomes thin, glistening, and dry. There is also a change in the chemical reaction from the normal acidity to alkalinity. These changes make the vagina more vulnerable to trauma and infection. Senile vaginitis is the result of such a condition and may be accompanied by a moderate vaginal discharge, with occasionally some tinging with blood. The most distressing symptom is the itching, which comes as the result of irritation of the sensitive and vulnerable skin about the vulva and rectum. These symptoms should be taken to the doctor, first for accurate diagnosis, and second because there are several ways of attaining a great measure of relief. One is by the use of local application of the estrogen hormone in creams, ointments, or suppositories.

The urethra, the small tube leading from the bladder to the exterior, also undergoes regressive changes. These at times may make the postmenopausal woman very uncomfortable by such urinary symptoms as increased frequency of urination, burning, and, most disturbing, incontinence. These symptoms also are relieved by local application of the hormone (which woman can be taught to apply by means of a specially sized suppository) and medication to control low-grade infection, which is so apt to be superimposed on the regressive changes.

The external genitalia also show the typical signs of aging. There is loss of subcutaneous fat in the mons and labia majora. The hair, which appeared at puberty, begins to drop out, and what remains becomes coarse and gray. The skin about the vulva undergoes the same changes as skin in general.

The reproductive organs are held in place by supportive ligaments for each organ and layers of muscles that form the floor of the pelvic basin. When these supportive structures are no longer adequate, displacement of one or more of the pelvic organs results. This more frequently is due to the excessive stretching and trauma of childbirth. The stress of lifting or pushing heavy objects, or even obesity, can aggravate and even sometimes initiate these abnormalities. Thus the bladder may protrude into the vagina (cystocele), the rectum may bulge forward (rectocele), or the uterus may drop down and even protrude far out of the vagina (prolapse, or fallen womb). Fortunately, with the high quality of obstetrical care that women receive today, extremes of these abnormalities, which used to be quite common, are rarely seen today. But mild conditions may become exaggerated in the later years by the aging of supportive tissues, which results in loss of their elasticity and strength. Usually, these conditions should be corrected surgically, for they are progressive and can become trying and even incapacitating.

The breasts, composed as they are of glandular tissue and fat, both of which had their growth and cyclic changes as the result of hormonal function, eventually show marked retrogressive changes. The fat decreases greatly, and the soft glandular tissue is replaced by fibrous cords, which are easily felt in the now sagging breasts. The nipple and areolar also decrease in size. Occasionally, in menopause and the years immediately thereafter, the breasts may seem to increase in size, feel swollen and tender, due to the hormone imbalance.

HOW OLD IS "OLD"?

Who can say, for *old* has many meanings. As applied to woman's material possessions, she calls them old or new according to their actual age, their competence or acceptability, or her sentiment toward them. Last year's hat is old regardless of its competence as a headpiece because it has been displaced by this year's fashion. She may refer to one dress as old when, in fact, it may be of fairly recent acquisition but does not measure up to her expectations. On the other hand, a particular dress that she likes she will cherish and refurbish, and she will not think of its age until its tired fibers no longer have the strength to hold together. She treasures each new electrical gadget because it provides the competence to do a better job quicker and with less expenditure of her own time and effort. But she also treasures an old pewter spoon because it is a family heirloom.

We have measured woman in the preceding ages in terms of her physical, mental, and emotional characteristics, her competence and perfection of these characteristics, and always her acceptability of and participation in the world of others. We may attempt to do the same for old age, although we have less factual information to provide the answers. The task is made more difficult because this age, unlike the preceding ones, which are fairly well defined as to time, has no time markers. A woman at 43 is undoubtedly an "old" torch singer, but she is a "young" scientist. In like manner, she is an "old" tennis champion, but a "young" grandmother.

It is obvious that some individuals are physically old at 40 and some young at 60 as measured by their physical abilities and activity. And that at 75 one individual is young and spry, while another is old and decrepit. Individuals have different rates of aging that do not correspond to the years they have lived.

Some people grow old sooner and faster than others because of the qualities of their heritage, their individual capabilities, and their experiences. A person becomes "old" at some particular age not because of any one of these determining factors, but by the interaction of all. For instance, a heart attack before the turn of the century was, more often than not, fatal. The person suddenly aged to the point of death. With the dawn of modern medicine, the person's chance of survival was increased, but he was sentenced to chronic invalidism because of the accepted medical practices of that time, with consequent loss of incentive, productivity, and participation. As a result of this, he aged rapidly and became old before his time. Now cardiac cases are returned to active life, although they are somewhat limited. Their life expectancy has been greatly prolonged but is less than that of a "well" person who has suffered no such stress and damage to a vital organ. He is therefore somewhat older.

The facts of psychological aging are not quite so obvious or easily measured because they concern what is actually happening to the woman's mental capabilities and what her feelings about it are. Both in turn are greatly modified by her physical health and her place in the world of others.

We measure psychological age in youth and maturity in terms of the person's ability to learn, to understand, to grasp facts, or to solve problems. We know the growth curve of mental ability reaches a peak at about thirty and levels off to a fairly constant level, which may be maintained throughout maturity and even far into the second age of maturity. Very little has been done toward measuring ability in old people, so we really don't know to what degree there is loss in the later years due to aging alone. The problem is made more difficult because such testing is dependent on the oldster's ability to see, to hear, to write—in other words, her physical abilities. Physical infirmities may interfere or impede their performance and give a false indication of psychological incompetence.

Psychological aging is not to be measured in terms of capabilities alone, but in the use to which they have been applied from early age through all the years of maturity. This consists of a blending of a desire to learn, the ability to wonder and to derive satisfaction and pleasure therefrom, a diversity of interests, and the will to make the necessary effort. Such full use of her mental capabilities will slow the process of aging and make it possible to adjust to the limitations that physical aging (which may include infirmities and loss of some particular ability) and the changes in her life situation (such as retirement and the loss of loved ones) impose on her activities.

Adjustment, however, does not mean blind and helpless resignation to one's losses. Rather, it means that a woman must regularly take stock of her assets and re-invest them for the greatest possible returns. She must also recognize the fact that the returns may not be either as great or of the same quality as formerly, but that they can be made to fill her needs. For example, retirement brings the loss of her occupation and the social status it has bestowed, which must be replaced by self-appointed tasks or projects. Or a widow must find satisfaction in less personal relationships with friends without expecting to fill the void completely. If a woman expects to retain the status quo of maturity, disappointment is in store for her. But if she accepts the changes and makes the most of what she has, the rewards can be rich and full, even though less spectacular.

Society says that the individual enters " old age " between the ages of sixty and sixty-five by setting the age of retirement when active work must cease. There are many things even now pointing to the fact that setting a date is unrealistic and may be detrimental to both the individual and society.

The meaning of " old age "—when it comes, what its qualities are, what to do with those who have attained it, and what they are to do with themselves—is one of the most pressing and unanswered questions of the day.

To attain old age thus becomes a challenge to each of us. To meet this challenge we must not only understand the meaning of aging, but our goals must be definitive, realistic, clear-cut, and worthy of the effort. This entails also a recognition of the obstacles that may stand in the way.

XXV

THE OBSTACLES

TODAY WE CAN BOARD a stratoliner to be whisked across the continent in a matter of a few hours with confidence that we shall arrive not only quickly but safely. Fresh and unfatigued we pursue the purpose of the journey, whether it be work or play. We may look back, only a few short years in the long span of human progress, with keen interest and pleasant nostalgia to the same journey traveled by wagon train. We forget how real the hazards of the journey were, how many were lost along the way, and how tired and worn the travelers were at the end of the trail. We may also look ahead, to the future of space travel, the obstacles of which now seem ominous and insurmountable and the goals unknown, mysterious, and of questionable value.

This change in man's mobility, his ability and success in journeying afar, is encompassed within this century. There has been a comparable change in the characteristics of his journey through life. We are approaching as never before the achievement of mankind's cherished hope for a long life, but we are as yet far from achieving serene old age as man's common destiny. Instead there are still many obstacles encountered all along the way. Some still prove to be insurmountable, and untimely death is the result. Others deprive him of his health and well-being.

Life has been lengthened largely by understanding the hazards and removing the obstacles that are the product of man's external environment. These obstacles were the diseases of infancy, childhood, and young adulthood. The outstanding examples are the conquest of some infectious diseases by prophylactic vaccines, and control of others associated with animal hosts, such as malaria, by the removal of these hosts. These achievements were coming to pass at the turn of the century and are now so well established that we take them for granted. Since then, health has been increased by the application of advanced knowledge of nutrition, maternal welfare, and child care. Other infections as causes of illness and death have been reduced. Appendicitis and pneumonia, once major causes of untimely death in young adults, are less often fatal because of better means for early diagnosis and treatment. The new wonder drugs, the sulfas and antibiotics, will now control most of the infections that still occur. (Other countries less fortunate than the United States are just now on the eve of removing these hazards to life and health.)

With the removal of some of the harmful agents in the external environment, man has added new things that are proving detrimental to his health, such as radioactivity, smog, and the dusts of particular industrial processes. With the changes in his way of life he has added stresses, which are proving harmful to his health and happiness. As he aspires to move into the new environment of space, he is confronted with other new factors, such as weightlessness, aloneness, and cosmic rays of the external environment. All are obstacles with which he must learn to cope.

As a result of the scientific advances, more individuals avoid or successfully surmount the hazards of childhood and early maturity only to encounter other obstacles, diseases of another kind or origin. Many of these disease processes of later years are so common and insidious that they are often wrongfully accepted as part of the aging process. Others seem to strike without warning and quickly destroy. But diverse as these illnesses may seem, they all have one thing in common—all have their origin from within the body. Changes in the internal environment or changes in the regulatory mechanism of some phase of body function leads to loss of control, decrease in efficiency, or loss of balance between functions. The result is such a change in structure of certain organs and tissues that they may no longer function efficiently and well. These diseases have been loosely classified together as the "degenerative diseases" or "metabolic diseases." They include such seemingly different processes as arthritis and other bone and joint diseases, high blood pressure, heart disease, senile dementia, and, lacking any other classification, cancer and other new growths. These obstacles provide the various kinds of stress that may rob woman of her health and vitality, and she too often arrives at the seventh age battered and worn, unfit to meet the challenge to make this truly an Age of Serenity.

We are living in a period in which there is acute consciousness of the threats of illness and the causes of death. We are confronted daily with the propaganda of the dangers and tragedies of disease. And we are appalled by the apparent rising toll in lives lost by "heart attack," "strokes," and "cancer," which suggests that these are the product of the age in which we live. They may be, in part. But they are the diseases of age (not caused by age), and more people are living to the age of particular vulnerability to such diseases. Furthermore, these are broad categories, each of which includes many specific disease entities. Some of these are mild, slow of progress; some can be controlled, some can be cured; and only some are the so-called killers.

It is true that we do not know the cause, we do not have a cure for, many of these diseases, but there is still a bright side. Even the worst killers do not strike a deadly blow each time. Nor will they strike everyone. And some of the killers can be cured. Much of the crippling can be prevented or ameliorated. Statistics can be helpful to us generally, if they encourage us to direct our energies and resources toward the support of research to find the cause and the means to cure or alleviate suffering. They may also be helpful personally if they induce us to meet our problems realistically by learning and applying the knowledge available for the preservation of our own health. They are harmful when they cause us to become apprehensive, introspective, preoccupied with illness, ever fearful of any suggestive sign or symptom. To meet the obstacles, each individual must find strength in her personal philosophy of life and her understanding of the meaning of health. Both are based on knowledge.

Cancer is, of course, not a disease of old age, for it is no respecter of time, age, or sex. It may be encountered at any age within any part of the body. It is considered here because it is a formidable obstacle to serenity. We shall consider it first to remove it from the continuity and context of the metabolic diseases that are associated with aging where it does not belong. To obtain a proper perspective on cancer, we must first understand the meaning of "new growth."

NEW GROWTH

Growth is an essential of life. Cells must divide continuously to form new cells. For health to be maintained, growth must follow a definite pattern, orderly and restrained. We have seen this action in the Age of the Unborn, where cells rapidly divided to form more and more cells, which take on different characteristics as tissues and organs are differentiated. The process is orderly, co-ordinated, and has its limitations and a specific goal. We have seen it in childhood, where growth had as its main purpose increase of the same kind of tissue for increase in size of the body. In maturity there is growth for a definite purpose, as in the menstrual cycle, and for continued replacement and repair, as in the skin. All of these are manifestations of growth that is normal. It has purpose. It is orderly, cells are replaced by similar cells to continue normal function. It is restrained; no more cells than are needed are produced. It is restricted in that the cells remain in the place that is normal for them; liver cells stay in the liver, bone cells in the bone, and endometrial cells in the uterus.

But there are times and places in the body when the growth process fails to be limited to the preservation of normal structure and function and does not meet the specifications of normal growth. New growths (neoplasms) are the result. "Tumor" is a general term applied to new growth, but it carries no special significance because it simply means "swelling" and may refer to mere increase in the size of an organ or the localized increase of cells in a tissue. I was quite startled for a moment when the word was used in such a general way. A doctor reported that Mrs. X, whom I had referred to him for further care, had "an expanding tumor of the uterus." He was facetiously confirming the diagnosis that Mrs. X was pregnant, and certainly her uterus was swelling with new growth. Usually "tumor" does not have such a happy portent, but neither does it forebode dire consequences.

"Tumor" encompasses the whole range of new growths and includes such diverse structures as moles on the skin, polyps, fibroids of the uterus, cysts of the ovary, all of which are benign; and cancer, which is malignant.

Benign Tumors

As a rule, benign means that a tumor is harmless to the host or at least does not threaten life. The cells grow in an orderly fashion, producing like cells of fairly normal structure corresponding to the cells of origin, and the tumor cells stay put in the site of origin. They are walled off and do not invade surrounding tissue. Thus a lipoma is a soft well-defined but excessive mass of fat, such as may occasionally be felt under the skin. A fibroma is a well-defined, usually hard nodule made up of connective tissue cells. Fibroids of the uterus are excessive amounts of a relatively normal type of tissues, the connective tissue and muscle.

Benign tumors are listed not because they are obstacles to health as a rule, but to emphasize that not all lumps are cancer. This does not mean that they should be ignored or self-diagnosed, but neither should the discovery of a lump create panic. There are a few instances in which a benign tumor may not be so benign but a threat to the health or life of the individual. One instance is the location in which the tumor occurs. A brain tumor, which may be a cyst or a neurofibroma, due to its increase in size and the fact that the bony cranium has little room for expansion of its contents may exert destructive pressure on the brain. Such a tumor is not malignant in the sense that cancer is malignant, but its effects may be just as deadly unless it is accessible to surgery. The second instance of a benign tumor being harmful is due to the kind of cells involved. Tumors made up of endocrine gland cells continue to secrete, and the quantity of the secretion becomes excessive for normal body function. We have met with hyperplasia (benign overgrowth) of the adrenal cortex, which results in virilism in the young woman. Adenoma of the pancreas may produce hypoglycemia or hyperinsulinism; and hyperplasia of the thyroid produces hyperthyroidism or exophthalmic goiter.

Malignant Tumors

Malignancy, as an attribute, characterizes its subject as being of evil disposition, malicious, disposed to do harm and inflict suffering. Malignant tumors have a dire portent because of the behavior of the cells that compose them. They will, if allowed to follow their course unchecked, destroy normal tissues of the body and life itself. "Cancer" has come to be the common name applied to all malignant new growths. Specific names are used to express the kind of tissue from which the cancer is derived. Thus carcinoma is a cancer that arises from epithelial tissues, such as the skin and vital organs of the body. Sarcoma is a malignant tumor that arises from the supportive tissues, such as bone and muscle. In blood, malignancy is exemplified in the leukemias.

In cancer, all the restrictions of growth are lost. The cells divide—sometimes rapidly, sometimes slowly—but they keep on dividing, piling up more cells that have no useful purpose. Cancer cells may arise from any tissue, but after a few generations of cell growth they lose much of the characteristic appearance of the parent tissue and take on the characteristics of malignancy. Growth is no longer orderly or restricted, but disorderly and unrestrained, and the cells of this new growth invade and destroy the neighboring normal cells.

Normal cells of an organ stay in the location where they are formed, pass their useful life, and are replaced by just the number needed to retain the integrity of that organ. Cancer cells have no such restrictions, they multiply, invade, and plunder. In the progress of their growth small blood vessels are damaged, and there is leakage of blood. When this occurs in the lining of organs, such as those of the digestive tract or the reproductive tract, the minute amount of bleeding may be detected. When the cancer cells have invaded larger vessels, veins and lymphatics, some may break off from the parent mass and be carried to other parts of the body. Even in this new territory they do not lose the capacity for wild behavior. They thrive just as well in different kinds of tissues and continue their unrestricted growth.

This transference of cancer cells from the point of origin to distant parts of the body is called metastasis (derived from the Greek meaning "taking up one's stand in a different place"). The time of occurrence of metastasis is the crucial moment in the life of the individual. It marks the dividing line between the cancer being curable and incurable. When the malignant growth is excised by surgery or destroyed by radium or X-ray before metastasis occurs, the individual may be cured. If some cells have already broken off and been carried to distant parts of the body, the cancer is usually incurable.

All cancers do not have the same degree of malignancy. How malignant any one will be depends on its rapidity of growth and its tendency to invade and to metastasize. Some cancers are slow growers and rarely metastasize, such as certain cancers of the skin. At the other extreme are those that grow rapidly and metastasize early before the tumor mass has achieved appreciable size. The degree of malignancy of a particular cancer may be recognized by the characteristic structure of its cells.

The Nature of Cancer Cells

Cancer cells are sick cells, and the sickness affects a particular part of the cell, the chromatin material within the nucleus. Among normal cells the control of the functions of the cell—life, growth, reproduction, and characteristics of behavior—resides within the nuclear material. Among cancer cells, their behavior is changed because the nuclear material is changed.

Modern sciences have not yet revealed the answers as to the cause and cure of this sickness, but perhaps they have already furnished the tools for some day finding those answers. All fields of science are contributing to the understanding of the sickness of cells. The electron microscope has provided means of studying the morphology of abnormal cells, radioactive isotopes are used to seek them out. Irradiation has been used to cause the sickness for experimental purposes and to destroy the abnormal cells. Histochemistry provides means of studying the details of intracellular chemical changes. Other disciplines, such as genetics, virology, immunology, and endocrinology, are contributing bits of pertinent information. Some day the pieces will all fall into place. Some have already been fitted into segments that have meaning.

Science not only is interested in the appearance and behavior of these sick cells (for the purpose of diagnosis and treatment) but is searching for the "how," and "when," and the "why" of these changes. The solution of the "why" may some day reveal the cause of cancer. But there are some interesting and useful facts that have already been established about the "how" and the "when," the life history of particular kinds of cancer.

Cancer has come to have such a terrifying connotation that the diagnosis of cancer seems to be an acute emergency. It seems to imply that "cancer has struck, heroic measures must be taken immediately!" Cancer doesn't suddenly "strike." The chances are that, when recognized, it has already been in existence for a long time. Cancer may start as the affliction of one cell or group of cells, and the development may be slow. There can be a long latent period, a matter of years in some instances, before the cancer becomes dangerous in the sense that it exhibits the destructive characteristic of invasiveness. Furthermore, some cancers after they have declared themselves are never very dangerous. The life history of each kind of cancer is different and depends on the kind of cells involved, the location in the body, the age of the individual. This does not mean that physicians have any inclination to temporize with any kind of cancer, but it gives them leeway to be selective in the treatment to be used.

Seeking the Cause of Cancer

The reason cells in some spot in the body go wild and wreak havoc on the rest of the organism has become the number one problem of medical research. There are many avenues of approach, all of which seem to be bringing the answer a little closer, but none supply the one way to truth—if there is only one way. There are groups of factors that undoubtedly affect cell behavior and seem to be likely implements in the various manifestations of cellular misbehavior. These include such different factors as heredity, irritants, hormones, and infective agents, particularly viruses.

The history of cancer in one's family is likely to be more meaningful as a cause of anxiety and concern than any other factor. A woman wonders if she is more likely to have cancer if her mother or some other member of her family had cancer. The increased frequency in some families and the apparent freedom of others suggests that there is a difference in susceptibility, but why or how this is transmitted we do not know. There is no way of determining how large a part it really plays or whether it plays any at all in the incidence of human cancer.

Irritants, as a possible cause of cancer, may include any factor derived from the external environment that threatens injury to the area to which it is applied. Many have been suspected as a cause of cancer. For instance, when a woman sustains a blow to the breast, she is frequently apprehensive that it may lead to cancer. And a woman who develops such a cancer may search back and usually remembers some such injury. The fact that there are far more women who also have had similar injury to the breast and do not develop cancer makes it improbable that there is any causal relationship.

We are now in the midst of the controversy as to the part that cigarette-smoking plays in the incidence of cancer of the lungs. Years ago, it was thought that pipe-smoking was far worse because of the increased frequency of cancer of the lip among pipe-smokers.

Hormones, particularly sex hormones, have received more than their share of notoriety in relation to cancer. It is understandable that they should come under scrutiny because they are stimulatory in their action. They cause growth, and they cause changes in cells in specific areas of the body. Sex hormones are essentially growth hormones as applied to the reproductive system. But it must be quite confusing to most laymen (as it is also to many doctors) to hear on the one hand that hormones are dangerous, that they cause cancer, and on the other that large doses of the same hormones are used to treat the same kind of cancer with some beneficial results.

In considering the organs of the female reproductive system and their hormones in relationship to cancer, there is one important fact to be remembered. The breast and the uterus, the most frequent sites of cancer, are *estrogen-dependent* tissues; they did not grow and develop until estrogen was supplied them, and they regress when estrogen is withdrawn. Cancer cells derived from these tissues have the same ability to respond. They may grow faster with hormone stimulation; they may slow down when estrogen is withdrawn (by castration) or suppressed (by androgen administration). But in either case cancer cells have the characteristic of wild growth, which will continue and gain momentum with time after hormone stimulation is removed, and they also overcome the suppression afforded by other hormones and resume their relentless destructive growth. There is no proof that the hormones cause the crucial change in cells from normal to malignant. The most that can be said is that these hormones change the environment in which cancer arises.

Each of these factors—heredity, irritants, and hormones—has appeared to be in some way associated with cancer with sufficient frequency to suggest a causal relationship. It might seem that where there is so much smoke, there must be some fire. But this is not necessarily so. There is no proof as to cause, there is only evidence as to incidence—the frequency with which they are co-existent. No one can say just how much each may have contributed to the fire. Any one may have provided only the dry tinder ready to ignite, added an inflammatory ingredient to the pile, or raised the wind to support and aggravate the conflagration. The source of the spark that sets the fire we do not know.

Infection is another likely suspect as the cause of cancer. Cancer cells in many ways behave as foreign elements, which fail to respond to the normal regulatory mechanism of the body and invade and destroy. Scientists have long searched for an infecting organism that could change the structure of the cell to produce this abnormal behavior. Viruses have come to be the most likely suspects. They live and reproduce only within living cells. One of the first experimental malignancies was produced by infecting a normal tissue with a virus.

The Diagnosis of Cancer

We are told that at present the one hope for the cure of cancer is early diagnosis. How is this to be achieved—by tests, by signs and symptoms, or by physical examination? Equally important: What constitutes early diagnosis?

The question is often asked: "Why hasn't some one devised a test for cancer?" And frequently, doctors have requests for a "cancer test." But such a request fails to recognize that testing requires two elements, a specific thing to be searched for and the appropriate tools for the search. In the days of the gold rush, prospectors found gold because they knew they were looking for heavy glittering yellow nuggets or dust, and they had the necessary tools in the pick ax, pan, and chemical assay. But they did not find uranium, for no one even knew that such a precious substance existed. Even after uranium was identified, finding it would have been difficult without the knowledge of one of its characteristics, radioactivity, and a tool, the geiger counter, to identify it by this characteristic.

There is no known physical, chemical, or even biological reaction that is peculiar to cancer. And until one is found, there can be no test for cancer. It has long been the hope of medical science to devise a test that would reveal the presence of cancer long before it had grown to the size that it would produce signs and symptoms. Many procedures have been tried, but none has proved to be reliable. The more recent investigations of cell structure in terms of its chemical components and their molecular structure, the enzyme systems, and immunological mechanisms have put new tools in the hands of researchers and made this hope seem more likely to be realized.

There are symptoms that occur with cancer, and it is important to know what these are and to be alert to their first appearance. But at best they are only circumstantial evidence to be investigated. They are not conclusive evidence that cancer is present. Not all lumps, pimples, or blemishes are cancer—the majority are not. Nor does bleeding necessarily mean cancer. All of the signs and symptoms can be caused by other processes, but they should not be ignored.

Many tests and procedures are useful in making the diagnosis of cancer, but there is no all inclusive list that must be used every time in a cancer check-up. Rather there are only two essential procedures, a detailed history and a complete physical examination. Thereafter the doctor must select the further procedures to be used to follow up suggestive findings. A person could not afford the time, would not relish the discomfort, or be able to pay the cost in a yearly check-up for all the procedures that are available. A doctor is not remiss when he does not order even a small number of these tests, and he is not necessarily giving the patient a thorough check-up when an imposing and expensive routine is followed.

The only means of diagnosing cancer has always been and still resides in the recognition of the characteristic morphology of the tumor. When the tumor is large, the structure of the mass itself may be suggestive. A lump felt in the breast may seem to be cancerous because it is hard, its outline not clearly defined; or a shadow in an organ on an X-ray, because of its shape and density, may seem to be cancer. But the actual definitive diagnosis can only be made by microscopic examination of the cells of the mass. This is usually accomplished by biopsy. A specimen is taken from the living tissue for examination.

In days gone by, investigation was often delayed until the mass by its size and the symptoms produced forced itself to the attention of the doctor and the patient. Now we are alert, and knowing where cancer is apt to occur, we look for small masses or changes that do not give the appearance of a mass at all. For example, the mouth of the cervix is one of woman's most vulnerable spots. Doctors do not wait until a characteristic mass is apparent, but investigate by biopsy any suspicious change. Biopsy is therefore the most useful diagnostic tool available today.

There are, however, two important aspects of the biopsy that should be emphasized. First, when a doctor proposes to do a biopsy, it does not necessarily mean that he will find cancer. Biopsy is a necessary precaution that he must take. And second, not all masses need to be biopsied. For example, the doctor may be able to identify tumors of the skin as harmless cysts, or fibromata, or the masses found on pelvic examination as inflammation of the tubes, cystic changes in the ovary, or fibroids of the uterus.

Exfoliative cytology has put another tool into the hands of the doctor, helping him to make an earlier diagnosis of cancer. Cells that line body cavities are constantly being shed as individual cells and maintain their characteristic structure, for a time at least, in the fluids within these cavities. Cancer arising in the lining, even while still a small mass, may also shed its cells. The presence of cells in the fluid may be recognized by microscopic examination.

The fluids accessible for such study include those of the vagina, the urinary tract, and the nose and throat. Material for study may also be obtained from internal organs such as the colon, rectum, stomach, and lungs by appropriate techniques. Fluids from cysts such as occur in the breast may be aspirated and examined. The findings of abnormal cells can only be taken as suggestive of cancer. The area from which the cells came must be located and a specimen for biopsy taken for a definitive diagnosis of cancer to be made.

The vaginal smear test is the most extensively used and widely publicized application of this technique. The taking of the test is quite simple and causes the woman no discomfort. The necessary material may be obtained by a swab introduced into the vagina. The technique of taking the smear and staining it affords no difficulty. But the reading of the slides and interpretation of the findings is not a routine laboratory test that any technician can do. It requires highly specialized skill. Some doctors have acquired this training and examine the slides they take, but most doctors prefer to send the slide to a pathologist for diagnosis.

The test is primarily a search for suspicious cells, which would indicate that cancer of the cervix may be present. Cancer of the cervix arises in the epithelium, the cells covering the surface or lining the canal. The most frequent site is the small area surrounding the opening where the stratified epithelium covering the vaginal surface joins the glandular lining of the canal. Cells are shed in very early stages of cancer into the vaginal pool. Cancer may occasionally arise from deeper areas within the canal from which exfoliated cells are not so readily obtainable. Only occasionally are cells found that have been shed from a cancer within the body of the uterus. And cancer of the vagina is very rare. Although this area from which suspicious cells may be obtained is very small, only about the size of the head of a match, it is one of the most frequent sites of origin of cancer in women.

Sometimes the articles on the cancer smear test presented for woman's consumption are misleading. Women are led to believe that they have had a test for cancer, and when the test is reported negative that they do not have cancer anywhere in their body. All this test reveals is the fact that suspicious cells have or have not been shed from one very small area. It tells nothing about cancer anywhere else in the body, and it is good for a limited time. The test should be repeated at yearly intervals.

The test is primarily a screening device whereby suspicion may be aroused when no other signs or symptoms are present. The frequency with which this occurs has been variously reported as one in 300 or 500 cases. This should lessen woman's fear that she harbors a cancer that has revealed no signs. A positive test is merely indication for further study. There are occasionally false positives. The test should not take the place of a careful physical examination but is merely one part.

Woman's Cancers

The difference in the life histories of specific kinds of cancer, the various techniques that must be used for diagnosis, and the potential danger to the individual are illustrated in the cancer of the female organs of reproduction. Not all organs are equally susceptible. Specific organs can be more vulnerable at particular ages and in special circumstances. Some are readily diagnosed, while others are elusive. Each requires individualized treatment.

Cancer of the uterus varies tremendously in its characteristics depending on whether it arises in the cervix or the body. Cancer of the cervix occurs most frequently during the reproductive life of women. It occurs more frequently among women who have borne children. Cervical cancer is characterized by its invasiveness. Arising as it does in the epithelium, it spreads into the wall of the cervix and then further to involve other nearby pelvic organs, the bladder and the rectum. Metastasis to distant organs is relatively late in occurrence. Cervical cells are frequently more sensitive to radiation (readily killed by application of X-ray or radium). Because of its usual accessibility, it should have a high incidence of diagnosis and cure.

Cancer of the body of the uterus occurs more frequently after the menopause and in women who have not had children. It also most frequently arises in the epithelium (endometrium), but encased in the thick muscular walls of the uterus, which has little tissue connection to other organs, it does not so readily invade and is also slow to metastasize. Although not as readily accessible to direct examination as the cervix, it frequently gives warning of its presence by minute amounts of bleeding, and it can be diagnosed early by a thorough curettage and cured by hysterectomy.

Cancer of the ovary is silent. It develops without the warning sign of bleeding or the symptom of pain. However, it occurs in older women. Therefore increasing size at a time that the ovary should be shrinking is a warning to the doctor that something is amiss. The chances of discovery early enough for cure are enhanced by the fact that ovarian cancer is usually slow of growth, slow to metastasize, and rarely invades.

Cancer arising primarily in the epithelium of the vagina is perhaps one of the rarest types of cancer in the whole body. Malignancy of other elements of the pelvic organs, such as the tubes, is also rare.

There are many abnormalities such as lumps, discolorations, and ulcers of the vulva, which a woman may see or feel—and fear to be cancer. They rarely are. Cancer in this area rarely occurs until after menopause. It has much the same characteristics as other cancers of the skin. It is slow in growing and slow to metastasize and has as its forerunner an aging process of the tissue, leukoplakia, in which the skin becomes thickened and white, with pearly nodules in some areas. The changes give rise to the discomfort of burning, itching, and later some slight bleeding. The cancer develops slowly and rarely invades or metastasizes until the original cancer is far advanced. Because these cancers can be seen and felt by the woman and are a source of discomfort, they can be diagnosed early and therefore are more often cured.

Thus cancer is in a sense a different disease in each of these organs. This fact serves to emphasize that there is no one symptom or sign, no one test for cancer. Rather the hope of early detection and cure lies in careful pelvic examination at regular intervals beginning in maturity and continuing into old age. X-ray examinations give little help in the diagnosis of pelvic cancer.

The breasts share with the cervix the greatest vulnerability to malignancy in woman, as well as accessibility for early diagnosis. Cancer of the breast usually arises from gland cells (adenocarcinoma). It grows to form a nodule or lump, which can be felt even when it is still quite small. There are characteristics of shape, consistency, and movability of nodules in the breast, which provide the doctor with suggestive evidence of whether or not they are malignant. The important thing is to discover the nodule before it has advanced to this state. Therefore all small nodules of the breasts should be suspect until proven otherwise. The woman who discovers a lump in her breast should see her doctor immediately. He alone can determine whether the lump is harmless or a threat to the woman's life. If a cyst is suggested by his findings on examination, he may insert a needle and draw out fluid, which may be examined for suspicious cells. Usually it is considered the safest procedure to remove a lump for microscopic examination. If it proves innocent of malignant qualities, nothing more is necessary. If the lump proves to be malignant, further measures must be taken to ensure that all the malignant cells have been removed.

The Treatment of Cancer

The control and cure of cancer depends on our ability to recognize these sick cells early and eliminate them before they have established a stronghold and increased in number. We may hope some day to cure them of their sickness, convert them back to normalcy before they have wrought havoc and destruction, or to immunize cells against this sickness. But such treatment must await the acquisition of knowledge and understanding of the sickness, which we do not now have. Even with our limited knowledge of cancer, how it starts and its various life histories, cancer can be cured. At present this depends on the removal of all the cancer cells in one location before they have had a chance to spread. This is most readily accomplished by surgery, although some kinds of cancer cells are removed by the lethal action of irradiation.

We are prone to take a pessimistic attitude toward the cure of cancer. This pessimism is engendered by the statistics of the incidence of particular kinds of cancer and the number of deaths and by our own personal experience and knowledge. This is not entirely justifiable, for a great deal of progress has been made. Before 1900 there was no particular effort or even means of diagnosing cancer early, and when the symptoms of the advanced stage became obvious, cancer was met with a rather fatalistic attitude that nothing could be done except to keep the person as comfortable as possible until the inevitable end. From the turn of the century to World War II there was no particular attempt to search out and make an early diagnosis of cancer, but when it was found, surgery and irradiation were extensively used in the effort to cure. In the time since then, tremendous changes have developed both in diagnosis and treatment and a dynamic search is under way for the cause of cancer.

The number of surgical cures has been increased by the advent of antibiotics and the acquisition of new tools and techniques (anesthetics, heart-lung machines, safer transfusions, new life-saving drugs, to name only a few). This applies particularly to areas that were previously inaccessible surgically. Also, more powerful means of irradiation have become available whereby tremendous doses may be delivered to pin-point spots without encroaching on the normal surrounding tissue. And selective irradiation can be administered by the radioactive isotopes.

The over-all number of cures has been greatly increased by the more intense search and early recognition of localized cancer and even precancerous lesions that is now going on. This number can be increased even more. Woman's two most frequent cancers, of the cervix and the breast, afford good examples.

Chemotherapy has come to be one of the most promising as well as the most extensively pursued fields in cancer research. It has long been the hope of medical science to find some drug that would search out cancer cells and destroy them or render them innocuous much as chemicals and antibodies act on infections. The difficulty lies in the fact that cancer cells and normal cells are too much alike in their requirements and susceptibilities. As a result, many of the drugs that might be lethal to cancer cells are also harmful to normal cells. Newer research is revealing the molecular structure of the components of the cells, particularly the nuclear material, and some differences are being found in the chemical requirements and metabolic processes between normal cells and cancer cells.

Chemotherapy of cancer has certain requirements as to safety and effectiveness. The chemical agent used must be lethal to the cells that take it from the bloodstream and attempt to use it in the metabolic processes. It must therefore be of such a structure that the normal cells will reject it. But it must be enough like a chemical that the cancer cell needs for the cancer cell to take it in and try to use it. In a rough way this is something like what happens when a weed-killer is applied to the lawn. The dandelions absorb it and die, the grass plants do not absorb it, and they live.

Chemotherapy affords the greatest hope for cure of cancer because its effects need not be localized but extend to all parts of the body, reaching cancer cells in whatever remote spot cancer may have arisen or been carried to. There is no expectation that one drug will be found for all cancers, but rather that many drugs will be discovered each of which will be useful in a particular kind of cancer.

Chemotherapy constitutes a large part of research on cancer therapy today. Thousands of drugs are being screened each year in the laboratories, applied to tissue cultures of cancer cells to determine their power to kill and to animals to test their effectiveness and toxicity. Of these, less than a hundred have been selected for clinical trial. A few give promising results. Some have already been found that control one particular type of cancer, others that are partially effective, that suppress or retard the growth of cancer cells (as in leukemia).

There have been important advances in other fields, especially immunology as related to cancer, which suggests the hopeful possibility of finding other means of controlling and perhaps curing, and even some day preventing, cancer.

Cancerphobia

This is a new word, and it might be called a new disease. Never have a people been so conscious of cancer and never have they been so fearful of it. It is like the plague, the black death of the dark ages, which swept over and wiped out large segments of a population. People trembled at the thought of the plague, and they fled from the area where it had struck. They did not know the cause of this affliction, they did not know the cure. They only associated it with death.

People's reaction to cancer today is very much the same. They fear, but they cannot run away, for cancer is an individual affliction, not an epidemic (as far as we know). Doctors are not immune; they too experience this urgency and unease. A doctor has no hesitancy in telling a patient that she has high blood pressure or heart disease, to explain the situation and recommend ways of treatment. But it is very difficult to tell a person that she has cancer. The very word terrifies.

Why are we so fearful? It may be that we have not yet achieved a positive concept of health, an important part of which is a healthy attitude toward illness and disease. We have come to be intolerant of all illness. And we have been conditioned in recent years to think too much of the horror of dying of cancer and little encouraged to think of living with cancer—that some cancer can be cured, life can be prolonged, suffering can be alleviated. This is partly due to unwarranted emphasis on the statistics of incidence and fatality of diseases. Too much of so-called education is really shock technique aimed at subjective reaction rather than realistic understanding. The disease becomes a monster lurking in the dark unknown, from which we as individuals cannot defend ourselves. We may only pay tribute in dollars and cents in hope that our particular dragon will not strike us.

In considering aging we are faced with the inevitability of death and the probability, as things now stand, of some form of illness. The important thing is not to try to hide from this thought but to integrate it into our way of thinking. We must make the most of what we have with the purpose of not only making life longer but also of making it good. This we cannot do if we are dominated by fear. Everyone should not be an expert on cancer, but each of us should know a few of the fundamentals, not for self-diagnosis, but for the recognition of signals of danger. We should use this knowledge with hope and confidence that there are things that may be done and with the realization that competent medical advice and care is essential. Cancer as well as illnesses of all kinds must be integrated into our maturity as part of the acceptance of things as they are and the attempt to make a proper adjustment on all the levels of our maturity—intellectual and emotional as well as physical.

RHEUMATISM

The news that an old lady has slipped and broken her hip is not surprising, for everyone knows that old people are quite likely to suffer a fracture on the slightest provocation. When we hear "Grandpa has his gout again," we must privately think that grandpa has been up to his old tricks of taking a few too many nips. On the other hand, "Grandmother's rheumatism is bothering her" elicits sympathy for the aching pain and stiffness of her poor old joints and most likely is accepted as something one has to expect and bear in old age. When a younger woman asks her doctor, "Do I have arthritis?" she is expressing her dread of a progressively crippling malady that she has seen in others, which may lead to distortion of her body and curtailment of her active life. All of these afflictions and many others that involve the bony and muscular framework of the body are summed up in one term *rheumatism*. And rheumatism, which conjures up the picture of a body bent and gnarled, creaking in the joints with slow and difficult motion, we are apt to associate with old age.

Rheumatism is not a single entity, nor is it the result of aging. It has its origin in the old humoral concept of disease, that certain kinds of humors or fluids characterized certain diseases. Today, diseases are classified as infections, metabolic, inflammatory, traumatic, hereditary, or allergic in origin, which leaves the causes of some diseases unknown. The framework of the body—bone, muscle, and soft tissue—may be the site of disease as the result of any one or combination of these factors. Thus rheumatism includes many different conditions: bursitis, fibrositis, myositis, sacroiliac strain, lumbago, gout, and rheumatic fever, as well as the different kinds of arthritis. They may be affected by age, but they are not caused by age. With this diversity in origin and in the part of the body that it may strike, it should not be surprising that rheumatism is the greatest crippler.

It would be inappropriate to discuss these diseases comprehensively, since our purpose here is to give knowledge and understanding of the normal, not of disease. It should, however, further this purpose to select a few that have either especial significance to women or a relation to endocrine gland function or hormone therapy.

Arthritis

"Arthritis" is a generic term that refers to diseases of the joints. It may be the result of any of the causative factors listed for rheumatism. We shall select only two types, osteoarthritis and rheumatoid arthritis. The female is no more vulnerable to osteoarthritis, than the male. Although she stands a good chance (70 per cent) of having some manifestations of it if she lives long enough, it will not cripple her. Rheumatoid arthritis is the type woman is more fearful of because it is the most crippling, and she is about three times more vulnerable than the male.

When a woman past fifty has pain and stiffness in her lower back, in one knee, then the other, or in the back of the neck, and these are due to arthritis, it will most likely be osteoarthritis. And when she notices knobbiness of the last joints of the fingers, which are hard and painful, she can be pretty sure they are Heberdeen's nodes, which are particularly feminine (90 per cent are found in women) and will do little else than hurt her vanity. Almost all individuals past middle age have some such changes, but only a few have symptoms that are disturbing.

Osteoarthritis, also called hypertrophic or degenerative arthritis, makes its appearance almost exclusively at middle age and thereafter and involves the large weight-bearing joints—the knee, the hips, and the spine. It is strictly a joint disease and has no systemic manifestation (as distinct from rheumatoid arthritis). It is due to wear and tear on the joint and the body's response. It starts between the ages of twenty and thirty and is very slowly progressive, although it may be precipitated by trauma or accelerated by faulty joint alignment, such as poor posture and obesity, which add stress to the joint. The first changes are in the articular cartilages, the antifriction surface and cushion of the joint, and consist of thinning, pitting, and splitting. Since the cartilage has no blood vessels, it is less able to repair the injury. Later there is progressive overgrowth of bone around the joint. There is also roughening and even breaking away of little particles into the joint, which can be felt in the knee as a peculiar vibration and can be heard in the neck as a crackling. Since osteoarthritis involves the weight-bearing joints particularly, it is most common in individuals chronically overweight. Weight reduction is one of the most effective ways of treating it, and it follows that maintenance of normal weight during maturity is one of the best ways of avoiding this type of arthritis.

The symptoms of osteoarthritis are limited to pain and stiffness of the joints involved. The onset of symptoms is insidious, beginning sometimes years before they become really bothersome. At first, after a day of strenuous exercise and night of undisturbed sleep, the woman on arising experiences difficulty in motion because of stiffness and pain, which quickly wears off. Later, as the process progresses, pain and discomfort occur with exercise. In the late years the symptoms are more or less unremitting. They may slow the person down or curtail her activities, but they do not cripple. The pain and stiffness are limited to the joints involved.

When the arthritic process involves the knee or hip, the symptoms are limited to that joint, as exhibited by pain on motion, but when the process involves the vertebrae, the picture is less clear because the spinal nerve may be involved and pain radiates to areas of distribution, causing various neuralgias. For example, when the vertebrae of the neck are involved, the pain may go to the head or may radiate to the shoulders or down the arms, frequently eliciting anxiety because it seems to resemble symptoms of heart trouble. When the arthritic process involves the lower back, pain may radiate around the abdomen or down the thigh.

The diagnosis by the doctor is usually not difficult. The history of its insidious onset, the age of occurrence of symptoms, the joints involved, and the lack of local reaction, usually indicate the nature of the underlying pathology. This can be verified by X-ray.

There is no cure for this condition, but there is much that can be done to relieve the symptoms. Reduction of excessive weight, moderate exercise with adequate rest, and correction of postural defects may be helpful.

Rheumatoid Arthritis

This form of arthritis, also designated infectious or atrophic, is a systemic disease and usually makes its appearance in young individuals. Eighty per cent of the sufferers are between twenty and fifty years of age. It is progressive, but the course is slow, and it may become crippling. Although it is apparently an infectious process, the cause is not known, and therefore there is no specific cure.

It is an inflammatory process accompanied by acute episodes of swelling, heat, and redness. It may involve any joint, but those of the fingers, wrists, and knees are most frequently involved. Eventually the function of the joint is destroyed, muscles around the joint atrophy and the skin covering becomes smooth and glistening.

It is of interest for two reasons. First, it strikes women three times as frequently as men—why, we do not know. Second, it is the type of arthritis that has responded most dramatically to cortisone (hormone) therapy. But it is not an endocrine disease. Cortisone is used as a drug to relieve symptoms, not as a hormone to relieve a deficiency. It does not cure, it merely holds the symptoms in abeyance.

The Fragile Old Lady

Woman has an almost complete monopoly on the type of bone disease that tends to make her the fragile old lady. This is called postmenopausal osteoporosis because it occurs after the ovaries have lost their efficiency in the production of estrogen and is characterized by the bones becoming light and porous.

Although we speak of "tired old bones," suggesting that they too, have vitality, we are more apt to think of bones as merely the framework, a rigid and fixed structure, which is not involved in body metabolism. The truth is, bone is a living tissue. It, too, has specific requirements for growth, replacement, and repair that are continuous throughout life and must be met to keep bones healthy.

Bone has a fibrous framework, the matrix, which serves both as a mold and as reinforcement for the hard material, calcium. Besides the fibers, the matrix also consists of different kinds of cells, which serve particular functions. Some cells are responsible for withdrawing calcium from the blood stream and depositing it within the framework, thus keeping the bone hard and strong. Others clear out the debris of wear and tear. The matrix of bone is a soft tissue and has physiologic requirements similar to other soft tissues, such as muscle and skin. Matrix consists largely of protein and therefore requires a constant supply of appropriate building blocks, the amino acids, for its synthesis. Vitamin C is essential for the formation of a particular component of the fibers, collagen. The matrix requires hormone regulation to keep the cells functioning at top efficiency. And it must be stimulated by an optimal amount of use (exercise or stress). Abnormal bone structure may result from the failure or lack of any one of these needs.

Osteoporosis is due to the failure of the matrix to use calcium, and not to an actual deficiency of available calcium. The result is that the bone, instead of being dense and heavy, is light and porous like a sponge. It is still hard, but it is fragile and easily crushed. Osteoporosis is thus quite different from the results of calcium deficiency, which leads to a softening of the bones (osteomalacia). Such bones remain tough. They will bend, but they do not break easily. The example that used to be common was rickets in children who had a deficiency of calcium and vitamin D. (We met this as a form of dwarfism.)

Postmenopausal osteoporosis is due primarily to hormone deficiency, although dietary deficiency and lack of exercise may be contributing factors. Estrogen deficiency results in osteoporosis in this manner. Estrogen provides the stimulus that maintains both a normal amount of matrix and normal structure of the matrix. This in turn assures normal and adequate function, which is active bone formation. When estrogen is deficient, there is just not enough matrix to do an adequate job. The result is that the bone is light and porous.

The deficiency occurs after the menopause when there is a gradual decline in the level of estrogen. It, of course, may never occur at all when the decline is gradual and the adrenals contribute sufficient estrogen and androgen, which has a similar stimulating effect on bone structure. It may also occur after surgical removal of the ovaries in young women. Then the loss of estrogen is abrupt, and therefore the bone changes may be more rapid and severe. The condition is more apt to occur or be made more severe by dietary deficiencies, especially protein deficiency. We are familiar with the atrophy of muscles that occurs when an arm or leg is immobilized for a long time in a cast. Bones also undergo atrophy when they are not used.

The symptoms of postmenopausal osteoporosis may be vague and insidious in their onset. Because the bones most frequently involved are the spine, pelvis, and upper end of the thigh, the symptoms are usually referable to these areas. In the early postmenopause, the complaints are vague aches and pains, particularly in the lower back. As time goes on, poor posture progresses to stooped shoulders and eventually the woman can no longer straighten up. She loses an inch or so in height. She appears older than her age. She prefers to be quiet rather than active, to sit rather than stand, partly because of weakness but also because motion, especially turning, twisting, and bending the back, is painful. Later these symptoms become more marked with more or less constant and severe pain in the back and hips.

In some instances the symptoms continue to be mild for years, and the first knowledge of the seriousness of the changes comes when the old lady slips and breaks her hip. Or the first sign may be sudden and severe pain in the back, which she experiences with some sudden jolting or a false step. This slight stress has been sufficient to cause the collapse of a vertebra.

In the treatment of postmenopausal osteoporosis, the most important thing is the recognition that it may occur, so that the necessary things may be done to prevent it. The next best thing is to recognize its presence before serious complications occur. Methods of treatment are simple and require only the administration of hormones and an adequate and optimal diet, high in proteins and vitamin C, and exercise. Estrogen is effective and efficient, and androgen, which will do the job quite well, very quickly relieves the pain, delays or stops the bone degeneration, and may help to restore, to a limited degree, normal bone structure. But when the condition has advanced and large doses are necessary, either may have unpleasant side effects. Estrogen will cause vaginal bleeding even in women sixty, seventy, or eighty years of age. Androgen will cause masculinization. The solution has been to combine the two. They add to each other in their therapeutic value but tend to nullify the unwanted side effects of each other.

One of the most gratifying findings in connection with the treatment has been reported from clinics that have used estrogen in a large number of women over a prolonged period of time, up to twenty years. Among these women there has been no increase in cancer of either the breasts or the uterus above the usual incidence of women of that age group. This should alleviate further the apprehension and fear that has been unduly aroused as to the danger of administering estrogen to woman for her menopausal symptoms.

A fractured hip in an old lady used to be equivalent to her death warrant. Old tissues heal very slowly, and even fractures properly set often fail to show much indication of bone regeneration. Furthermore, the old lady was immobilized in a plaster cast for weeks. Immobility is an old person's worst enemy. She needs to be up and about to maintain her circulation, her appetite, and her other body functions. But especially she needs contact with people to keep her alert, active, and interested.

Immobilized in bed, withdrawn from the world of activity, the tired old body slows down and loses whatever efficiency might have been left, and interest and hope give way to despair.

Doctors have found means to circumvent this by surgery and by strengthening the bones with a nail or bone splints. This is usually not too difficult an operation, and the fragile old lady is up and about again in a few weeks, perhaps not as good as new, but with a repair that will serve her adequately for her remaining days.

HEART DISEASE

The welfare of the body—each organ, each tissue, each cell—is dependent on the supply of nutrients and oxygen brought to it in the blood, unremittingly and without stint, with each heart beat. Sudden and complete deprivation of this supply brings the organ to a sudden standstill, and if this persists too long, function cannot be resumed. When this involves such vital structures as the heart or certain areas of the brain, the result is death of the whole organism. Chronically inadequate supply of blood to any organ or tissue results in decreased efficiency of function, loss of resiliency and ability to meet stress, reduced margin of safety and degree of adaptability, and degenerative changes in the cells and tissues.

The hazards to health and to life arise from the failure of the heart to pump or the blood vessels to transport efficiently. These we recognize as heart trouble and high blood pressure and the more serious consequences as heart attack and stroke.

It is not our purpose to discuss all the possible disturbances in structure and function of the cardiovascular system. Rather we shall use one to illustrate certain broad principles that are applicable to all the metabolic or degenerative diseases.

The Heart and Its Vessels

The heart is a most rugged organ. It functions from early in the age of the unborn to the last heart beat sixty, seventy, or ninety years later, steadily and continuously, with a slight pause between each heart beat as its only period of rest. It slows down when the body is at rest, and it is ready to respond by increased rate and force in times of need. It does not lose this efficiency with aging. There is little change in the structure of its tissue; there is little change in function. Anyone who has seen an oldster stand the stress of surgery and that of the accompanying illness that made surgery necessary, or has watched a body waste away with an incurable disease, cannot but wonder at the continued strength of this magnificent organ.

The heart comes by this strength, this durability, in part by heritage just as other structural components of the body do, and in part by the manner in which it is called on to develop and maintain its potentialities starting in childhood. One cannot expect a competent response to such strenuous exercise as mountain climbing at age sixty in an individual who has led an indolent physical life all the years before.

There are some changes in competency with advancing age. The heart does lose some of its resiliency, some of its strength, and some of its ability to react adequately to stress, just as do all other aging tissues. These are usually compensated for by the fact that in old age fewer demands are made on it by such things as sudden or strenuous activity or exposure to extremes of heat or cold. The heart fails when stress has been too long or too great or when it has suffered injury that has reduced its efficiency of performance.

The diseases of the heart are the result of insults heaped on it. Such injury may first be dealt in the Age of the Unborn or in any of the succeeding ages, and the type of injury varies with the different ages. Those of early life are due to failure in development (congenital defects) or infections, particularly rheumatic fever. These forms of heart disease are rapidly decreasing in frequency and severity, as we have learned the cause and prevention of some of them and ways of correcting many by surgery.

The kind of heart disease that makes its first appearance in middle age is the real obstacle to health and longevity, for it is the cause of crippling, of decrease in life expectancy, and of sudden death. It may occasionally be a carryover from childhood injury. Most frequently it is a complex entity in which the primary factor is disease (structural change) of the blood vessels that supply the heart.

What Is a "Heart Attack"?

An attack implies a sudden and dangerous assault on the normal function of the heart. The point of attack is the coronary artery, which has been rendered less competent by disease. Most attacks cause pain, but they are not all equally painful or equally serious. Accordingly, there are two main types of attack, angina (coronary insufficiency) and coronary occlusion.

Angina pectoris (meaning pain in the chest or heart pain) is the mildest and least serious. It is a particular kind of pain that is located under the breast bone, over the region of the heart, and frequently radiates down the left arm. It is apt to be brought on by exercise, which places an increased demand on the heart's activity. Angina is not necessarily the precursor of serious heart disease. A person may suffer anginal attacks for years and never have a serious heart attack. And a person may and frequently does have a more serious heart attack without the premonitory sign of angina.

"Coronary attack" is the familiar name applied to the more serious condition. More exactly it is due to coronary occlusion or coronary thrombosis, the first meaning that the vessel has been completely closed and the second that a blood clot has obstructed the channel of the vessel. Such conditions occur in vessels that are the site of atheromatous changes, and the result is complete stoppage of blood flow through the particular vessel involved. The severity of the attack depends on where the obstruction occurs, which will determine how much and what part of the heart will be deprived of its blood supply. If occlusion occurs in a large artery or in an already damaged heart, the result may be sudden death. But this major catastrophe is not nearly as common as smaller accidents, from which recovery can and frequently does occur.

The immediate result of occlusion is that a portion of the musculature of the heart is put out of commission. If the demands placed on the heart are not too great, it can carry on. With rest and time a wonderful healing process occurs, which may restore the heart to nearly normal function and may enable the individual to resume also nearly normal physical activity. This healing consists of two processes. One, fibrosis, is a patching up of the damaged area with tough scar tissue; the other is the growth of new blood vessels into the area to provide adequate blood supply.

Why Does a Person Have a Heart Attack?

We are frequently confronted with the situation in which a person seemingly in good health (he may only recently have had a physical examination and been pronounced well) is suddenly struck by a heart attack. Why should this be so? Why are there no warning signs that the doctor can detect? Why do attacks occur?

The immediate cause of the attack can be accounted for by stress placed on an already damaged heart. It may have been some unusual strain such as shoveling snow, or intense excitement over good or bad news or anger; or it may be only slight exertion, a heavy meal that provides the proverbial last straw of a long period of excessive demand. The nature of the crippling, the damage to the heart, we also know, although its presence may not have been recognized until the attack occurs. The underlying pathology is atherosclerosis of the coronary arteries that began years before and passed through various stages of change, the climax being reached when the vessel is occluded. So the question is not why does a person have a heart attack, but what started the changes toward the abnormal structure of the blood vessels in the first place? What made it a progressive process that led to hidden crippling and made the heart vulnerable? There is no one answer.

Medical science has come to realize that the so-called degenerative diseases or diseases of metabolic origin do not have one cause. Rather the answer must be sought in three areas, which are distinct but mutually interrelated and interdependent. These areas are: the individual and his own particular vulnerability; the internal environment, the body's ability to adapt to stress; and the external environment and the stresses it imposes. These are successfully integrated in health. Failure or faults in one area have repercussions in others, and the result is illness or disease.

There are two physical factors (perhaps more) that determine in part a person's vulnerability to heart disease,—sex and heritage. Woman just because she is woman is far less vulnerable to coronary disease than man.

During the years that her own particular endocrine glands are functioning at a high level she has a high degree of immunity. Coronary artery disease in women is rare before the age of fifty and occurs occasionally between fifty and sixty; but after the menopause women lose this advantage and in old age are almost as vulnerable as men. Thus it averages out that coronary attacks for all ages are four times more frequent in men than in women.

Heritage also plays a part in vulnerability. It is a frequently observed fact that heart trouble occurs more frequently in some families than in others. But heart disease is not inherited. What is inherited is the type of cardiovascular system that is more vulnerable. Just as we inherit color of hair and eyes so also do we inherit a particular type of body build. The short stocky individuals (as compared to others of the same racial background) are more susceptible to cardiovascular difficulties than tall thin persons. This may be increased by the acquired characteristics of culture, physical activity, dietary habits, and psychological drive.

Considerable evidence has been brought forward to indicate that the quality of the diet, particularly the amount of fat, is a significant factor in the incidence of heart disease due to atherosclerosis. Intense research is being devoted to determining how, why, and to what degree this is so. Authorities are as yet not agreed as to the significance and validity of the vast amount of data that has already been presented.

In recent years, cholesterol has become a familiar term frequently assumed to be an important factor in heart trouble. Patients are requesting of their doctors a "cholesterol test." Hearty eaters are admonished to watch their cholesterol, and the crash technique of cholesterol-free diet is advocated to ward off trouble. How is it that a chemical compound that is a normal component of the body has taken on such sinister guise? Just what part, if any, does it play in atheroscelrosis and heart disease?

We have a peculiar quirk in approaching any problem of wanting a name and a number and of being satisfied with these without recognizing that both are only tools, ciphers of shorthand. The name is a means of expressing a whole host of qualitative characteristics. The number is not absolute but merely indicates a quantitative relationship of considerable variability. This is true whether we are considering intelligence and I. Q., hypothyroidism and BMR, or diabetes and blood sugar. It is also true for heart disease and cholesterol. And here cholesterol is both a name and a number.

Incrimination of cholesterol is based on two facts: atheromatous plaques (the early changes in the blood vessels) consist of deposits of cholesterol esters; and individuals who have heart attacks, strokes, and other vascular accidents frequently have high blood cholesterol levels. But proof is not to be found in examining just one element in the abnormal changes in the blood vessels and one element in the blood. Further investigation must be made.

Research has indicated that it is not only how much fat is in the diet, but how many calories, what kinds of fat. Fats are compounds of fatty acids, and they circulate in the blood stream in combination with other substances, mostly proteins. There are two groups of fatty acids—the unsaturated, which include the essential fatty acids, and the saturated fatty acids. The unsaturated fatty acids are derived in the diet largely from the vegetable oils (corn, soybean, and cottonseed, but not cocoanut, oil). The saturated are the solid fats of animal origin (fats of meats and dairy products). The body does not use these in the same way. For example, ingestion of an excessive amount of saturated fatty acids may raise the blood cholesterol level while equal amounts of unsaturated may lower it. So the questions arise: Where is the error in fat metabolism? What is its cause? There are many things being considered—the total amount of fats, the ratio of saturated to unsaturated fats, the kind of lipoproteins formed, other lipotropic factors, the roles played by hormones and vitamins. There is as yet no answer.

Exercise is also an important factor in the incidence and development and treatment of atherosclerosis. A heart attack is often attributed to exercise, and for the specific incident it may be. But proper exercise is perhaps one of the best means of preventing a first attack or a recurrence.

The incidence of coronary artery disease is three times more frequent in men leading a sedentary life (professional or white collar workers) than in those whose work involves a certain amount of physical activity (farmers, for example). But this is not purely a case of exercise versus no exercise at a particular age. Rather a long-range view should be taken. Both types of adults were active youngsters. But the sedentary adult slows down in the amount of his physical activity as he grows older.

At the same time he continues his early dietary habits and may also acquire the bad habits of too rich foods and irregular eating. The college athlete does not ensure himself superb good health in later years, unless he also adjusts his diet to his new (and reduced) activities and continues an adequate amount of exercise.

It used to be that a coronary attack meant chronic invalidism with all exercise prohibited. Doctors are now stressing the importance of a return (how soon and how far depends on the extent of the injury to the heart) to some degree of physical activity or even the taking up of exercise that had previously been slighted. Thus exercise is not only permissible, it is also necessary for two reasons: it speeds the recovery and helps maintain the regulatory mechanisms of total body health; and pleasant out-of-doors exercise is one of the best cures and preventatives of neuroses, especially cardiac neurosis.

We are led to believe that heart disease of middle age and later is the result of the stress and strain of everyday living and a product of our particular kind of civilization. Some go so far as to say that it is purely psychosomatic and portray the "coronary personality" as one with insatiable drive, with never any pause for satisfaction in accomplishment, never any relaxation but always a striving for still another goal of achievement, with complete disregard for the needs of physical health and well-being. Those who do not agree with this concept point out that such heart disease also occurs in individuals who lead a placid existence and is by no means the universal common destiny of those who do not know the meaning of serenity.

What Can Be Done about Heart Attacks?

In the past heart attacks were accepted with a fatalistic attitude. A person died, or if he survived, he was condemned to a life of invalidism, deprived of participation in any physical activity, and lived with the constant dread of another attack, which might prove fatal. Now, with the modern means of accurate diagnosis of the extent of damage and the modern tools of treatment (drugs, diet, and surgery), many more people are surviving the initial attack, and, what is perhaps more important, they are being encouraged to return to active life. The public is coming to recognize that a cardiac case should not be deprived of work, but rather that work should be found commensurate with his ability, which may be considerable. Perhaps with time other techniques will become available by which the damage or crippling can be made even less.

Meanwhile, the problem of prevention falls on the shoulders of the individual. It becomes his responsibility to make use of the knowledge of the contributory factors that is now available. Obviously, there is nothing that he can do about the vulnerability that comes with heritage. So he must concentrate on the things that he can do something about— his nutrition, exercise, and equanimity. These become especially important to those who do have the heritage of greater vulnerability.

Good nutrition requires first of all that he understand and subscribe to the principle of normal nutrition, which will assure him of getting all that he needs of the protective foods—proteins, minerals, and vitamins. The consensus of authorities seems to be that for a normal individual of normal weight who subscribes to a balanced diet, there need be and probably should not be any reduction of the percentage of fats in the diet. If an individual is overweight, he should reduce by lowering his daily caloric intake, and the easiest way to do this is to reduce the amount of fat in the diet. Certainly individuals should not subscribe to any crash method and attempt to eliminate all or a greater part of fats from the diet. The elimination should be selective and under medical direction.

It is important to find time for pleasant stimulating exercise out of doors if possible. It should be regular and not limited to a few strenuous hours on the week end or to an effort to recoup an indolent year by packing into a two weeks' vacation strenuous and unaccustomed exercise.

Avoidance of stress means avoidance of subjecting the body to too much work, too little rest, too little recreation, and too much food and drink.

Equanimity requires a degree of maturity, which the woman must achieve for herself. No little part of this is facing up to problems as they present themselves and accepting situations that cannot be changed without being overwhelmed by them. Perhaps most important to the individual is finding satisfaction in what is hers, whether it be material goods, status in her work or community, her own talents, or her relationship to other people.

Women can play a peculiar, particular, and important part in the prevention of heart disease. Since coronary artery disease is so much more frequent in men than in women, a woman's role becomes that of lending a helping hand to her husband, encouraging and assisting him in meeting the problems of his health, which for some obscure reason he often seems so reluctant to do for himself. She can do much in guiding his dietary habits, encouraging him to find time for more leisure, recreation, and exercise. And since so often he is striving to make a name, establish status, and achieve security, she can help him arrive at the true meaning of security, which is not to leave her a wealthy widow but to continue to be, in perhaps more moderate circumstances, a life-long companion. Perhaps she can bring him to do what more and more women are accepting as a simple routine, to visit his doctor regularly. She also will profit by these shared experiences of good nutrition, healthful exercise, and equanimity.

Heart disease (which includes all of the vascular system) now stands at the top of the disease list as the number one killer. As such it is the object of many fields of research. This is fine, for the more we know about health and the cause of ill health, the greater becomes the possibility of achieving a healthy, happy, and long life. But this fact has generated fear and apprehension, which in itself is a major deterrent to the goal that we are seeking. It has led to the belief that there is one killer whose identity can be tracked down and annihilated. If we just give enough money to provide scientists facilities for research, the breakthrough will be quickly achieved. But research does not work that way. No one researcher is going to find one simple answer. One may find the keystone that fits the arch, but it will be effective only when the whole arch has been built strong and sturdy by the long and patient accumulation of truths and by the discarding of faulty material by many workers in many seemingly unrelated fields.

Scientists can detect the cause of failure in even the most complicated man-made structures, such as rockets and missiles, because they know how they are made and how they work. This is far from true for scientists concerned with success (health) and failure (death) in living organisms, particularly the human body, because we are still far from knowing all the facts of the structure of the human body and even further from knowing the laws that govern its function.

Aging and death are part of life. Decrepitude and senility come partly as a result of this and partly due to the injuries and insults dealt to different parts of the body, including the heart. As science has removed the previously lethal agents from the environment—infections, malnutrition, and rigors of climate and terrain—and new forms of violent death have been substituted for old, internal changes become the more frequent causes of death. This is emphasized by the fact that the recording of cause of death now seeks to be more specific, and we find "cardiovascular failures" listed instead of "senility," "natural causes," or "old age." The fact is, it can be very difficult to say what caused death, even when autopsies are performed. At one extreme, little pathology of a specific nature may be found, while at the other extreme, there is so much that it is surprising the old machine held together so long, for there are found a dozen things that might seem to be sufficient to cause death.

There is another reason for caution that should be brought to bear in evaluating the figures that place heart disease in the number one position. Heart disease has always been high on the list because the heart is the most vital organ. We associate life with the heart beat and death with its cessation. We can do without some organs, and life continues; we can lose a part of some organs, and the remaining part will compensate. One kidney can be removed, and the other does an adequate job. The removal of a good portion of the liver, or the injury to certain areas of the brain are not incompatible with life. When such organs as the endocrine glands are removed, we have the means of meeting their deficiency. But the heart structure must remain intact. It has some power of compensation by hypertrophy to carry the heavier load, as in high blood pressure, healing injury with scar tissue, establishing collateral circulation (new vessels to replace injured ones). But all these mechanisms must come from within the heart itself. Actually, heart failure is the ultimate cause of all death since life is said to be present as long as the heart beats and to depart when the heart becomes silent.

This is not meant to belittle heart disease and its importance as a health problem. Rather it is for us to accept it and govern our lives accordingly with the best knowledge that is available and leave to the professionals the business of finding the cause and the cure and the wrangling with statistics. Only by this can we be free to spell out our allotted time in a constructive, rewarding, interesting way.

PREMATURE AGING

The challenge of the Age of Serenity is life extended at least to the traditional three score years and ten and perhaps in future generations to well past the century mark. But years alone are not the measure of success. The ideal of aging is continued physical fitness and life adjustment within the limitations imposed by the years of living. Premature aging occurs when these qualities of health are lost.

Premature aging may present many different appearances, and it may be due to many different causes. There are individuals who are old far beyond their years, and others who seem never to grow old. There are some who have risen above all kinds of difficulties, and others who have succumbed to less, and some who never had what it takes to meet life. Premature aging occurs within many life situations, but it is not the inevitable result. It may be insidious in its onset and slow of progress. It may seem to start abruptly and lead to rapid deterioration.

The obstacles that lie in the path to long life and a healthy old age have been presented as individual entities, disease processes that, for the most part, arise from within. Only examples of the most frequently occurring diseases have been discussed—cancer and heart disease because they have the potentiality of cutting life short and rheumatism because it can cripple. There are, of course, many other diseases of equally distinct identity and other, less clearly defined, degenerative processes. All may be debilitating to various degrees. These examples serve a useful purpose in helping us to understand the causative mechanism of a particular disease, which may rob an individual of health or life. It would, however, create a false impression to stop with that. In all disease processes, the effects are not confined to one organ or one system but involve the total personality. They accelerate in varying degrees the aging process.

The Rate of Aging

The rapidity of the aging process must always be measured in terms of the total personality. It will be determined by the balance that is maintained between two opposing forces—the vitality of the individual and the stress to which he is subjected.

Vitality refers to the individual as a whole—the ability to live and to function effectively. It is the sum total of the body resources, the health of the individual. Thus it may be said that "living" is the expenditure of energy; "vitality" is the amount of energy available at a given time; and "aging" is the irreversible loss of energy, which produces structural and functional changes.

We are endowed at the beginning of life, at conception, with a life force, which with an optimum rate of expenditure should last a long but limited time. This life spark, vitality, is our storehouse of energy. We have to use it at a rapid rate to get started in the business of living, to differentiate and to grow from one cell into a human being. Then we are able to coast along through infancy and childhood with less expenditure for our internal affairs. Adolescence calls for more rapid and skillful expenditure as we branch out to the more complicated activities of being an adult. Maturity brings stability, when expenditure can be slow, steady, and orderly, and the available supply can be made to last through second maturity and to ripe old age.

The human body is not like an alarm clock that is wound up, runs, strikes the hours for the allotted time and then stops. It is more like a dynamo, which generates energy at the same time that it is using energy. In the process some energy is lost; there is wear and tear and decline in efficiency.

The body possesses potentialities beyond those of any machine. It has a great amount of reserve power. There are regulatory mechanisms whereby energy is conserved and restored. The body is able to change the way energy is used under different conditions of need and the amount used. These components of vitality do not break down with age. They are damaged by abuse and disease. It is the individual's responsibility to keep them in good working order.

We have seen these in action in each of the preceding ages. Furthermore, we explored in detail in the Age of Maturity the basic requirements for the conservation of vitality. We found that physical health depends on proper nutrition and the balance of the optimum amounts of exercise, rest, and relaxation. Mental health also was found to be a dynamic quality which required nurture and exercise of all its components such as initiative and the ability to be happy and to attain satisfaction. The indissoluble interrelationship of the two provides the psychosomatic concept of health. These same qualities are also the determining factors in the process of aging. They are however modified by another factor that alters vitality, and that is "stress."

Stress has many meanings and often is used loosely to express any situation in which living is made more difficult. It may apply to a nonliving object, in which case it is a disturbing force, that threatens change in the structure of the object. Under too great a stress a piece of cloth will tear, a blow will dent a piece of metal or crush a fragile figurine. Stress occurs, the damage is done, and there is no way the object can regain the integrity of its structure.

Stress applied to living organisms has a different meaning. When anything in the internal or external environment of a living organism threatens it, there is a reserve power that can be called into use to sustain the organism. It makes changes through its regulatory mechanisms to meet the new demands, and when the situation is prolonged, it adapts itself to the new and altered circumstance in such a way as to maintain as nearly normal function as possible.

Causes of Premature Aging

Aging is an inevitable consequence of living in which there is a depletion of vitality. Under optimum conditions the rate is slow and provides for continuous and adequate vitality even into mature old age. There are many ways in which the rate of aging may be altered, vitality rapidly depleted, squandered, or dissipated. We may group these according to heritage, the physical and psychological factors of health, and the kind and amount of stress. And we shall see that in every case of premature aging all have contributed.

1. Heritage—Unfulfilled

We are apt to think of the positive aspects of heritage as material possessions and the negative in terms of physical abnormalities and to believe that there is nothing that one can do to change either. This is an unreasoned, thoughtless appraisal of heritage.

We each possess as our individual heritage qualities of mind and body, our own particular mixture of strength and weakness. It is important to know what these qualities are, but it is more important how we handle them. We cannot choose our ancestors or change our heredity, but we can analyze our assets and liabilities and govern ourselves accordingly.

Whether the quality of longevity will be realized at its maximum, or marred and lead to premature aging depends on how well the assets of health are cherished and invested and on the recognition of our own particular vulnerabilities. It is important to recognize the obvious but sometimes ignored fact that there is no rigidity, certainty, predestination. Traits run in families, but they do not appear in every individual. Some diseases are more common in some families, but not every member will inherit this particular vulnerability, and there is much that those who do can do about it. For example, in heart disease we have seen that some individuals have the heritage of body build and vascular structure that seems to be particularly vulnerable to atherosclerotic changes. But with proper attention to health one may hope to, and probably can, avoid sudden catastrophe.

We all have two assets of heritage for longevity and serenity, which we may not recognize and almost always fail to use to the fullest. These are derived from our cultural heritage. The first is the vast storehouse of knowledge of health—how to attain and keep it. Mothers use it for the health of their children but fail to avail themselves of its beneficent attributes for their own health and long life. The second is the vast wonderland of general knowledge that is ours to explore and enjoy, and there is more than enough to keep each of us busy, interested, and eager for many lifetimes. Here are to be found the ingredients of the magic elixir of life. To partake is to stay young; to abstain is to stagnate and to age prematurely.

2. Stress—Excessively Applied

Healthy aging does not deprive the body of the capabilities to withstand stress within physiological limits. When stress is too strenuous or too prolonged, exhaustion occurs, and the result may be slow degeneration in structure and function or death. Too continuous demands on the body's reserves and ability to adapt lead to deterioration in structure and function. As an example, the body can stand an occasional overindulgence in food with only some passing discomfort. But when the excess, even moderate in amount, is of long and continuous duration, the result is obesity with decrease in efficiency of body function, personality changes, and eventually changes in structure with increased vulnerability to disease processes.

When we examine the so-called "diseases of stress" in a world-wide aspect rather than in our own particular environment, we find evidence that throws doubt on the validity of the name. These diseases exist in cultural environments that do not contain the elements of stress as we identify them. For example, peptic ulcer we associate with the business executive constantly under pressure of jangling telephones, deadlines to meet, big deals to put across, or the vagaries of the stock market. But peptic ulcer is not his affliction alone; it occurs more frequently among the oriental laborers in rice paddies.

Stress is looked upon as a product of the times in which we live. This is true only to a limited extent and then because we allow it to be so. It is doubtful that our time is any more stressful than any other. Certainly the time when plagues were common and swept through a land were times of stress. And those times when human life had no value and the individual was suffered to live only at the whim of the absolute ruler of his land were also times of stress. In the history of our own country stress has been a repetitive factor in our progress. An unknown and hostile environment provided the stress of everyday life for the early pioneers as they struggled to establish a foothold, supply themselves with food, shelter, and protection, and push the frontier across a vast continent. And always there have been threats that had to be met to preserve the right of the individual to live in dignity and freedom with equality and justice. The same stresses are present today in a different guise perhaps. But they are not the cause of our individual problems, the obstacles to our individual quest for health, old age, and serenity.

Stress undoubtedly plays an important part in our state of well-being, or lack of it, and the production of illness. This stress comes from within. It is of our own making. The drive to get ahead, to achieve status, to ensure security, and the abuses that we heap on our bodies are the real destructive forces. They go unchallenged and are accepted as virtues. We hear much of stress but little of satisfaction, a pause to relish achievement, to appreciate the good things, and to value the vast storehouse of treasures that has come to us as our heritage.

Freedom from stress alone will not lead to healthy old age, nor is excessive stress the only cause of rapid aging. It is aided and abetted by lack of attention to the positive requirements of health.

3. Health—Unattended

When acute and severe illness strikes or accidents occur, a certain amount of damage is visited on the body to either a part, an organ, or a system, and a certain amount of vitality is lost. But the body has great reserve power to stand this particular kind of stress, and if it can be tided over the sudden emergency period, normal health can be restored. These, therefore, do not necessarily speed the aging process. There are many familiar examples, such as surgical operations, injury, hemorrhage with excessive loss of blood, acute specific infections.

The more frequent and the more important way in which vitality is lost and aging speeded up is in the day-by-day squandering of our reserve. This we may do by using it in excess—long hours of activity, physical stress unrelieved. More often it is the result of failure each day to attend to the needs of health—proper nutrition, proper rest, relaxation, and exercise. We do not have to choose wearing out or rusting out. Rather we must guard against excessive wear from overuse in one element and rust from disuse or no use in another.

Most of the degenerative diseases have as part of their causative mechanism lack of attention to the necessities of good health habits. We have seen this in the example of heart disease; a heart attack may seem to come suddenly, but the vitality of the vascular system, its ability to stand stress, has been undermined by years of lack of attention to the basic requirements of health.

Premature aging does not have a sudden onset at some specific time in later maturity. We could go back further in life to the age of infancy or youth and detect the incipient causes of premature aging.

Woman only a generation ago was old before her time, worn out by too frequent child-bearing, the hard work of caring for her family, the lack of rest and relaxation. To these may be added an unbalanced diet, which led to obesity, and malnutrition, and perhaps just as important, psychological malnutrition and starvation.

4. Equanimity—Unachieved

Equanimity is not passive acceptance of life, but a dynamic quality of living compounded of initiative, interest, curiosity, participation, productivity, and satisfaction in accomplishment. These need never be lost with aging. As a matter of fact there is greater need for these qualities and they can be put to more fruitful use as the years go by. Some individuals may never have known and therefore never have achieved equanimity. Others may have allowed illness, hardship, sorrow, or frustration to rob them of it. There are other stumbling blocks to serenity—ignorance, fear, apathy, and indifference in relation to disease.

The obstacles to serenity should be viewed in a positive way. They all lead to premature aging with loss of health, loss of ability to perform, and loss of enjoyment of life. As a public health problem our prime purpose should be prevention. This applies to all illnesses and diseases and can be accomplished only by the dissemination and application of the knowledge that we now have about the positive aspects of health and by the furtherance of that knowledge by research.

We must not fall into the error of concentrating on the horrors of this disease or that disease and the search for its cure, lest we defeat our purpose by generating fear rather than teaching health. Better means of curing disease is, of course, important and always will be. But we must not lose sight of the fact that many diseases have been wiped out because we have found the cause and the means of prevention. Others have been made controllable, the symptoms have been ameliorated, the damage lessened.

Finding the cause and providing the means of control will not solve the problem of the disease processes that lead to premature aging. They will not automatically wipe out heart attacks or even reduce their incidence. Success or failure will depend on the efforts of the individual.

We tend to be unrealistic about diseases. On the one hand we allow unreasonable fear to dominate, disturbing our thinking and behavior, and on the other hand we are indifferent about learning of the means of protecting our health and applying the knowledge available. The case of poliomyelitis is a good example. We knew that polio was a killer and a crippler caused by a virus. Before the vaccine was found, there was great fear, anxiety, and sometimes panic when the season for polio approached, and cases began to be reported in increasing numbers. And the wail spread over the land—why can't "they" do something about this disease that is crippling our children.

When the effective and safe vaccine was first found, and the quantity was limited, there was great impatience on the part of parents to have their children immunized. Sometimes there were instances of scandalous means being employed to get it. Now, only a few years later, we are apathetic, large numbers of the susceptible age group have not availed themselves of this simple, inexpensive way to protect their health—and polio is still a menace to health. If this is true of infection that is comparatively simple as to cause and means of prevention, how much more true is it of the diseases of internal origin.

The greatest deterrent to mature old age has its origin in the age of maturity. When the individual is shortsighted and so involved in the affairs of the age that she loses sight of the needs of health and fails to plan for the future, then stagnation, boredom, and loss of vitality are the inevitable consequences. We must evaluate our needs and capabilities and set our goals high. Of course there is no certainty that we shall all attain them, but we cannot expect to achieve goals that we do not even try for. Occasionally, an individual disregards the needs of health and achieves great age. But for every one who does, there will be millions who do not.

We must not seek the attainment of serenity by emphasizing the negative aspects of health. Knowing the obstacles that may be encountered is important, but it is not enough. Our efforts must be directed toward discovering the true pathway, the surest and safest route, to positive goals.

XXVI

THE GOALS

AS WOMAN STANDS at the threshold of this second age of maturity, she may pause and wonder what lies ahead for her. Will she achieve the longevity that is becoming the lot of so many more people every year? If so, what will it be like to be an old woman? If she is wise, she will realize that she has not yet reached the final goal, that there are others to be achieved. Her problem is to understand what these goals are, what can be done to assure their achievement, and with this knowledge to direct, or re-direct if necessary, her way of life so that old age will bring fruition, not obsolescence, decrepitude, and despair. She cannot foresee what changes the years will bring to her personally, she can only visualize them in terms of her acquaintance with old age as it has come to others.

She recognizes Whistler's portrait of his mother as the quintessence of serene old age in its delineation of character, its inspirational beauty, its quietness and simplicity. But such a portrait of old age cannot be the goal of modern woman. She would reject the idea of being relegated to a rocking chair with a cap on her head to symbolize her age, her hands folded in idleness. The utter stillness, the resignation, and above all the aloneness, make it unacceptable as her ultimate goal.

Nor would the proud and domineering matriarch who ruled her family by sheer force of her personality, confident in her own omnipotence, unmindful of the needs of youth, perhaps hardened and embittered because of her own misfortunes, or crotchety because of her infirmities, be modern woman's goal. She is a favorite character in fiction that portrays life in the days gone by when family unity was more universally revered and in the psychological excursions into the abnormal by modern writers. She has her counterpart on a smaller scale in modern life, but this is a type that is representative of only a few and is the symbol of what not to be. Then there is the little old lady in lavender and old lace. She is a fragile figurine, devoid of life responsibilities, an object to be protected and cherished. It might require little effort to be such a person in modern days, but she is hardly the goal of a mature personality.

The modern version of "mother growing old" is no more realistic than the portraits of by-gone days. Today woman is pictured as well-groomed, youthful, smiling, happy in her assurance of a steady income, and free from responsibility, work, and dependence on others. She can follow her dream to far-away places and to carefree and contented living. Actually, such a portrait is a negation of growing old and the substitution of perennial youth for the attributes of maturity—a meaningful life in the world of others.

Among modern woman's acquaintances with old people, there are some who still enjoy a life of activity and are self-respecting and respected. There are also many who have lost their goals and their status. They have become the displaced persons of our present-day culture without work, home, family, health, hope, or future. The portrait that brings only fear and dread of old age is that of chronic invalidism, in which a life of usefulness is past, and woman has become a burden to herself and her family. Most disturbing is the specter of senility, the deterioration of her faculties, in which she becomes at best garrulous and boring, and at the worst demented.

Each of these portraits has some element of reality, but the true picture of old age should be of a dynamic person in the world of people. As such, woman would continue to use her capabilities to the fullest and to derive satisfaction therefrom, and she would be accorded a respected place in society. She cannot achieve these goals alone. She needs the help of the community and of science. Her goals, if she is to fulfill her need, are to belong, to be healthy, and to be serene.

THE NEED TO BELONG

We have defined the ages of woman as changing aspects of maturity separated because of her relationship to others. Our modern culture has accorded her some degree of equality with the male in exploiting her potentiality for maturity, and in the last age she shares with him society's evaluation of the oldster, which at the present date is not always a very happy one.

The place accorded by the community to persons of old age has varied through history from veneration or the ancestor worship of the orientals, to the practice of primitive people of abandonment, even extermination, of those who could no longer contribute to the physical work of the tribe. In our culture, within the past hundred years, old age has experienced moderate versions of these two extremes.

Before the turn of the century, there was a respected place for the old-sters in the social and economic structure of our homes and communities. Then the structure was largely that of individual enterprise and the population was largely rural or small town. Individuals were allowed to work as long as they liked or were able, no matter what their age. Age was respected for its qualities of wisdom and skill acquired by experience and of reliability proved by the years. At that time, family life had greater stability. There was the old homestead or the ancestral home, which had been owned and cherished through many generations. Family ties and family responsibility were real and strong. There was always a place for the old person and if she was not venerated, usually she was respected and provided for within the unit of the family. The burden of the old person was infrequent, however, because relatively few reached ripe old age. Woman, whose place was strictly in the home, had a life of continuing meaningfulness and security. There was always a place with respect, work, and some responsibility for Grandmother and maiden Aunt Susie.

There have been revolutionary changes in our social structure since the turn of the century that have resulted in the loss of status for the old person. The lengthening of the life span has produced a constantly increasing number of individuals who are living to old age and has decreased to almost the vanishing point a place of respect and a use for them. Thus we are faced with the problem of old age, a peculiar paradox in which a normal age of life (which is beginning to constitute a large fraction of the total life span) has become a problem. It would seem that we have learned to extend life, but are at a loss to know what to do with it. The situation as it exists today is not one that makes growing old attractive. Both the individual and the community have contributed to the creation of this dilemma, and both must contribute to its solution.

The oldster has suffered loss of status on the individual level as family ties have become less meaningful. Children no longer grow up in the old homestead, marry, and settle down in the same community. Rather, the family breaks up early, children move to distant places, and their marriages more frequently than not do not unite two families long known to each other.

Members of the modern family, part of the industrial society, are mainly city dwellers living in small quarters. Even for those who wish to meet their responsibility to the old members of the family and to maintain closer family relationships, there are many obstacles. The old person may have to be moved from familiar places and friends to live among strangers, with nothing to occupy her time. The care of the old person, especially if she is infirm, is a problem often difficult to meet. Old people are farmed out to rest homes or left to shift for themselves. They are thus denied the privilege of being a functioning part of the family. For those who are so incapacitated physically or mentally as to require special care, it may be better for all concerned that they be placed in institutions equipped to provide such care.

The old person has lost status on the social level, the right to be a functioning part of the community as long as she is able. As a culture we are youth-worshippers. There are few occupations in which age is not a detriment. The few exceptions include elder statesmen and retiring top brass of the armed forces (who are not really old, as their age may be anywhere from 45 up). Even these are not immune to the pressure of "youth," and once out, only an occasional one makes a comeback. The vast army of workers, including professionals, white collar workers, and the salaried labor force, have the specter of replacement, retirement, and the loss of status and income always before them. The unfortunate who loses her job many years before the retirement age finds it difficult to get another job because she is " too old." This is especially true of women. When the " age " arrives, little thought is given to what the past performances of these workers have been or what contributions they have made and are still able to make. They are summarily brushed aside to make way for youth.

This is not to say that youth should not have a chance or should wait for the oldsters to die off. But the system is short-sighted on two counts. The first is that nonproductive older persons will soon constitute a large part of our society for whom the necessities of life must be provided, and if they are not permitted to work, youth must support them. The second is that the youth of today fails to recognize that they will be the oldsters of tomorrow, and they have the opportunity to prepare a better status for themselves by doing something to better the lot of the older person today.

The problem of what to do with these old people became serious at the time of economic depression. To assure jobs for younger individuals, forced retirement from work at a specified age was resorted to. Recognizing that some provision for the livelihood of these people was necessary, " social security " with its regulations and small benefits came into being. We are only beginning to recognize that retirement and social security are neither realistic nor the most beneficial way of handling the situation, from the standpoint of either the community or the individual. It is true that some favored few in the professional groups and independent business continue to work, to be independent, and occasionally are graduated to the status of the elder citizen, adviser, or member of the board. But the vast majority find that there is no longer a place for them. They are no longer useful, productive members of the community. If they depend on social security, they are prohibited by law to earn an amount that will provide a decent existence.

The social problem of old age is broad and complex and beyond our scope as it involves the need of providing food, shelter, clothing, and medical care for the aged who can no longer provide these things for themselves. The solution is the responsibility of the agencies of government and the medical and social sciences as well as the individual. Some recognition of the enormity of this problem on the national level is evident in the President's White House Conference on Aging and in the work of the Center for Aging Research at the National Institutes of Health.

Scientists are pointing out that age alone does not render an individual valueless. What she loses in manual dexterity and strength can be compensated for by skill, judgment, and stability. Older persons can continue to be contributing members of society, but there must be changes that will make it possible for them to continue to be self-supporting and self-respecting citizens as long as they are able. Thus, they will not be a drain on the public purse, and they will maintain a better state of health.

The community has the responsibility of recognizing these needs of its older citizens, but this is not the duty of the community alone. The individual has a responsibility also. Woman must recognize that the day will come when she no longer has the qualities of youth and be prepared to use the talents that can come with age.

When the problem of growing old is applied specifically to woman, the same general principles hold true, but there are important differences and added difficulties. Women have come to be a large part of the labor force. But woman's employment has been restricted to the little jobs. She has not been trained to use or encouraged to recognize her talents. Consequently, there is not a chance in a million that the average woman will become an elder citizen or a member of the board. She holds a job usually to help the family, not as a matter of choice but of necessity. She may be ready to retire, but the years have brought little experience that will enable her to assume another role so that she may continue to belong.

For the woman who has devoted her years of maturity to the rearing of a family, retirement comes first when the children leave home. Later she shares the problem of retirement with her husband, with a reduction of income and a man around the house who does not know what to do with himself. And four out of five will be widowed.

Woman needs to be prepared, so that she can continue to be an active part of the family and community. To accomplish this, she needs to be well, and she needs to have progressed in her maturity of personality. This is not as hard as it might seem, for women have an advantage over men in that they may have been holding two jobs all along, business and home, and they find greater satisfaction in personal relations. With training and experience, woman's contribution could be increased and her personal satisfaction made greater.

THE NEED TO BE WELL

Merely to grow old, even to be provided for, is not enough. The goals also include enjoyment of a healthy old age. The advances that have occurred in our culture have removed many of the hazards of life in infancy, childhood, and early adulthood and have made it probable that the individual will live to the full three score years and ten or more. To assure the health of these elder citizens, a new discipline in medicine, geriatrics, is developing.

The word " geriatrics " was coined in 1909. At first it was a branch of medicine to deal with the illnesses of old age, just as pediatrics was developing as a specialty that dealt with the diseases of childhood. With the conquest of infectious diseases, pediatrics assumed a more positive goal, that of the "well child," which endeavors to understand and supply the needs for healthy growth and development and the prevention of illness. Geriatrics also has come to mean the science that seeks to understand the process of aging, what is necessary to healthy aging, and the prevention of the illnesses so frequently associated with aging. (Gerontology deals with the experience of aging of all things from the planetary system to the atom. As applied to humans, it includes the physical, psychological, medical, social, economic, and philosophical aspects of aging.)

The search for knowledge to enhance health and prolong life has always been a part of medical science, and some of the basic concepts now recognized as important go back as much as six or seven centuries. Even then, there was some understanding of change in the needs for good health, to provide proper nutrition and ways to preserve eyesight. There was also recognition of the fact that individuals had different rates of aging associated with different mental occupations and physical careers, and these hastened aging more than illness did. Perhaps the most significant observation was that old people who enjoyed young people profited by the experiences of their company with better health of mind and body.

The aim of geriatric medicine is a positive wellness that means that an individual not only manages to survive, but also reaches old age with maximum efficiency of function of all the aspects of her personality. We have reviewed the obstacles to this goal and found that each one represents a process that arises within the individual. The beginnings are obscure; many are due to stresses, insults, and injuries of early years, and their effects are cumulative. We do not know the cause or the cure, but we do know that many can be avoided by proper attention to health in the years long before old age.

Geriatrics has demonstrated that the obstacles are not hopeless situations. Most of them are slow in developing and give some warning of their presence, and there is much that can be done to stay their progress. Some faults can be corrected. Surgery, for example, is no longer denied an individual because of age alone. Perhaps most encouraging is the fact that some of the old people in mental institutions are being salvaged and returned to useful life. This is being accomplished through the recognition that there are things that they can do or be taught to do, and the doing gives them a sense of belonging. The benefits derived from tranquilizers suggest that mental deterioration is not an inevitable part of the process of aging.

Geriatrics recognizes that illnesses in the aged have their peculiar characteristics. The body responds to stress, illness, or injury in a different way than it did in earlier years. In the old person, the body does not exhibit obvious signs of stress. The physical signs of illness are muted and vague. A child with a simple cold may run a high fever, while an oldster with pneumonia may have no such obvious signs as chills, fever, or severe cough. Perhaps this is the reason pneumonia has been called the old man's friend—it came, silent as the night, and carried him away.

Geriatrics has also brought recognition of what illness means to the old person in terms of her ability to work and to continue to belong. A heart attack out of the blue may seem to the person to be the end of life. Her whole personality may suffer a violent dislocation, as she envisions herself a chronic invalid, dependent, unable to perform, and in constant danger of another attack and sudden death. Her heart may withstand the damage and recover adequate function, yet she may be reduced to a life of invalidism.

The constructive aim of geriatrics in the field of public health is not just sickness insurance, hospitalization, and homes for the aged and incurables, but a positive attack on the problem of prevention. The largest areas of research in medical sciences are devoted to the causes and means of control of these obstacles. But the application of this knowledge will be the responsibility of the individual.

Woman is made more conscious of the physical aspects of her being by the feminine functions of menstruation and childbearing. They may serve as a barometer of her normalcy and health to a certain extent. She should know from her own experience the quality of wellness and should appreciate its significance. But she gets little encouragement or direction to experience the full degree of wellness that can be hers, and she is given much information concerning the abnormalities of mind and body. Such information, which is not based on sound knowledge of physiology with appreciation and understanding of the normal, can be the source of anxiety and fear rather than of serenity. The illnesses that become the obstacles of healthy old age are insidious. Woman will recognize their symptoms only if she knows the meaning of wellness, based on a sound foundation of good nutrition, exercise, rest, and relaxation.

Woman's capability of achieving the goal of serenity has as its bulwark her physical health. And for the most part she does not have the degree of health that she is capable of. Woman often reaches the Age of Serenity with the scars of previous illnesses, some of which she was not responsible for. But she is responsible for the abuse and neglect that she has heaped on herself. Impairments are not the result of one insult but are the accumulation of years of bad habits.

To maintain wellness, avoid illness, and slow the process of aging, a woman should take advantage of all that medical science has to offer. One of the most important steps is a regular and complete physical examination. Many of the catastrophies that seem to strike without warning have in reality been in the making for some time previously and might possibly have been avoided had the early signs been recognized and proper measures taken to correct them. There are, of course, some that have no such signs or that cannot be corrected. This periodic examination should be a health examination, not just a search for some particular abnormality. Many women seek medical assistance only when frightened by such an experience as a friend having a heart attack or dying of cancer, or finding in themselves symptoms they fear indicate a specific disease. They make the mistake of selecting the type of examination they think they need and go for a specialist's examination.

The ideal concept that must guide both a woman and her doctor is that health involves her whole personality, and she should be examined as such. This is not as formidable as it may seem. It does not necessarily involve a rigid array of many tests, X-rays, and other diagnostic procedures. Neither is it a simple test for a specific disease, such as a cholesterol test for vascular disease or a smear test for cancer. Rather it is an evaluation of her health as a whole person. A careful history and physical examination and a few routine laboratory tests will serve as the basis for selection of further investigation deemed necessary. Having her own doctor to whom she goes regularly will make such examination simpler and more meaningful. And having some one she knows will mean that she is less likely to put it off. Her own doctor will be familiar with her problems, medical and personal, through the years, and useful data thus will have accumulated and will not have to be ascertained with each examination. Her doctor will recognize early changes, for her past history gives a basis for comparison. It does not matter whether her doctor is the family doctor, her gynecologist, or an internist as long as he considers her whole physical health. He can refer her to a specialist if some finding warrants further investigation.

Aging, we have said, is a normal process, not a disease, and senescence is a normal part of life not characterized by chronic invalidism. If this be true, why then do not all people have a serene old age? It is a consummation devoutly to be wished but as yet rarely attained. We do not know the answers; perhaps we have only scratched the surface. But we are not using all the knowledge that is available about how to make this a longer, healthier, and happy age. There is no magic formula for healthy old age. Health during this age depends on the degree of health a person brings to the age, the stresses that are inherent in the age, and the diseases that are common to old age.

THE NEED TO BE SERENE

To grow old gracefully is to accept and adapt to the changes that age will bring, but it also requires preparation. Grace implies harmony, or an innate charm, qualities that have been nurtured with knowledge, understanding, and skill perfected through sustained effort, discipline, and training. Woman grows old gracefully, achieves the goal of serenity, in proportion to the quality of her preparation for, and the assiduous attention to, all the aspects of her mature personality, physical and psychological.

Physical Basis

The physical basis of serenity is health, and it is doubtful whether many women know what it is like to be really well. They may have glimpses of it on occasions but to understand it woman must go back to youth when exercise was a joy, there was no limit to her energy, appetite and sleep were no problem, and life was filled with enjoyment of today enriched by the hopes and dreams of tomorrow. Years need not rob her of these, but only change the means and modes of their expression.

What woman should know about the physical basis of health has been the aim of this book—to acquaint her with the normal, to lead her to appreciate the wonderful mechanism that is her body, and to instill in her the desire to keep it working for her at the peak of efficiency. This is, of course, only an outline, but it is hoped that it will have opened vistas and stimulated her interest to seek further information with firm determination to apply this knowledge. It should serve as a guide in her pursuit of positive wellness. She must know what aging means, accept the limitations, and adapt to them. But she must also appreciate and use the benefits that age bestows.

Psychological Aspects

The psychological aspects of woman's personality in the Age of Serenity consist, as they did in the first age of maturity, of her mental capabilities and emotional components and indeed are the outgrowth of these. Whatever maturity and serenity she will achieve in this age depends on the degree to which she has developed these in the earlier ages. It is important to realize that preparation for the first age of maturity is also preparation for the second age of maturity. This may seem obvious, but it is a fact frequently overlooked. It is important that her training be aimed also at her fulfillment as a person, so that she will be prepared when the needs of fulfillment in the feminine role cease to dominate the picture.

THE MYSTERY AND THE LEGEND

Woman is still the eternal mystery. We have pursued knowledge and understanding in terms of her structure and function and the changes that take place as she advances through the seven ages. We have seen the ages emerge as distinct and characteristic phases of her maturity, as her relationships change within her world of other people. But the final solution of the mystery is not yet at hand, for therein lies also the meaning of life and love, which do not belong to her alone but to all mankind. Nor do we really need or want to find the solution in scientific facts alone, for it is from the mystery that our ideals and inspiration arise and our dreams are made.

But concerning the ingredients that go into the making of woman, we may inquire into the ancient legend of her creation and qualities attributed to her in terms of the maturity that modern woman is capable of giving them. We may accept her virtues—the grace and beauty of her being, the joyousness and warmth of her personality, her sensitivity and fidelity—as still ideals to be cherished. And we may find even in her shortcomings elements that can be made to contribute to the rich fulfillment of life.

Her vanity need not be empty pride of appearance or attainments. It can be a love and respect of self, which she must have if she is truly to love and respect others. It can be self-assurance, which brings peace within herself and frees her to participate and contribute harmoniously in the world of others.

Fickleness may mean instability or changeableness without reason. But ability to change is an asset if used to adapt to the vicissitudes of life, to express dissatisfaction with mediocrity, and to seek always things truly better.

Woman is curious. But curiosity becomes a virtue when it changes its direction from meddlesomeness to the ability to wonder and the desire to learn more of the beauty of the world and to have a sympathetic interest in the problems and achievements of others.

In the ancient legend woman chattered incessantly. But in terms of modern woman's maturity speech is one of her most precious possessions. The ability to communicate is the fountainhead of knowledge. It is the means of sharing life's experiences with others. She can give a word of encouragement, sympathy, or understanding, of apology or of courtesy, and occasionally of advice, that can contribute not only to the happiness of others but also to that within herself.

Woman's timidity suggests a shying away from people and problems, but it may mean a sensitivity to the rights of others wherein her modesty, dignity, and humility give meaning to aggressiveness and hostility. Woman is sentimental. But sentimentality is never a vice when it sees beyond the material and sets higher values on love, hope, and dreams and cherishes the memories of these in past experience. Even woman's idleness can be a virtue when it means a halt in a life of activity to savor and appreciate the blessings that are hers.

There are many questions left unanswered about maturity and serenity, their meaning and their achievement. But one truth stands crystal clear and its corollary is obvious. To be a woman is a privilege with peculiar and profound responsibilities. To become an old woman can be a pleasure of fulfillment.

INDEX

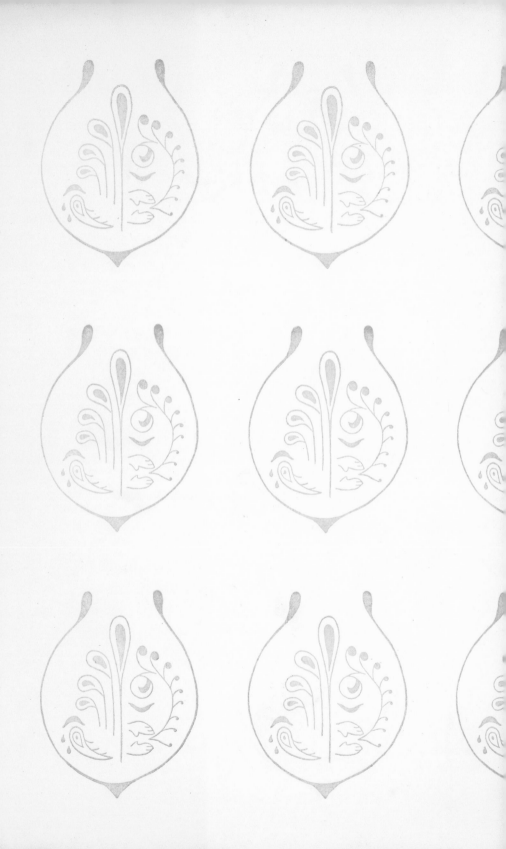